CANCER AND CHEMOTHERAPY

Volume I

CANCER AND CHEMOTHERAPY

CANCER AND CHEMOTHERAPY

Volume I

Introduction to Neoplasia and Antineoplastic Chemotherapy

Edited by

Stanley T. Crooke, M.D., Ph.D.
Archie W. Prestayko, Ph.D.

Research and Development
Bristol Laboratories
Syracuse, New York
and
Department of Pharmacology
Baylor College of Medicine
Texas Medical Center
Houston, Texas

Editorial Assistant

Nancy Alder

1980

ACADEMIC PRESS
A Subsidiary of Harcourt Brace Jovanovich, Publishers
New York   London   Toronto   Sydney   San Francisco

ACADEMIC PRESS, INC.
111 Fifth Avenue, New York, New York 10003

United Kingdom Edition published by
ACADEMIC PRESS, INC. (LONDON) LTD.
24/28 Oval Road, London NW1 7DX

Library of Congress Cataloging in Publication Data
Main entry under title:

Cancer and chemotherapy.

Includes bibliographies and index.
CONTENTS: v. 1. Introduction to neoplasia and
antineoplastic chemotherapy.
1. Cancer——Chemotherapy. 2. Antineoplastic
agents. I. Crooke, Stanley T. II. Prestayko,
Archie W. [DNLM: 1. Neoplasms——Drug therapy.
2. Antineoplastic agents. QZ267 C214]
RC271.C5C285   616.99'4061   79-8536
ISBN 0-12-197801-X (v. 1)

PRINTED IN THE UNITED STATES OF AMERICA

80 81 82 83   9 8 7 6 5 4 3 2 1

CONTENTS

PART II   CARCINOGENESIS

PART III   ANIMAL MODELS OF HUMAN CANCER: THEIR USE AND LIMITATIONS

PART IV   IMMUNOTHERAPY OF CANCER

PART V ANTINEOPLASTIC DRUG DEVELOPMENT: APPROACHES, DESIGN, AND EVALUATION

LIST OF CONTRIBUTORS

Numbers in parentheses indicate the pages on which the authors' contributions begin.

S. C. Barranco (123), Department of Human Biological Chemistry and Genetics, University of Texas Medical Branch, Galveston, Texas 77550

William T. Bradner (221, 313), Antitumor Biology Department, Bristol Laboratories, Syracuse, New York 13201

Harris Busch (21), Department of Pharmacology, Baylor College of Medicine, Houston, Texas 77025

Stephen K. Carter (343), Northern California Cancer Program, Palo Alto, California 94303

Michael A. Chirigos (263, 285), Virus and Disease Modification Section, Laboratory of Chemical Pharmacology, Developmental Therapeutics Program, Division of Cancer Treatment, National Cancer Institute, Bethesda, Maryland 20014

Charles A. Claridge (327), Antitumor Biology Department, Bristol Laboratories, Syracuse, New York 13201

Yerach Daskal (137), Department of Pharmacology, Electron Microscopy Unit, Baylor College of Medicine, Houston, Texas 77030

Terrence W. Doyle (295), Medicinal Chemical Research, Bristol Laboratories, Syracuse, New York 13201

Benjamin Drewinko (95), Department of Laboratory Medicine, The University of Texas System Cancer Center, M.D. Anderson Hospital and Tumor Institute, Houston, Texas 77030

Ferenc Gyorkey (137), Department of Pathology, Veterans Administration Medical Center, and Department of Pharmacology, Baylor College of Medicine, Houston, Texas 77030

Phyllis Gyorkey (137), Department of Pathology, Veterans Administration Medical Center, Houston, Texas 77030

Lawrence Helson (229), Memorial Sloan Kettering Cancer Center, New York, New York 10021

Archie W. Prestayko (3), Research and Development, Bristol Laboratories, Syracuse, New York 13201

Fred Rapp (197), Department of Microbiology and Specialized Cancer Research Center, The Pennsylvania State University College of Medicine, Hershey, Pennsylvania 17033

Paul Siminoff (249), Department of Immunology, Bristol Laboratories, Syracuse, New York 13201

James E. Strong (77), Department of Pharmacology, Baylor College of Medicine, Houston, Texas 77025

I. Bernard Weinstein (169), Cancer Center, Institute of Cancer Research, Columbia University College of Physicians and Surgeons, New York, New York 10032

GENERAL PREFACE

With the rapid development of new chemotherapeutic approaches and new agents used in the treatment of patients with cancer, a basic instructional workbook describing in some detail the drugs currently employed, current therapeutic approaches, and agents in development is essential. However, to understand fully cancer chemotherapeutic agents and their use, one must understand various aspects of anticancer drug development, the molecular and cellular biology of malignant disease, and the clinical characteristics of the most common neoplasms. Only with this information can a detailed discussion of anticancer drugs be presented.

It was with these thoughts in mind that Cancer and Chemotherapy was developed; the goal: to provide in a single source the information necessary for a detailed understanding of the major antineoplastic agents. Thus, Volume I is designed to provide the fundamental information concerning the molecular and cellular biology of cancer, carcinogenesis, and the basics of anticancer drug development. Volume II will provide clinical information relative to the most common human malignancies and discusses the use of chemotherapeutics in the treatment of those diseases. In Volume III the antineoplastic agents will be discussed. It contains reviews of all the major anticancer drugs and a review of agents in development. Furthermore, in two sections—the molecular pharmacology of selected antitumor drugs and the clinical pharmacology of selected antitumor drugs—significantly more detailed discussions of certain drugs are provided. These drugs were selected because they have interesting characteristics, and adequate data are available to allow a more detailed discussion. These two sections should be of particular value to individuals who have an interest in certain aspects of particular drugs.

Stanley T. Crooke
Archie W. Prestayko

PREFACE TO VOLUME I

The term "cancer chemotherapy" can be used broadly to refer to all chemical agents used in treating cancer. These include the cytotoxic drugs, hormones, and immunotherapeutic agents. Volume I of *Cancer and Chemotherapy* discusses the biochemical basis on which each of these classes of agents is utilized. The unique aspects of the cancer cell are discussed and a rationale for various chemotherapeutic treatments is presented.

Because it is well documented that various chemicals and viruses can cause or enhance the development of cancer, a discussion of both chemical and viral carcinogenesis is also presented.

Chemotherapeutic agents have been obtained from microbial culture broths, plants, and biotransformation and chemical syntheses. The first detection of anticancer activity of these agents must come from various prescreening tests and antitumor screening tests. A discussion of the approaches to and design and evaluation of various agents in animal tumor models is presented.

Inasmuch as the final test of the utility of an anticancer chemotherapeutic agent is the effect on a tumor in a patient, it is appropriate that the concluding chapter in this volume discusses clinical trials needed to establish such clinical efficacy and drug-related toxicity in patients with cancer.

Stanley T. Crooke
Archie W. Prestayko

Part I
The Molecular Biology
of Cancer

1
MACROMOLECULES AND THEIR SYNTHESIS
Archie W. Prestayko

I. INTRODUCTION

Most of the anticancer drugs employed clinically exert their antitumor effect by inhibiting nucleic acid (DNA or RNA) or protein synthesis. This inhibition can occur through cross-linking of bases in DNA (e.g., bifunctional alkylating agents) or binding to and inactivation of enzymes necessary for the synthetic processes. It can also occur by substitution of bases in nucleic acids with inactive analogs or through breakage of DNA by antitumor drugs such as bleomycin. Whatever the mechanism might be, it appears quite clear that DNA, RNA, and protein molecules and/or the processes involved in their syntheses are important cellular targets for anticancer agents.

It is important, therefore, to understand and to study these synthetic processes as they relate to the antitumor activity and toxicity of antitumor drugs. New drug development has as its major goal the enhancement of therapeutic activity of a drug, i.e., maximizing antitumor activity and minimizing toxicity. Since the historical landmark discovery by Watson and Crick (1953) of the double helical

CANCER AND CHEMOTHERAPY, VOL. I

structure of DNA, much information has been obtained on the "central dogma" of molecular genetics, i.e.,

$$DNA \to {}^1DNA \to {}^2RNA \to {}^3protein$$

These events referred to respectively, (1) replication, (2) transcription, and (3) translation, will be described in this chapter. Excellent detailed information on this subject has been published by Watson (1975) and Lehninger (1975).

II. NUCLEIC ACIDS

A. Building Blocks

1. Bases

Deoxyribonucleic acid (DNA) and ribonucleic acid (RNA) are large molecules which store and transfer genetic information in cells. They are composed of a

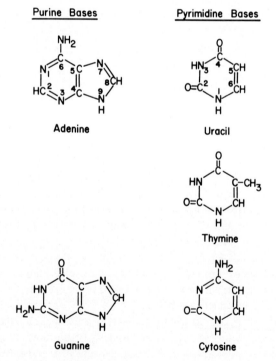

Fig. 1.   Chemical structures of purine and pyrimidine bases of nucleic acids.

polymeric structure of nucleotides which are composed of a nitrogenous base, a pentose sugar, and phosphoric acid. The bases present in DNA and RNA are shown in Fig. 1. The purine bases adenine and guanine are present in both DNA and RNA. The pyrimidine bases cytosine and thymine are found in DNA, while cytosine and uracil are present in RNA.

2. Nucleosides

Nucleosides consist of a purine or pyrimidine base chemically linked to a pentose sugar. In DNA the pentose sugar is 2-deoxy-D-ribose, while in RNA the sugar is D-ribose. The bases are attached to the sugars at the carbon-1 position.

3. Nucleotides

The attachment of a phosphate to the carbon-5 position of the pentose of a nucleoside yields a nucleoside monophosphate or nucleotide. The nomenclature of the various ribonucleotides and deoxyribonucleotides is given in Table I. Addition of one or two phosphates on the existing 5'-phosphates of mononucleotides yields di- and triphosphonucleotides, respectively. The utilization of these compounds in the synthesis of DNA and RNA will be described in Section II,B. The polymerization of the nucleotides into a polynucleotide or DNA strand is shown in Fig. 2. The polynucleotide structure for RNA is the same except that the sugar is D-ribose instead of 2-deoxyribose, and the base thymine is substituted by the base uracil. However, two DNA strands combine to form the double helical DNA molecule, while RNA exists primarily as a single strand.

TABLE I

Nomenclature of Ribonucleotides and Deoxyribonucleotides

Ribonucleotides	Deoxyribonucleotides
Adenosine-5'-phosphoric acid (adenylic acid, AMP)	Deoxyadenosine-5'-phosphoric acid (deoxyadenylic acid, dAMP)
Guanosine-5'-phosphoric acid (guanylic acid, GMP)	Deoxyguanosine-5'-phosphoric acid (deoxyguanylic acid, dGMP)
Cytidine-5'-phosphoric acid (cytidylic acid, CMP)	Deoxycytidine-5'-phosphoric acid (deoxycytidylic acid, dCMP)
Uridine-5'-phosphoric acid (uridylic acid, UMP)	Deoxyuridine-5'-phosphoric acid (deoxyuridylic acid, dUMP)

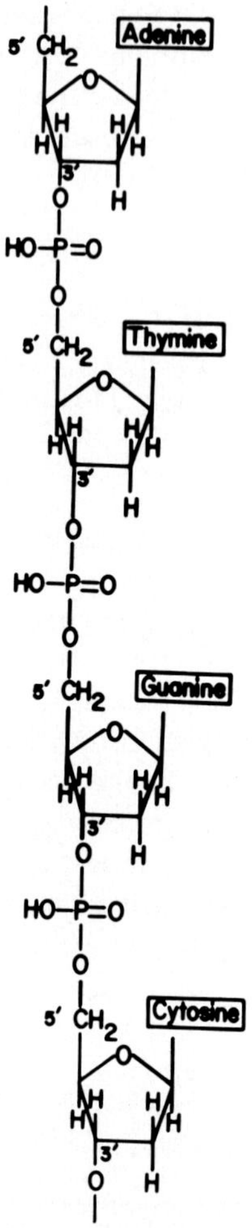

Fig. 2. Polymerization of deoxyribonucleotides into a polynucleotide strand of DNA. Phosphate–deoxyribose residues form the backbone structure of DNA.

B. DNA Replication

1. Genetic Consistency

The basis for transfer of genetic information from a parent cell to a daughter cell is the duplication of DNA. Replication of DNA followed by cell division and separation of identical sets of DNA molecules into each daughter cell ensures that, when cells grow and divide, they maintain their genotype. Figure 3 illus-

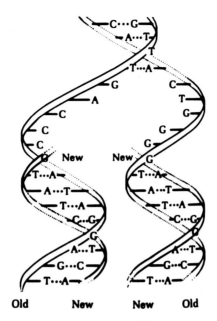

Fig. 3. Replication of DNA. Both parent strands of DNA are replicated to form a new strand with complementary base sequence. (From Watson, 1975.)

trates the replication of a new strand of DNA from an existing strand. Since both strands of DNA are reproduced, each daughter cell receives the parent strand of DNA and the newly synthesized strand which now form the double-stranded duplex DNA molecule.

The maintenance of specificity of base sequence resides in the fact that adenine (A) and guanine (G) bases in the old strand form hydrogen-bonded pairs with thymine (T) and cytosine (C) bases, respectively, in the new strand. Hence, A–T and G–C base pair specificity accounts for the precise reproduction of the base sequence in the new strand complementary to that in the old strand of DNA.

2. Enzymes in DNA Replication

Although the physical state of DNA in bacterial cells and eukaryotic cells is vastly different (*Escherichia coli* cells contain a circular tightly packed DNA which is relatively protein-free compared to eukaryote chromosomes which contain many proteins associated with the linear DNA), the enzymes (polymerases) that carry out the DNA replication process are quite similar. Considerably more information has been obtained on these processes in bacteria than in nucleated cells, and, therefore, the general mechanisms presented here are those which have been worked out for *E. coli* cells.

DNA Polymerase

$$dNTP + (dNMP)_n \underset{DNA}{\overset{Mg^{2+}}{\rightleftharpoons}} (dNMP)_{n+1} + PP_i$$

Bacteria	eukaryotes
I	α
II	β
III	γ

Fig. 4.   DNA polymerases in bacteria and eukaryotes and their generalized function.

DNA polymerase I (or α in eukaryotes) catalyzes the addition of deoxyribonucleotide residues to the 3' end of the DNA chain shown in Fig. 4 (Kornberg, 1960). Deoxytrinucleotides (dATP, dGTP, dCTP, and dTTP) react at the 3'-hyroxyl of the terminal deoxyribose of the DNA in the presence of magnesium and polymerase I. The attachment of the nucleotide causes the release of inorganic pyrophosphate (PP_i). Pure DNA polymerase I is able to add about 1000 nucleotides/minute/molecule of enzyme at 37°C. Polymerase I was also shown to possess 3' → 5'- and 5' → 3'-exonuclease activity, i.e., it could sequentially cleave off single nucleotides from either terminus of the DNA polynucleotide chain.

The other two enzyme molecules DNA polymerase II and III were discovered by Gefter (1974) and Kornberg and Gefter (1972), respectively. These enzymes have stringent requirements for activity and are believed to be important in maintaining the fidelity of DNA replication. Another enzyme DNA ligase (joining enzyme) has been shown to catalyze the synthesis of a phosphodiester bond between a 3'-hydroxyl at the end of one chain and a 5'-phosphate at the end of the other.

3.   Proposed Steps in DNA Replication

From the many separate investigations, a scheme for bacterial DNA replication has been proposed (Figs. 5a–c). In the initial step, specific initiator proteins recognize an initiation point on DNA. At this point, DNA-directed RNA polymerase binds to produce an RNA primer for the new DNA chains. Unwinding proteins bind close to the initiation site and open up the two strands of DNA which then allows the RNA primers to be synthesized. This process occurs antiparallel on both strands of DNA.

DNA polymerase III, using RNA as a primer, is capable of adding deoxyribonucleotides onto the RNA primer to form a short DNA chain. The primer RNA is then excised leaving the short DNA fragment (Okazaki *et al.*, 1968). The Okazaki DNA fragments are joined through the action of DNA

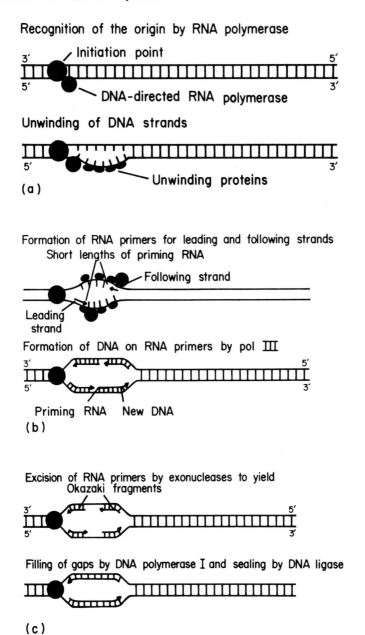

Fig. 5. Proposed steps in DNA replication in bacteria. (a) Recognition of initiation points and unwinding of DNA. (b) RNA priming and formation of DNA on RNA primers. (c) Excision of RNA primers and joining of short DNA fragments. (From Lehninger, 1975.)

polymerase I and DNA ligase to form complete long-chain DNA strands. From this replication fork two new DNA strands are formed in opposite directions.

Although much less information is available in eukaryotic cells, there is evidence supporting the formation of Okazaki fragments and the utilization of similar enzymes. This process is complicated by the presence of chromosomal proteins such as histones and nonhistone proteins (Busch *et al.*, 1975).

C. Transcription—RNA Synthesis

1. RNA Polymerases

The transfer of genetic information from DNA to RNA occurs through a process termed transcription. This process also involves enzymes (RNA polymerases) capable of polymerizing ribonucleoside 5'-triphosphates into an RNA polynucleotide chain which has a base sequence complementary to that of the strand of DNA upon which it was synthesized. This DNA-directed RNA polymerase reaction is shown in Fig. 6. This reaction is very similar to that which occurs in DNA synthesis. However, RNA polymerases in bacteria and eukaryotes have less similarity than do the DNA polymerases.

Burgess (1971) described the bacterial enzyme as a protein of 490,000 molecular weight with α, β, β', and σ subunits. The σ subunit is believed to be important in the initiation of RNA synthesis and is, therefore, considered a regulatory factor. The polymerase with only the α, β, and β' subunits is still capable of polymerizing ribonucleotides into a polynucleotide chain.

In nucleated cells, at least three different RNA polymerase enzymes have been identified. Polymerase I (A enzyme) is found only in the nucleolus of the cell and is involved in ribosomal RNA synthesis. Polymerase II (B enzyme) and polymerase III (C enzyme) are found in the extranucleolar portion of the nucleus and are involved in the synthesis of messenger RNA and transfer RNA. Polymerase I and II have different ionic requirement for optimum activity.

RNA Polymerase - Transcription

$$NTP + (NMP)_n \underset{RNA}{\overset{Mg^{2+}}{\rightleftharpoons}} (NMP)_{n+1} + PP_i$$

Bacteria		eukaryotes
one enzyme with	I	(A) nucleolar
α, β, β', σ	II	(B) nucleoplasmic
subunits	III	(C) nucleoplasmic

Fig. 6. RNA polymerases in bacteria and eukaryotes and their generalized function.

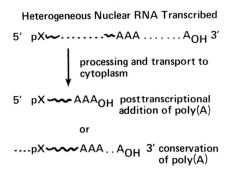

Fig. 7.   Synthesis and processing of heterogeneous RNA (direct transcript in the nucleus) through cleavage or addition of polyadenylic acid residues.

Polymerase I is only slightly more active in the presence of manganese than magnesium, while polymerase II has a definite manganese ion requirement (Roeder and Rutter, 1969, 1970).

2.   Messenger RNA

The most diversified species of RNA in the cell is messenger RNA (mRNA). A separate mRNA is required for synthesis of each different protein. The mRNAs are synthesized in the nucleus and processed and transported to the cytoplasm where they associate with ribosomes to form polyribosomes on which protein synthesis then takes place. Figure 7 illustrates some important features of the synthesis and processing of mRNA.

Messenger RNA is transcribed from DNA in the nucleus as a heterogenous molecule (Darnell *et al.*, 1973). It contains regions of polynucleotides that do not code for proteins. One of these regions contains polyadenylic acid [poly(A)]. This poly(A) occurs on the 3' end of the RNA (Fig. 7). As the nuclear RNA is processed and transported to the cytoplasm, the number of adenylic acid residues is decreased. The exact function of the change in poly(A) residues between nucleus and cytoplasm is unclear. It is possible that some poly(A) may be added posttranscriptionally. With the appropriate processing and transport from the nucleus, the heterogeneous RNA now becomes cytoplasmic mRNA ready for directing synthesis of proteins by polyribsomes.

3.   Ribosomal RNA

The nucleolus is the site of synthesis of the precursors of ribosomal RNA. The synthesis of ribosomal precursor RNA and its processing into cytoplasmic RNA has been extensively studied Warner (1974). Figure 8 summarizes these series of events. The DNA gene in the nucleolus which codes for ribosomal RNA is transcribed by RNA polymerase I into a large RNA molecule which has a

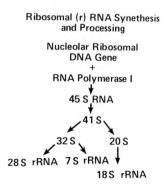

Ribosomal (r) RNA Synethesis
and Processing

Nucleolar Ribosomal
DNA Gene
+
RNA Polymerase I
↓
45 S RNA
↓
41 S
32 S   20 S
28 S rRNA 7 S rRNA
18 S rRNA

Fig. 8.   Processing of nucleolar ribosomal precursor RNA into cytoplasmic ribosomal RNA.

sedimentation coefficient of 45 S, as determined by sucrose density gradient centrifugation. This large RNA is complexed with proteins and cleaved into a smaller 41 S RNA by special ribonucleases. Further cleavage to 32 S and 20 S RNAs give rise to the cytoplasmic mature 28 S and 7 S RNAs in the large ribosomal subunit and 18 S RNA in the small ribosomal unit.

The overall process of RNA synthesis, cleavage, binding to preribosomal proteins, and maturation of ribosomal particles is summarized in Fig. 9 (Prestayko *et al.*, 1974). This is a complex process and many more studies are required to define the exact mechanisms that are involved. The transport into the the nucleus and nucleolus of ribosomal proteins which are synthesized on cytoplasmic polyribsomes and the transport out of the nucleus of ribonucleoprotein

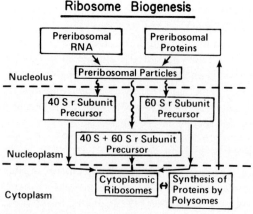

Ribosome Biogenesis

Fig. 9.   Schematic representation of events involved in the synthesis and transport of ribosomes in eukaryotic cells. (From Prestayko *et al.*, 1974.)

particles (ribosomal precursor complexes of RNA and protein) must be a dynamic and regulated process which responds to the needs of the growing cell. Resting cells have a much slower rate of ribosomal RNA and protein synthesis than do actively growing tumor cells, which have a large polyribsome population actively synthesizing proteins.

4. *Transfer RNA*

Transfer RNAs (tRNA) or low molecular weight soluble RNAs have an important function in polymerizing amino acids into polypeptides (proteins) on polyribosomes. There are many of these RNAs in a cell, each with a specificity for a particular amino acid. Like messenger RNA and ribosomal RNA, transfer RNAs are synthesized as precursor RNA molecules in the nucleus by extranucleolar RNA polymerase. They are transported to the cytoplasm where they exist in a soluble form, readily available to bind to an amino acid.

The structure of a representative tRNA molecule from yeast which is specific for the amino acid alanine is shown in Fig. 10. The complete nucleotide sequence of this molecule was first established by Holley *et al.* (1965). The secondary structure of tRNA possesses some interesting features. The C–C–A terminus of tRNA is the site of attachment of the amino acid. Two nucleotide loops are present which contain pseudouridine (Ψ) and dihydrouridine (hU), respectively. The anticodon loop contains the trinucleotide which serves as the recognition site for binding to the appropriate nucleotide sequence in messenger RNA; hence, the specificity for amino acid polymerization into protein resides in the triplet

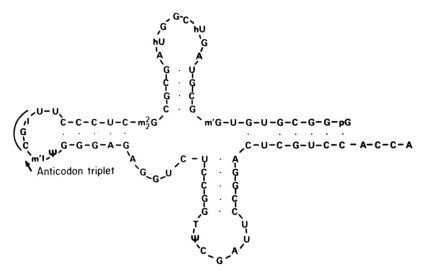

Fig. 10.   Amino acid sequence of alanine-specific transfer RNA from yeast.

codon–anticodon recognition between messenger RNA and transfer RNA. Section III will discuss in greater detail the joining of amino acids into polypeptide chains.

III. PROTEINS

A. Building Blocks

Proteins, which form the structural basis of every living cell, are composed of amino acids joined together by peptide bonds. The 21 natural amino acids listed in Table II are found in a wide variety of common proteins. The reaction which

TABLE II

The Natural Amino Acids

Name	Formula
Neutral amino acids	
Glycine	$H_2N \cdot CH_2 \cdot COOH$
Alanine	$H_2N \cdot \underset{\underset{CH_3}{\mid}}{CH} \cdot COOH$
Valine	$H_2N \cdot \underset{\underset{CH(CH_3)_2}{\mid}}{CH} \cdot COOH$
Leucine	$H_2N \cdot \underset{\underset{CH_2 \cdot CH(CH_3)_2}{\mid}}{CH} \cdot COOH$
Isoleucine	$H_2N \cdot \underset{\underset{CH_3 \cdot CH \cdot C_2H_5}{\mid}}{CH} \cdot COOH$
Phenylalanine	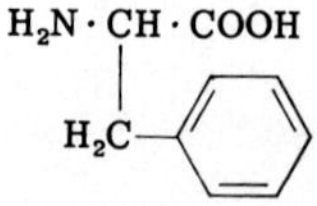
Proline	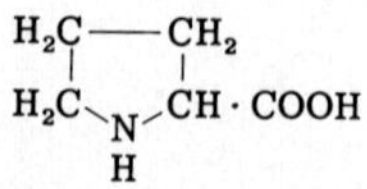
Tryptophan	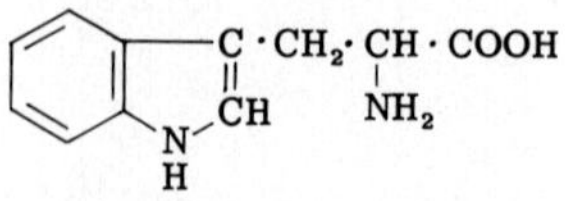

TABLE II (*Continued*)

Name	Formula
Serine	$H_2N \cdot CH \cdot COOH$ $\quad\quad\ \ | $ $\quad\quad CH_2OH$
Threonine	$H_2N \cdot CH \cdot COOH$ $\quad\quad\ \ \|$ $\quad\quad CHOH \cdot CH_3$
Methionine	$H_2N \cdot CH \cdot COOH$ $\quad\quad\ \ \|$ $\quad\quad (CH_2)_2 \cdot SCH_3$
Cystine	$HOOC \quad\quad COOH$ $\quad\ \| \quad\quad\quad \|$ $H_2N \cdot CH \quad CH \cdot NH_2$ $\quad\quad \| \quad\quad\ \|$ $\quad H_2C \cdot S \cdot S \cdot CH_2$
Asparagine	$H_2N \cdot CH \cdot COOH$ $\quad\quad\ \ \|$ $\quad\quad CH_2 \cdot CONH_2$
Glutamine	$H_2N \cdot CH \cdot COOH$ $\quad\quad\ \ \|$ $\quad\quad CH_2 \cdot CH_2 \cdot CONH_2$
The acidic amino acids Aspartic acid	$H_2N \cdot CH \cdot COOH$ $\quad\quad\ \ \|$ $\quad\quad CH_2COO^-$
Glutamic acid	$H_2N \cdot CH \cdot COOH$ $\quad\quad\ \ \|$ $\quad\quad CH_2 \cdot CH_2 \cdot COO^-$
Tyrosine	$H_2N \cdot CH \cdot COOH$ $\quad\quad\ \ \|$ H_2C—⟨benzene ring⟩—O^-
Cysteine	$H_2N \cdot CH \cdot COOH$ $\quad\quad\ \ \|$ $\quad\quad CH_2 \cdot S^-$
The basic amino acids Histidine	$H_2N \cdot CH \cdot COOH$ $\quad\quad\ \ \|$ H_2C $\quad\ \ \diagdown$ $\quad\quad C = CH$ $\quad\quad \| \quad\quad \|$ $\quad\ HN \quad NH$ $\quad\quad \diagdown C \diagup {}_+$ $\quad\quad\ | $ $\quad\quad H$
Lysine	$H_2N \cdot CH \cdot COOH$ $\quad\quad\ \ \|$ $\quad\quad (CH_2)_4 \cdot NH_3^+$
Arginine	$H_2N \cdot CH \cdot COOH$ $\quad\quad\ \ \|$ $\quad\quad (CH_2)_3 \cdot NH \cdot C = NH_2^+$ $\quad\quad\quad\quad\quad\quad\quad \|$ $\quad\quad\quad\quad\quad\quad\quad NH_2$

POLYPEPTIDE STRUCTURE

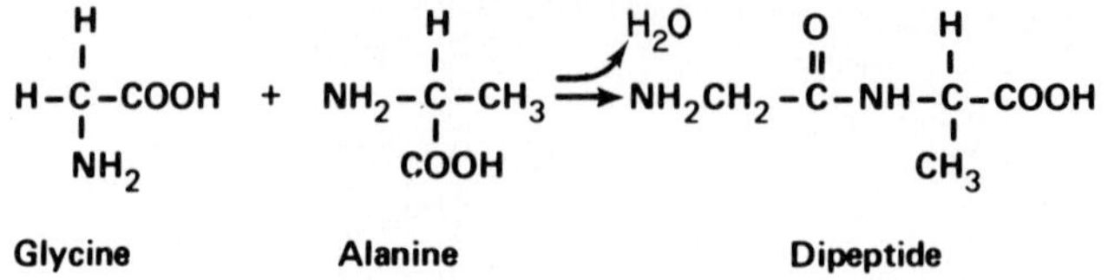

$$H-\underset{\underset{NH_2}{|}}{\overset{\overset{H}{|}}{C}}-COOH \quad + \quad NH_2-\underset{\underset{COOH}{|}}{\overset{\overset{H}{|}}{C}}-CH_3 \quad \xrightarrow{H_2O} \quad NH_2CH_2-\overset{\overset{O}{||}}{C}-NH-\underset{\underset{CH_3}{|}}{\overset{\overset{H}{|}}{C}}-COOH$$

    Glycine   Alanine   Dipeptide

Fig. 11. Formation of a peptide bond between two amino acids.

forms a peptide bond between two amino acids in a protein is shown in Fig. 11. The carboxyl group of one amino acid forms an amide linkage with the amino group of another amino acid resulting in a continuous chain of amino acids or polypeptide molecule.

B. Translation—Polypeptide Synthesis

The synthesis of proteins by ribosomes involves several specific biochemical processes shown in Fig. 12. These events have been extensively studied in bacterial cells and are similar in both bacterial and eukaryotic cells (Revel *et al.* 1973).

1. Activation of Amino Acid

The attachment of an amino acid to the C–C–A terminus of a tRNA is termed "activation of amino acid" (Fig. 13). Aminoacyl-tRNA synthetases are enzymes which catalyze this reaction. Each amino acid and tRNA have specific activating enzymes. The initial reaction of an amino acid with adenosine triphosphate (ATP) occurs between the α-phosphate of ATP and the carboxyl group of the amino acid forming the aminoacyl–adenylic acid and pyrophosphate. The second reaction transfers the amino acid to the terminal adenosine of the respective tRNA. The tRNA–amino acid complex is then available for the formation of a peptide bond.

ACTIVATION OF AMINO ACIDS
↓
INITIATION OF POLYPEPTIDE
↓
ELONGATION OF POLYPEPTIDE
↓
TRANSLOCATION OF POLYPEPTIDE
↓
TERMINATION OF POLYPEPTIDE

Fig. 12. Steps in protein synthesis.

$$\text{ATP + amino acid} \underset{}{\overset{\text{activating enzyme}}{\rightleftharpoons}} \text{(aminoacyl}$$

adenylate) + pyrophosphate

$$\text{(aminoacyl adenylate) + tRNA} \underset{}{\overset{\text{aminoacyl-tRNA synthetase}}{\rightleftharpoons}}$$

aminoacyl-tRNA + adenylic acid

Fig. 13.   Activation of an amino acid.

2. *Initiation of Polypeptide Chains*

The synthesis of proteins in bacterial cells begins by attachment of the *N*-formylmethionyl-tRNA (fMet-tRNA) to the initiation codon AUG in mRNA (Fig. 14a and b). Various initiation factors (IF-1, IF-2, IF-3) bind to the ribosomal subunits and facilitate binding of the fMet-tRNA to the messenger RNA on the 30 S ribosomal subunit. This initiation complex then combines with the 50 S ribosomal subunit to form the 70 S ribosomes and the fMet-tRNA is attached to the P site on the 50 S subunit.

3. *Elongation, Translocation, and Termination*

A second aminoacyl-tRNA (A_1-tRNA) attaches to the A site on the 50 S subunit and a peptide bond is formed between the fMet and A_1. The result is a dipeptidyl-tRNA at the A site. Translocation of this dipeptidyl-tRNA to the P site replacing the discharged fMet-tRNA, leaves the A site open for another aminoacyl-tRNA (A_2-tRNA). By this method the amino acid chain is elongated to the point where the protein molecule is complete and must be terminated. The termination process is not clearly understood, but it appears that a specific termination codon is recognized and specific proteins (release factors) dissociate the polypeptide chain from the ribosome. Similar protein initiation factors, elongation factors, and release factors have been described in eukaryotic cells. Initiator methionyl-tRNA rather than *N*-formylmethionyl-tRNA has been described and AUG appears to be the initiator codon in these nucleated cells.

IV. DISCUSSION

Although synthesis of molecules, such as lipids and carbohydrates, may be targets for cytotoxic drugs, most of the information available points to the synthesis of purines and pyrimidines or the polymerization of purines and pyrimidines or amino acids into DNA and RNA or protein as the most common

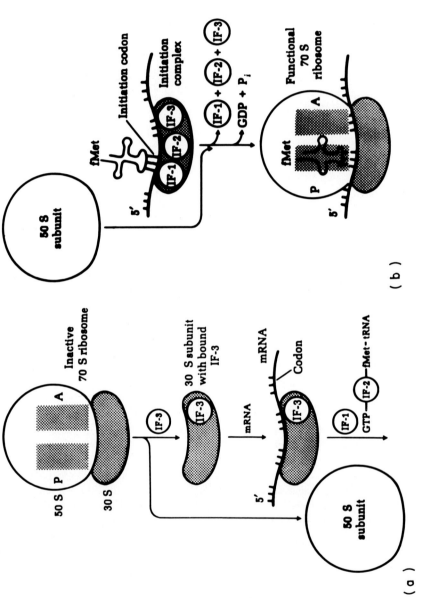

Fig. 14. Initiation of polypeptide chains. (a) Binding of messenger RNA and initiation factors (IF) to the small ribosomal subunit. (b) Formation of the fMet–tRNA–small ribosomal subunit initiation complex, binding to the large ribosomal subunit and formation of the first peptide bond between the peptidyl (P) site and aminoacyl (A) site. (From Lehninger, 1975.)

targets of anticancer drugs. It is clear from the information presented that these biochemical reactions are very complex, and much more investigation is necessary before the precise sites of action of the various anticancer drugs can be accurately identified.

The selection of an anticancer drug for treatment of a tumor depends on a number of factors, including metabolism of the drug, penetrability into the cells, acquired resistance to the drug, growth rate of the tumor cells, vascularity of tumor, and toxicity of the drug. These factors, in addition to the cytotoxic effect on tumor cells via inhibition of nucleic acid or protein syntheses, are important considerations in the design of new antineoplastic drugs.

REFERENCES

Burgess, R. R. (1971). *Annu. Rev. Biochem.* **40**, 711–740.

Busch, H., Ballal, N. R., Olson, M. O. J., and Yeoman, L. C. (1975). *Methods Cancer Res.* **11**, 43–121.

Darnell, J. E., Jelinek, W. R., and Molloy, G. R. (1973). *Science* **181**, 1215–1221.

Gefter, M. L. (1974). *Prog. Nucleic Acid Res. Mol. Biol.* **14**, 101–115.

Holley, R. W., Apgar, J., Everett, G. A., Madison, J. T., Marquisee, M., Merrill, S. H., Penswick, J. R., and Zamir, A. (1965). *Science* **147**, 1462–1465.

Kornberg, A. (1960). *Science* **131**, 1503–1508.

Kornberg, T., and Gefter, M. L. (1972). *J. Biol. Chem.* **247**, 5369–5375.

Lehninger, A. L. (1975). "Biochemistry," 2nd ed. Worth, New York.

Okazaki, R., Okazaki, T., Sakabe, K., Sugimoto, K., Kainuma, R., Sugina, A., and Iwatsuki, N. (1968). *Cold Spring Harbor Symp. Quant. Biol.* **33**, 129–143.

Prestayko, A. W., Klomp, G. R., Schmoll, D. J., and Busch, H. (1974). *Biochemistry* **13**, 1945–1951.

Revel, M., Grover, Y., Pollack, Y., Scheps, R., and Berissl, H. (1973). *Ciba Found. Symp.* 1 [NS] 69–85.

Roeder, R. G., and Rutter, W. J. (1969). *Nature (London)* **224**, 234–237.

Roeder, R. G., and Rutter, W. J. (1970). *Proc. Natl. Acad. Sci. U.S.A.* **65**, 675–682.

Warner, J. R. (1974). *In* "Ribosomes" (M. Nomura, A. Tissieres, and P. Lengyel, eds.), pp. 461–488. Cold Spring Harbor Lab., Cold Spring Harbor, New York.

Watson, J. D. (1975). "Molecular Biology of the Gene," 3rd ed. Benjamin, Menlo Park, California.

Watson, J. D., and Crick, F. H. C. (1953). *Nature (London)* **171**, 737–738.

2

THE CELL AND ITS FUNCTION
Harris Busch

I. INTRODUCTION

Virtually every cell type in the human body represents a highly specialized structure whose phenotype contributes to the elegant functioning of the physiology and adaptability of the individual. Cancer cells have a dysplastic phenotype, represented by (a) uncontrolled cell growth and division, (b) invasiveness, and (c) metastasis which is transmitted genetically or epigenetically to the daughter cells (Busch, 1974, 1978a). The evidence is clear that a single cancer cell is sufficient to produce cancer in susceptible hosts and that cancer represents a disordered state of biochemical genetics (Figs. 1–3) (Furth and Kahn, 1937; Hosokawa, 1950; Ishibashi, 1950).

CANCER AND CHEMOTHERAPY, VOL. I

Clinically, cancer (like such diseases as syphilis) appears to be "many disease states" depending on the phenotype of the tissue of origin (Busch, 1974). In studies on neoplastic disease, it is clearly important to distinguish between the manifestations of the disease and the fundamental pathological events. For example, patients presenting with severe hypoglycemic states as a result of insulinomas may not exhibit any late effects of cancer at all. In this case, the organ-specific phenotypic changes related to the neoplastic process dominate the clinical picture. However, the underlying cancerous disease state is the same as in the other human neoplasms.

Moreover, in neoplasms of any given tissue, there is a broad range of quantitative variants. Insulinomas are a good example of variants from high levels of insulin production and secretion to very low levels or none at all. Accordingly, the investigator has the problem of defining those events that are critical to the disease process and directly related to it and differentiating those that either are results of indirect events of the process or are totally unrelated.

II. THE RELATIONSHIP OF CYTOPLASMIC PROCESSES TO THE CANCER PHENOTYPE

All of the common lethal characteristics of cancer cells (Figs. 1 and 2) are related to cytoplasmic functions, particularly invasiveness (Figs. 3 and 4) and metastasis (Fidler, 1979). Of course, many biosynthetic activities involved in growth are carried on by cytoplasmic systems. For the most part, none of the mechanisms involved in these biosynthetic reactions appear to differ from those of the nontumor systems. Accordingly, a key question is where is the locus of the cancer lesion in the neoplastic cells or in what way is there a differentiation of the neoplastic cells, so that they exhibit their special common features.

There are no major properties of cancer cells that are not exhibited by nontumor cells in ontogeny (Busch, 1976a). For example, growth is a property of all cells, invasiveness is a property of several types of white cells, and metastasis is a common embryonic phenomenon (Figs. 4–8). Although production of abnormal chromosomes is an uncommon and pathological event in nontumor cells and generally leads to destruction of the affected cell, alterations in chromosome number such as polyploidy commonly occur in liver cells with maturation and aging (Sandberg and Sakurai, 1973).

As recently pointed out in studies from many laboratories (Fishman and Sells, 1976; Fishman and Busch, 1979), the "tumor antigens" of human cells and nonviral animal tumors frequently represent fetal gene readouts (Fig. 6) ranging from late fetal stages to as early as elements of sperm and ovum. Simply expressed, along with neoplastic transformation, there frequently is a fetal gene activation which is apparently quite random in terms of the "biological clock."

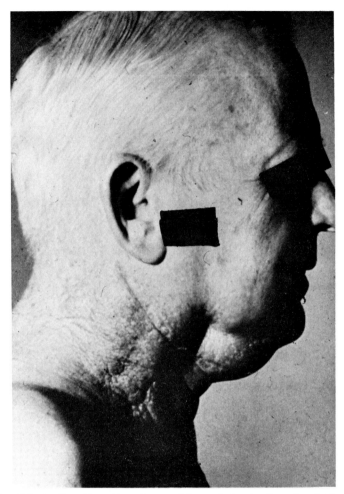

Fig. 1. Patient with epidermoid carcinoma of the neck showing line of partial healing after resection.

Of course, it is by no means proved that such fetal gene readouts have any more to do with meaningful neoplastic processes than do the activation of genes for production of the many isozymes reported to exist in various tumors (Sato and Sugimura, 1974; Weinhouse, 1972).

The concept that fetal genes are active in the process of neoplasia is an attractive one (Busch, 1976a). If one considers the genome to be a large mass of potential gene readouts (Fig. 4) which are subject to the influence of factors and various stimuli that may act through receptors intermediates or directly on the

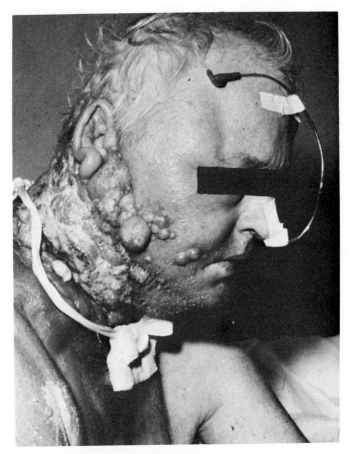

Fig. 2. Same patient as in Fig. 1, 3 hours premortem. The ulceration of the surface and presence of fibrin are apparent as well as local metastatic lesions. The patient also suffered from mediastinal penetration of the tumor.

genome, it may be considered that in each cell (Fig. 5) a limited population of genes is operative. Their products, which are mRNA species of various types, interact with ribosomes that originate in the nucleolus to form the polysomes, which are the units of protein synthesis in the cytoplasm. These are involved in the production of specific proteins (P1-P3, R1, etc.) that define the phenotype of

Fig. 3. (A) Light microscopic view of the cancer cells stained with Azure C. The pleomorphism of the nucleoli is apparent. (B) Electronic micrograph of a Novikoff hepatoma showing the enlarged nucleolus and the enlarged nucleus with the large ratio of nucleus to cytoplasm. Note the microvilli find on the cell surface. Labeling with tritiated uridine for short times shows partial localization to the nucleolus.

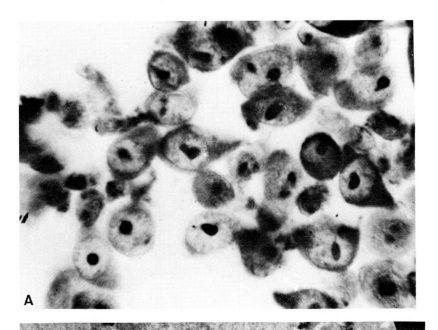

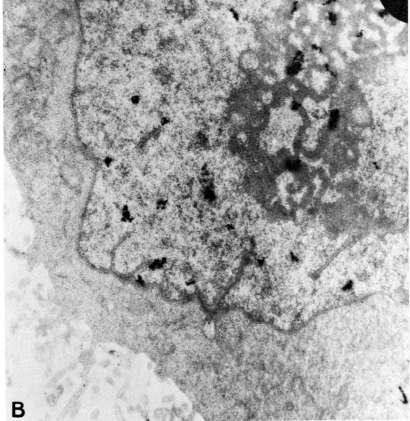

RESTING OR GROUND STATE

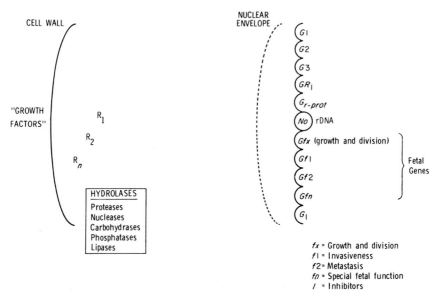

Fig. 4. Elements of cellular response to external stimuli in the resting or ground state. It is envisioned that growth factors and other stimuli are almost continuously present in the cellular periphery in equilibrium with intracellular elements. The symbols are R_1–R_n, cytoplasmic receptor proteins; $G1$–GR_1, structural genes including genes for receptor proteins (GR_1); $Gf1$–Gfn, fetal genes with functions indicated; G_1 inhibitor genes; No, rDNA genes; and $G_{r\text{-}prot}$, genes for ribosomal proteins.

the specific cell. The key point is that the fetal genes are "silent" in these mature cells of normal individuals.

In fetal cells (Fig. 6) there is a complex series of events in progress, related largely to the time point on the biological clock. As Fig. 6 indicates, the fetal cells operate with their own set of signals, which are coupled with special readouts that produce the incredible number of events that not only involve growth, specialization, and migration of cells but also specify organization with an incredible order of accuracy. As many have noted, special events occur in ontogenesis which do not recur during normal life. For example, the processes involved in limb bud formation, including initiation, elongation, and termination of growth, can be interfered with by thalidomide to result in the arrested states characteristic of phocomelia. Even if the drug is removed, there is no repetition of the phenomenon, i.e., the limb buds do not continue to grow. Accordingly, there is only a defined "time window" during which limb bud growth and development occur.

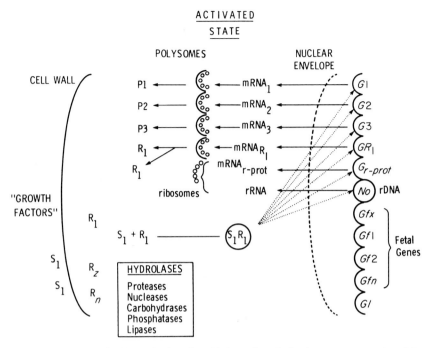

Fig. 5. Response of cells to stimulus (S_1) with formation of stimulus–receptor complex (S_1R_1) which impinges upon a group of genes (Gl–GR_1, $G_{r\text{-prot}}$, and $G_{No\text{-}rDNA}$), to produce a series of mRNAs, ribosomes, and polysomes that in turn synthesize specific products, including R_1. The "battery" of fetal genes is not involved in these normal responses. P1–P3, protein readouts. (See Fig. 4 for other symbols.)

Needless to say, these special time points in the biological block must be under control of special "start" and "stop" signals which are probably active only during the specific phases of ontogenesis. There is a rigid timing of these events in embryogenesis; either a series of feedback loops, or specific inhibitors must exist that "turn off" specific fetal functions. Among the types of shut-off mechanisms that could exist are (a) loss of fetal "stimulus" factors (S_f) or (b) the inhibition by fetal factors of the function of S_f (Fig. 6). If, in cancer cells, some special fetal genes are activated (Figs. 7 and 8), suppression of function may not occur in the adult because associated factors have long been inoperative. It is thus conceivable that a variety of functions of neoplastic cells could be controlled if specific fetal control elements were available (Illmensee and Mintz, 1976).

Figure 7 indicates that, at the time of exposure to carcinogens, three and possibly more major effects may occur in which a carcinogen may interact with receptors, activators, cellular or chromatin enzymes or other proteins, or directly or indirectly with the genome. The carcinogen may exert a direct effect on the

FETAL

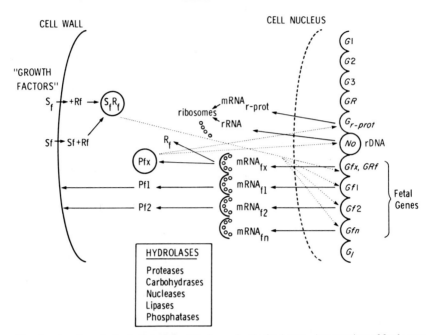

Fig. 6. A pattern similar to that of Fig. 5 is shown for the fetal state when a variety of fetal genes are activated by stimulus S_f (fetal "stimulus" factors) and receptor Rf to form S_fR_f, which acts in the same way as the factors controlling structural genes of the adult. (See Fig. 4 for other symbols.)

Fig. 7. Effects of carcinogenic agents on cellular responses. It is envisioned that carcinogens permit structural genes to function in production of normal products; but that, through several mechanisms, fetal genes are activated to produce a variety of fetal products, including Pf1 and Pf2, which are important to invasiveness and metastasis. The carcinogen may act with a fetal receptor to directly interact with the genome or may cause a new stimulus within the cell to interact with a receptor that will interact with the genome. Alternatively, the carcinogen may interfere with degradative reactions that are involved in normal growth controls. Ca, carcinogen. (See Fig. 4 for other symbols.)

Fig. 8. This diagram indicates the expression of cancer as a continuous production of gene products involved in growth, invasiveness, and metastasis. Such cells no longer produce R1, R2 (blocked, $\mathbb{R}_1$, $\mathbb{R}_2$), or others that may have phenotypic specificity. It is envisioned that these gene products and their derepressors are produced or maintained in high concentration through mitosis and keep these genes activated during new cell formation. Moreover, the lack of fetal extracellular regulatory mechanisms do not permit these genes to be inactivated as they would be during fetal growth and development. (See Fig. 4 for other symbols.)

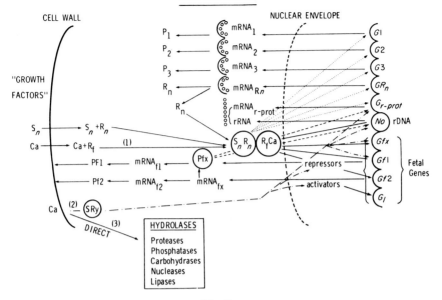

Fig. 7.

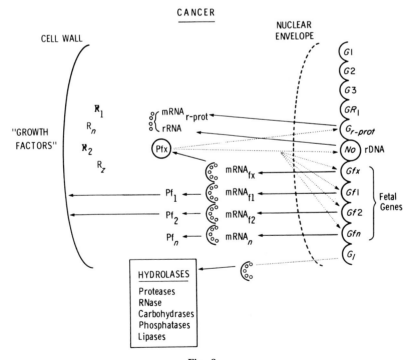

Fig. 8.

genome (Fig. 7). The primordial cell that becomes a cancer cell is thrown into genomic disarray that leads to the dysplasia referred to by Sugimura (1976). Carcinogens may destroy most affected cells. Others undergo a wide variety of phenotypic alterations ranging from total loss of phenotypic function to excessive production of specialized production of specialized products. At some crucial time, the genome becomes "set" for its altered functional activity in which both fetal and specialized genes are expressed (Fig. 8). In recent studies, it appears that in cancer cells the genome "set" occurs even before telophase has been completed (Busch *et al.*, 1979).

The cancer cells that emerge from the oncogenic event have a fundamental fixed mechanism that includes operation of fetal genes. In these cells, many normal receptors are deleted (Fig. 8). Other receptors may be produced, R_n or R_z. However, the key genes, *Pfx, Pf1,* and *Pf2*, that are depressed, represent those fetal gene elements that are the key to the biology of cancer, including cell growth and division, invasiveness, and metastasis. The cellular mechanisms involved and their control are the primary interests of the following elements of our cancer research (Busch, 1976a).

III. THE RELATIONSHIP OF THE CELL NUCLEUS TO THE CANCER PHENOTYPE

Much new information has accumulated on the structures (Figs. 9 and 10) and products of the cell nucleus (Tables I and II) (Busch, 1974, 1978a,b,c; Elgin and Weintraub, 1975; Stein and Kleinsmith, 1975).

For the purpose of the present chapter, the topic is segregated into the general divisions of (a) the structures and contents of the cell nucleus; (b) chromatin, its constituents, and the synthesis of mRNA; (c) the nucleolus and synthesis of rRNA; and (d) some special features of the nucleolus of cancer cells.

In any consideration of the nucleus, it should be recalled that whether it represents a small structure in large cell or a giant structure in a relatively small cell, there is always a layer of cytoplasm, no matter how small, between it and the cell's plasma membrane. That structure plays an important role in the feedback interactions of the nucleus with the whole array of stimuli to which the cell is exposed (Figs. 3B, 4, and 9). In this sense, the nucleus is part of an integrated system by which cells of various organs respond to extracellular and intracellular stimuli (Fig. 5). These stimuli interact with the nuclear informational system to produce specific products (Table II) that permit response of the cytoplasm to the environment and its functional demands. The charm of the cell nucleus rests in the remarkable variety of its potential products which alter cellular function so remarkably from tissue to tissue and organ to organ (Busch, 1974).

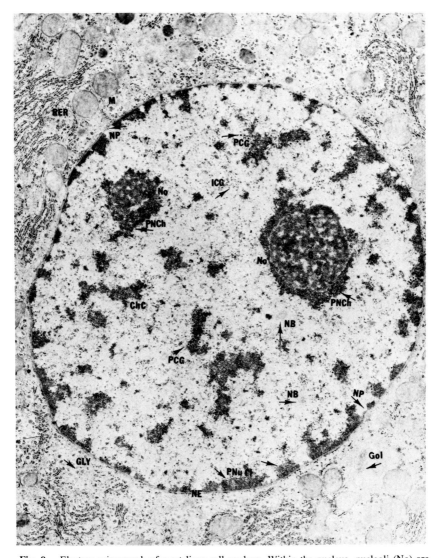

Fig. 9. Electron micrograph of a rat liver cell nucleus. Within the nucleus, nucleoli (No) are surrounded by perinucleolar chromatin (PNCh). The nucleoli consist of granular (G) and fibrillar (F) elements. Chromocenters (ChC) are distributed randomly within the nucleoplasm. Frequently, perichromatin granules (PCG) are associated with these chromocenters. Within the nucleus occasionally nuclear bodies (NB) and interchromatin granules (ICG) are seen that are apparently cross sections of the nuclear ribonucleoprotein network. The inner layer of the nuclear envelope (NE) surrounds a conspicuous layer of dense chromatin (PNuCh). The clear areas within this heterochromatin layer usually mark the location of the nuclear pores (NP). In the cytoplasm, glycogen elements (GLY) are present. Mitochondria (M) and rough endoplasmic reticulum (RER) are distributed throughout the cytoplasm. Occasionally Golgi (Gol) complexes are seen around the nuclear periphery. Lead citrate–uranyl acetate staining. ×18,000. (Courtesy of T. Unuma and Y. Daskal.)

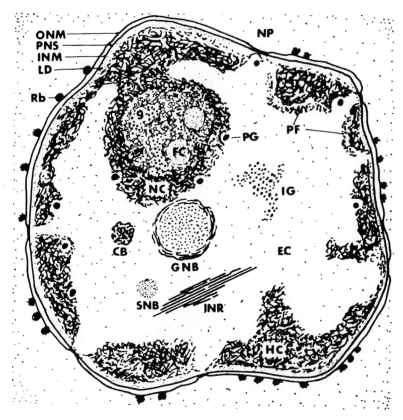

Fig. 10. Ideal section of a nucleus, showing all the main components. The nucleus is surrounded by the outer (ONM) and inner nuclear membranes (INM) that enclose the perinuclear space (PNS), which is a part of the rough endoplasmic reticulum and has ribosomes (Rb) attached. Between the chromatin and the inner membrane lies the lamina densa (LD), which is thinner in front of the nuclear pores (NP). The chromatin is found as heterochromatin (HC), nucleolus-associated chromatin (NC), and euchromatin (EC). The nucleolus shows the granular (g) components, and fibrillar centers (FC). In the borderline of the chromatin, many perichromatin granules (PG) and a layer of perichromatin fibrils (PF) (of which only a portion has been drawn) are to be found. Finally, in the interchromatin space, a cluster of interchromatin granules (IG), a granular nuclear body (GNB), a simple nuclear body (SNB), a coiled body (CB), and an intranuclear rodlet (INR) have been drawn. (From Bouteille *et al.*, 1974.)

A. The Role of the Cell Nucleus

The nucleus is the major repository of genetic information—chromatin, which contains DNA and its associated proteins. Very small amounts of DNA are in the mitochondria, and if there is a significant amount of DNA in the cell membrane or the endoplasmic reticulum, it is at such a low level that, thus far, reports of its

TABLE I

Nuclear Structures

    I. Nuclear envelope
        A. Outer layer—continuation of the endoplasmic reticulum
        B. Outer layer
        C. Nuclear pores
        D. Juxtaenvelope chromatin
   II. Chromatin—chromosomes
        A. Interphase chromatin
           1. "Euchromatin"—dispersed chromatin
           2. Heterochromatin—condensed chromatin
        B. Meiotic chromatin
           1. Chromatin in various states of condensation
           2. Defined metaphase chromosomes
  III. The nucleolus
        A. Nucleoli in various stages of cell function
        B. "Nucleolar chromosomes"
        C. rDNA and its controls
        D. Preribosomal RNA
        E. Interlocks of rRNA and ribosomal protein synthesis
        F. The nucleolar channel system
  IV. Nuclear ribonucleoprotein network
        A. Perichromatin granules
        B. Interchromatin granules
        C. Nuclear bodies
        D. Nuclear rodlets
        E. Nuclear inclusions
        F. mRNP precursor particles (informosomes)

---

presence have not been uniformly reproducible. The genetic information of the cell nucleus becomes operational in the form of polysomes which contain messenger RNA (template RNA), ribosomes, and associated biosynthetic elements (Table II).

A major question in cell and molecular biology is what is the nature of the control systems that regulate the genome. Since the DNA is the same in virtually all cells of an individual (red blood cells and haploid cells excepted), it remains totipotent throughout the life of the cell (Gurdon, 1974). The substances that govern the gene readouts must be derived from the cytoplasm or external cellular milieu directly, or by interaction with appropriate "receptor" or "carrier" molecules that interact with gene loci. The mechanisms of transport and function of these substances are discussed later.

Many very beautiful light microscopic studies have been made on nuclei and nucleoli (Busch and Smetana, 1970; Montgomery, 1898). Recent elegant advances in scanning and electron microscopy have provided improved two- and

TABLE II

Nuclear Products

   I. DNA
     A. Complete DNA replication during cell division
     B. Gene amplification or repetition
  II. RNA
     A. Messenger RNA
       1. mRNA sequences
       2. poly(A) 3′ termini
       3. The 5′ cap (? nucleus)
     B. rRNA
       1. 28 S rRNA
       2. 18 S rRNA
       3. 5.8 S rRNA
       4. 5 S rRNA
     C. tRNA
       1. tRNA nucleotide sequence
       2. Many modified tRNA nucleotides
     D. Low molecular weight nuclear RNA
       1. Uridine-rich nuclear RNA U1. U2. U3
       2. Other species including $4.5 \text{ S RNA}_{I-III} \cdot 5 \text{ S RNA}_{III} \cdot 8 \text{ S RNA}$
     E. Precursor processing reactions for each RNA species
 III. Ribonucleoprotein particles
     A. mRNP particles
       1. Informosomes
       2. Polysomes
     B. rRNA particles
       1. Granular nucleolar elements
       2. Completed ribosomes

---

three-dimensional analyses of the nuclear structures as well as their spatial inter-relationships (Table I). The fundamental structure of the cell nucleus is rather simple. As seen in Figs. 9 and 10, isolated nuclei essentially consist of a highly permeable, double-layered envelope which circumscribes a semihomogeneous structure. The basic nuclear framework is the ''nuclear ribonucleoprotein network'' (''nuclear matrix''), the hub of which is the nucleolus (Fig. 9). The nuclear envelope and the ''nuclear matrix'' provide both the basic elements of nuclear structure and the sites of attachment of critical nuclear elements (Figs. 9 and 10). In general, the nucleus may be considered to be a unit structure containing an internal matrix surrounded by a double-layered envelope of high porosity (Franke and Scheer, 1974).

Although at one time the nucleus was thought to be an amorphous structure with the exception of the nucleoli, improved methods have shown that it contains a series of particulate structures (Bouteille *et al.*, 1974) that serve special and important roles in its function (Figs. 9 and 10).

B. The Double-Layered Nuclear Envelope

The nuclear envelope (Fig. 5) consists of two portions: the outer layer, which is frequently covered by ribosomes and is in intimate contact with the cytoplasm and endoplasmic reticulum, and the inner layer, which is composed of "membrane" and is in turn in contact with chromatin and the nuclear elements. The two layers regularly join at the nuclear pores which are shown in cross section and on end in Fig. 11. These structures are not simply holes in the nuclear wall (like holes in a whiffle ball) but rather, have been shown to contain a number of elements that are arranged in a highly ordered form (Franke and Scheer, 1974). Many studies are in progress on the nuclear envelope in the hope of discerning more about its semipermeable character with respect to substances being added to the nucleus and the mechanism of penetration of the large particles and other elements out of the nucleus into the cytoplasm. While the nucleus is continuously "sensing" cytoplasmic activity, its response is in the form of large particles that must pass through the "retaining wall" of the nuclear envelope. Presumably, the nuclear pores would serve the function of permitting such large "packages" to

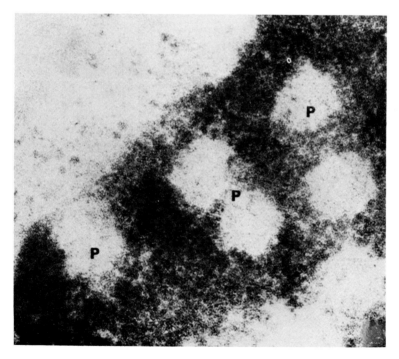

Fig. 11. Vertical section through the nuclear envelope at the nuclear pores (P). (From Franke and Scheer, 1974.)

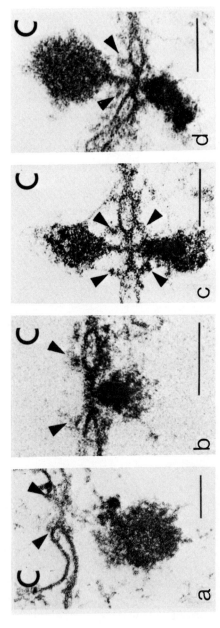

Fig. 12. In (a)–(d) the possible sequence of events is shown for penetration of the pore complexes (some annular granules are denoted by arrowheads): the large globule approaches the pore complex and becomes connected to it by thin filaments (a); it then reaches the pore center (b) and elongates into a 100–150 Å broad rod; the material passes the pore center in this rodlike form, transitorily assuming a typical dumbbell-shaped configuration (c); then the material rounds into a spheroid particle (d); and is deposited on the cytoplasmic side; for some time still revealing fibrillar connections. C, Cytoplasmic side. (a) ×83,000. (b) ×135,000. (c) ×110,000. (d) ×100,000. Scale indicates 0.1 μm. (From Franke and Scheer, 1974.)

migrate out of the nucleus into the cytoplasm. Some electron microscopic pictures support this suggestion (Fig. 12).

Chromatin is a complex of nuclear DNA, its associated proteins, RNA, and small molecules (Busch *et al.*, 1975). Chromatin is the interphase state of the chromosomes (Figs. 13 and 14): it has enormous complexity and unusual properties. The basic problems in manipulation of chromatin relate to the difficulties of the handling of chemical evaluations of molecules of such enormous size as DNA, which are now generally believed to be as long as the chromatids.

The task of sorting out a specific DNA cistron in an intact form from such

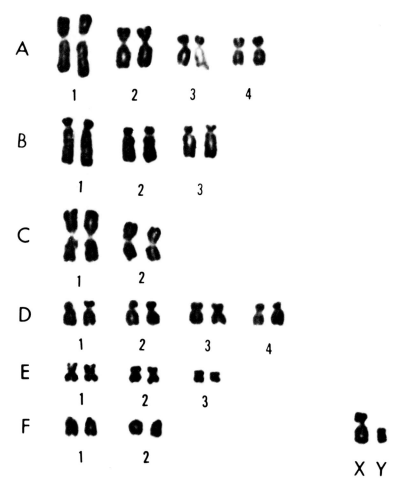

Fig. 13. Normal karyotype showing metacentric chromosomes (A,C, and E), achrocentric chromosomes (B,D, and F), and chromosomes X and Y.

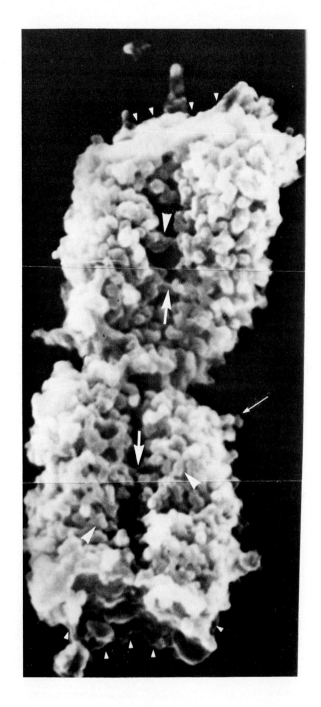

Fig. 14.

structures has challenged many investigators, and except for rare cases, such as the "amplified" and segregated rDNA found in some "satellites," individual DNA species have not been isolated from chromatin.

The histones in chromatin are approximately equal in weight to the DNA, and, further, DNA is closely associated with histones in somatic cells. Accordingly, it appeared that the histones had some critical structural or stabilizing role, particularly since the number of charges that were positive on the histones were roughly equal to the number of negative charges on the DNA.

This very interesting equivalence has been subjected to much reappraisal in recent years by virtue of the demonstration that there were significant interactions between histones which are sufficient in themselves to produce small nuclear bodies referred to as "nu bodies" (Olins and Olins, 1974). These "nu bodies" are apparently composed of histone subunits, i.e., two molecules each of histone 2A, 2B, 3, and 4, and further, they may be related to structures also containing histone 1. The nu bodies were originally reported to be "beads on a string" (Fig. 15) in extended chromatin structures. Many studies have led to the development of the model (Fig. 16) which shows that the nu bodies are composed of one and one-half DNA turns surrounding the core octamer of the four histones noted above (Pardon and Richards, 1979).

The role of the nu bodies is undefined. There is a random distribution of nu bodies in both transcribed and untranscribed chromatin. Moreover, virtually all the liver sequences transcribed into mRNA are present in nu body-associated DNA. Accordingly, nu body formation is random with respect to DNA sequence, and the nu bodies in any specific DNA region do not restrict transcription.

C. Nonhistone Nuclear Proteins

The definition of nuclear proteins, although apparently obvious, has been the subject of considerable methodological evaluation. Needless to say, what will be called a "nuclear protein" is dependent upon the technique employed for isolation of the nuclei (Fig. 17). It is well recognized that most nuclear proteins (if not all) are synthesized in the cytoplasm and must be present there in small amounts at some point (Comings and Tack, 1973). The early controversy about "contractile" proteins, that have been reported to be present in the cell nucleus (Douvas *et al.,* 1975; LeStourgeon *et al.,* 1975); had arisen from the failure of some

---

Fig. 14. Scanning electron micrograph of whole-mount isolated CHO metaphase chromosome 2. Membranous platelike structures (small arrowheads) connects both chromatids only at their distal ends. Multiple interchromatidal connections (large arrows) are seen in the interchromatidal furrow. Highly coiled topical "microconvules" (large arrowheads) and axial coilings (small arrows) are present. ×65,000. (From Daskal *et al.,* 1976.)

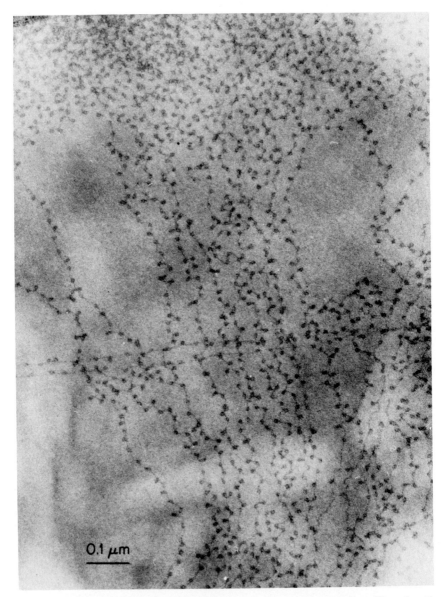

Fig. 15. Nu bodies. Chromatin fibers streaming out of a rat thymus nucleus. The spheroid chromatin units (nu bodies) exhibit local variations in arrangement and separation, possibly due to differential stretching of the fibers. Negative stain 0.5% ammonium molybdate, pH 7.4. ×326,000. (From Busch *et al.*, 1975, courtesy of D. E. and A. L. Olins.)

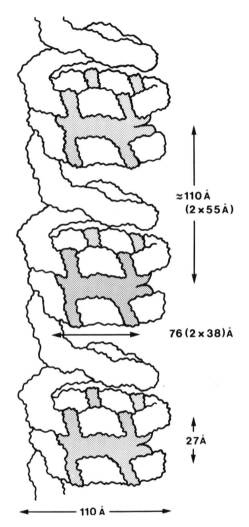

≈110 Å
(2×55Å)

76 (2 × 38)Å

27Å

110 Å

Fig. 16. Diagramatic representation of interrelation of nucleosomes in chromatin. (From Pardon and Richards, 1979.)

groups to isolate nuclei in satisfactory form. As a result, proteins limited to the cytoplasm have been reported to be present in nuclei. The failure to employ satisfactory procedures for nuclear isolation (Busch and Smetana, 1970) results in preparations that confuse the complex problems of nuclear protein chemistry (Comings and Harris, 1975).

It became clear in 1963 (Steele and Busch, 1963) that the nonhistone proteins are a very heterogeneous series of molecular species, including proteins of the

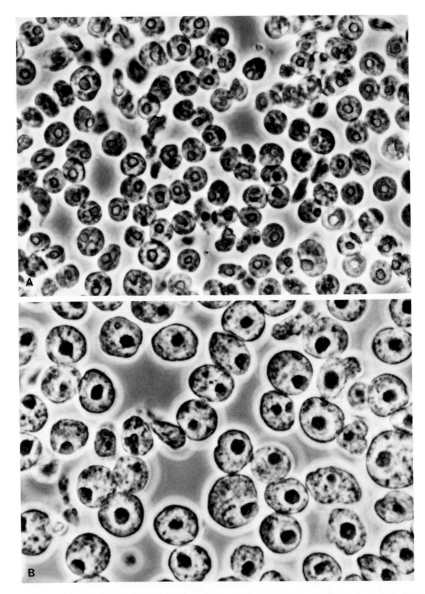

Fig. 17. Phase microscopy of a preparation of isolated nuclei of Morris hepatoma 9618. (A) ×600. (B) ×1100. (From Busch and Smetana, 1970.)

nuclear envelope, the nuclear sap, the chromatin, and the nucleolus (Table III). In each of these groups there are a number of important subgroups that include various enzymes, phosphoproteins, processing enzymes and transport elements (Busch *et al.,* 1975; Busch, 1965).

The greatest interest in recent years has centered on the proteins that are "chromatin associated," largely because of the findings of Paul and Gilmour (1966a,b, 1968), and subsequently many other workers, that the "gene control

TABLE III

Nuclear Nonhistone Proteins

    I. Nuclear membrane proteins
        A. Structural proteins
        B. Transport proteins
        C. Processing enzymes
        D. Nuclear pore proteins
   II. Nuclear sap proteins
        A. Cytonucleoproteins
            1. Receptors, normal and modified
            2. RNP particle proteins
                a. Small U1 and U2 RNA
                b. Samarina particles
        B. Phosphoproteins
        C. Enzymes
  III. Chromatin-bound proteins
        A. Solubility classification
            1. Acid solubility
                a. Acid soluble
                b. Acid insoluble
                    i. Solubilized by DNase
                    ii. DNase residue
            2. Soluble in dilute NaCl
            3. Solubility in concentrated NaCl
                a. Soluble in 2 *M* NaCl
                b. Soluble in 3 *M* NaCl 7 *M* urea
            4. Soluble in phenol
            5. Soluble in sodium dodecyl sulfate
        B. Structural proteins
        C. Gene control proteins
        D. Phosphoproteins
        E. Enzymes
  IV. Nucleolar proteins
        A. Ribosomal precursor proteins
        B. Structural proteins
        C. rDNA control proteins
        D. Phosphoproteins
        E. Enzymes

TABLE IV

Evidence for Specificity on Nonhistone Proteins (NHP)[a]

Test system	References
Organ-specific transcription of chromatin	Paul and Gilmour (1966a,b; 1968)
Tissue-specific restriction of DNA	Richter and Sekeris (1972); Kamiyama et al. (1972)
Tissue-specific binding of progesterone receptor	Steggles et al. (1971)
Mechanism of action of female sex hormones	Jensen and DeSombre (1972)
NHP in chromatin—organ specificity	Gilmour and Paul (1970)
Tumor transcriptional specificity; regenerating liver specificity	Kostraba and Wang (1972a,b; 1973); Kadohama and Turkington (1973)
Tissue specificity of NHP	Barrett and Gould (1973); Orrick et al. (1973); Yeoman et al. (1973a,b)
Antigenic specificity of chromatin	Chytil and Spelsberg (1971); Spelsberg et al. (1971c); Zardi et al. (1973)
Specificity of mitotic proteins	Rovera and Baserga (1971); Rovera et al. (1971); Stein et al. (1972)
Phosphoproteins in gene regulation	Teng et al. (1971)
Stimulation of synthesis by phytohemagglutinin	Levy et al. (1973); Pogo and Katz (1974)

[a] From Busch et al. (1975).

proteins'' are present in these fractions (Table IV). The evidence that the gene control proteins are in chromatin was obtained by preextraction of ''citric acid'' nuclei with dilute salt solution (0.15 M NaCl–0.1 M Tris), followed by distilled water to swell the chromatin. Following these extractions, the residue called ''chromatin,'' was demonstrated to exhibit ''fidelity'' of transcription by analysis of products produced after incubation with RNA polymerase and appropriately labeled nucleoside triphosphates. The products produced were then hybridized in competition studies with RNA of specific tissues.

The key demonstration was that on reconstitution of the chromatin initially disassociated with high salt (2 M NaCl, 5 M urea, 0.01 M Tris, pH 8.3) and reconstitution with histones, DNA, and nonhistone products in interrupted gradients of salt and urea, the RNA readouts were characteristic of the tissue or origin of the nonhistone proteins, and not the DNA or the histones. Many subsequent findings have supported and extended these conclusions.

The studies on the binding of hormones to nonhistone proteins have been most interesting in this respect. The studies of Jensen and his associates (Jensen and DeSombre, 1972) on estrogen–receptor interaction initiated the series of studies in this field. The recent studies (O'Malley and Schrader, 1976) in O'Malley's group (O'Malley and Means, 1974) have shown a relationship between the steroid hormone–receptor complex and the production of special mRNA related to oviduct proteins.

TABLE V

Nuclear Enzymes

---

1. RNA synthesis and processing
   RNA polymerases A, B, etc.
   RNA modification enzymes: methylases, formation of modified bases
   RNA trimming or special cleavage enzymes
   RNases: exo- and endonucleoytic
2. DNA synthesis
   "True" synthesis
   Ligases
   Excision enzymes
   Terminal addition enzymes
   DNases
   Modification enzymes: methylases, etc.
3. Other modification and synthetic enzymes
   Histone phosphokinases, methylases, acetylases, deacetylases, proteases
   Nonhistone protein kinases and methylases
   Nucleoside kinases
   NAD pyrophosphorylase
4. Dehydrogenases
   Steroid dehydrogenase
   Cytochrome oxidase
   Glycerol-3-phosphate dehydrogenases
   Glyceraldehyde-3-phosphate dehydrogenases
   Succinate, malate, isocitrate, lactate, NADH, NADPH, glucose 6-phosphate,
      phosphogluconate
5. Transferases: glycosyl for glycogen phosphorylases and branching enzymes
6. Enzymes of uncertain function
   ATPases
   Carboxylesterases
   Phosphatases
   5'-Nucleotidases
   Phosphodiestrase

The nonhistone proteins serve very important enzymatic functions (Table V), and some have interesting nuclear localizations as suggested by Vorbrodt (1974). Evidence that some of these proteins bind to mRNA has been accumulating.

D. Links between the Nonhistone Proteins and the Histones

The two-dimensional gel electrophoresis methods for nuclear proteins (Figs. 18–20) led to the unequivocal demonstration that there are very large numbers of these molecules, i.e., in excess of 400 species (Busch *et al.*, 1974; Orrick *et al.*, 1973; Peterson and McConkey, 1976a,b; Yeoman *et al.*, 1973a,b). The continuing efforts to isolate and identify individual nuclear proteins has led to the demonstration of new HMG molecules (high mobility proteins) by Goodwin *et*

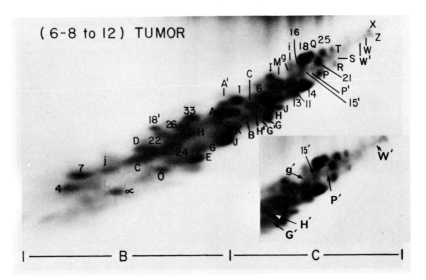

Fig. 18. Two-dimensional polyacrylamide gel electrophoresis patterns of chromatin proteins (Busch *et al.*, 1974). The horizontal dimension is on 6% acid–urea gel and the vertical dimension is an 8% SDS gel. In the insert, the tumor related spots are labeled.

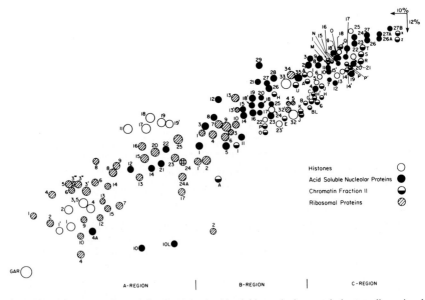

Fig. 19. Composite picture of separation of acid-soluble nucleolar protein by two-dimensional gel electrophoresis (Orrick *et al.*, 1973). 10% acid–urea horizontal dimension, 12% SDS vertical dimension.

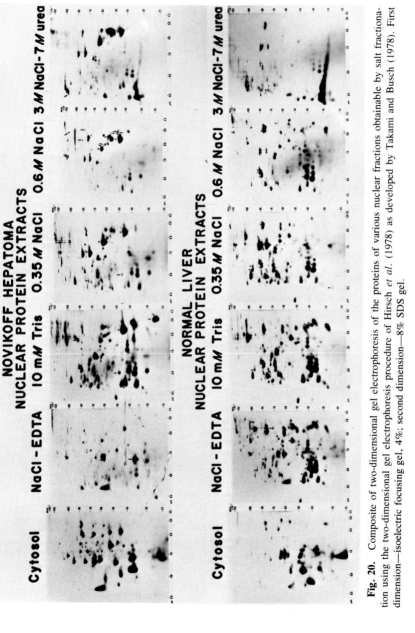

Fig. 20. Composite of two-dimensional gel electrophoresis of the proteins of various nuclear fractions obtainable by salt fractionation using the two-dimensional gel electrophoresis procedure of Hirsch *et al.* (1978) as developed by Takami and Busch (1978). First dimension—isoelectric focusing gel, 4%; second dimension—8% SDS gel.

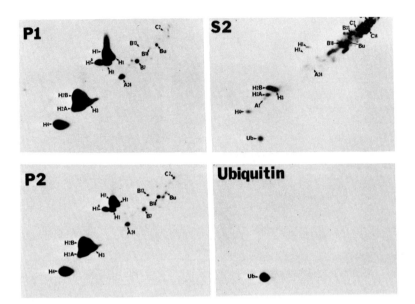

Fig. 21. Two-dimensional polyacrylamide gel electrophoretic fractionation of 500 μg each of 0.4 N H$_2$SO$_4$-soluble proteins and 25 μg of ubiquitin. The gels were obtained using proteins from pellet (P1 and P2) and supernatant (S2) chromatin fractions as well as known samples of purified ubiquitin (lower right). Electrophoresis was from right to left in the first dimension and top to bottom in the second. (Courtesy of I. L. Goldknopf.)

al. (1975, 1978). A particularly interesting protein, A24 (Fig. 19), named on the basis of migration on two-dimensional gel electrophoresis, is a conjugated form of histone 2A, with ubiquitin bound to it in an isopeptide linkage (Goldknopf *et al.*, 1977; Olson *et al.*, 1976).

Although the functional role of this protein is not yet known, it seems possible that the nonhistone ''arm'' (ubiquitin) of this protein may be cleaved off the 2A histone in the course of gene activation (Fig. 21).

Fig. 22. (A) Two-dimensional autoradiogram of normal rat liver nuclear 0.15 M NaCl-soluble proteins. Samples were run in the first dimension on 9.5-cm tube gels of 6% acrylamide, 4.5 M urea, 0.9 N acid at 120 V for 5.5 hours. The second dimension was 8% acrylamide, 0.1% sodium dodecyl sulfate, 0.1 M phosphate (pH 7.1) slab gel. Gels were stained with Coomassie brilliant blue R after 15 hours of electrophoresis at 50 mA/slab. After destaining, the gels were subsequently dried under vacuum and exposed to X-ray film for 5 to 15 days. After development, the stained spots were matched with spots on the film. Numbers followed by p indicate radioactive spots that do not comigrate with stained spots. (B) Two-dimensional autoradiogram of Novikoff hepatoma nuclear protein soluble in 0.15 M NaCl, 0.01 M Tris, 0.001 M phenylmethylsulfonyl fluoride. The dashed line separates regions B and C of the gels which are defined in Fig. 27.

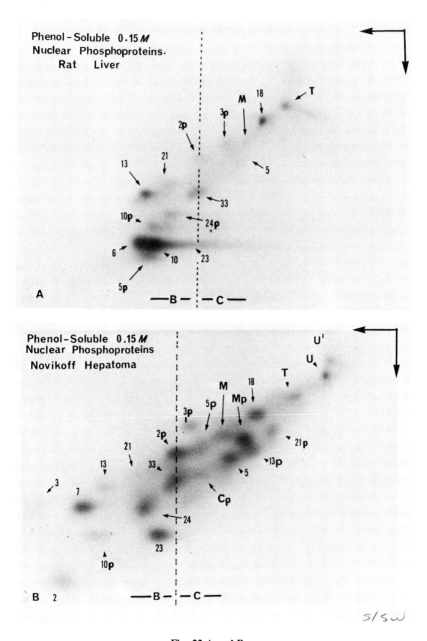

Fig. 22 A and B

The functions of nonhistone proteins have not yet been completely evaluated. Important developments in this area include two-dimensional gel electrophoresis using diagonal systems which showed the presence of unique proteins in experimental tumors (see Fig. 18, inset arrows) and extended studies on the system differentiated between histones, extranucleolar nuclear proteins, ribosomal proteins, and proteins of chromatin fraction 2 (Fig. 19).

More recently, using another two-dimensional technique (Hirsch *et al.*, 1978), it has been possible to separate over 400 nuclear proteins (Fig. 20) of various cells (Takami and Busch, 1978). The proteins have been separated in part by salt fractionation of the nuclei.

Additional techniques, such as labeling with ^{32}P, have permitted identification and demonstration of separable tumor phosphoproteins (Fig. 22).

E. The Nucleolus

The portion of the nucleus that synthesizes about 85% of all cellular RNA is the nucleolus (Fig. 23), which plays an essential role of production of new ribosomes (Busch and Smetana, 1970). The nucleolus is the product of nucleolus organizer regions of chromatin (Fig. 24), which apparently contain the rDNA and the specific sites of structural organization for interlocking nucleolar protein and RNA products.

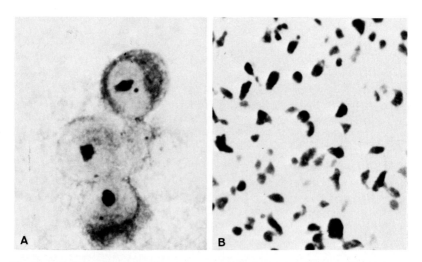

Fig. 23. (A) Smear of nuclear preparations from Walker tumor stained with toluidine blue. The nucleoli and the cytoplasmic basophilic structures are stained intensely. × 1600. (B) Smear of isolated nucleoli from Walker tumor. × 1600. (Courtesy of Dr. K. Smetana.) (C) Electron micrograph of liver nuclei showing nucleolar structure. (D) Isolated liver nucleoli showing morphological similarities to nucleolus in (C).

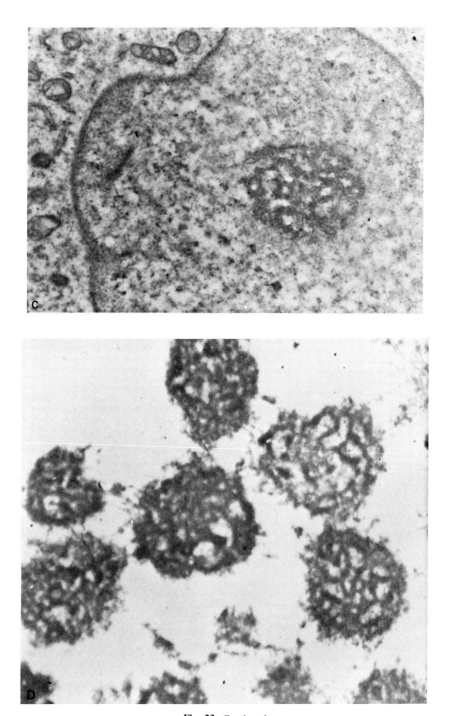

Fig. 23. *Continued*

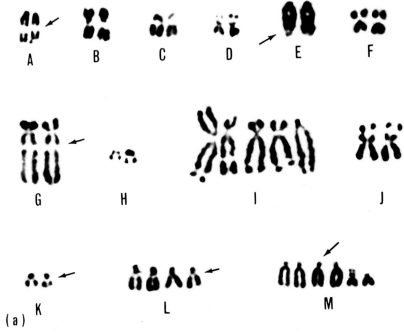

Fig. 24. (a) Chromosomes of a number of species with secondary constrictions. The arrows represent the positions of the constrictions. Top row from left to right: A, *Spilogale putorius* (spotted skunk); B, *Mephitis mephitis* (striped skunk); C, *Mustela putorius* (ferret); D, *Felis catus* (domestic cat); E, *Cervus canadensis* (elk); F, *Sus scorfa* (domestic pig). Second row: G, *Carollia perspicillata* (fruit bat); H, *Pipistrellus subflavus* (Eastern pipestrelle); I, *Tamiasciurus hudsonicus* (red squirrel); J, *Chinchilla laniger* (chinchilla). Third row: K, *Tupaia glis* (tree shrew); L, *Alouatta caraya* (black howler); M, *Homo sapiens* (man). (Courtesy of Dr. T. C. Hsu, M. D. Anderson Hospital, Houston, Texas.) (b) Silver stained Novikoff hepatoma cells showing nucleus in metaphase containing nucleolar NOR doublets. Another nucleus contains rows of three or more of nucleolar dense granules.

The nucleolus is the sole cellular location of some very specific cellular and nuclear components (Table VI). One of the most remarkable facets of nucleolar function is the production of the enormous nucleotide chains (12,000) of 45 S nRNA which are synthesized with great rapidity by RNA polymerase I (Chambon *et al.*, 1974; Roeder and Rutter, 1969, 1970) on repetitive genes, and also, are methylated, cleaved, and modified as the molecules are formed. In addition, the nucleolus is a site of protein binding to the newly synthesized RNA to form the nucleolar granular elements (Fig. 9). These granular elements are the RNP products of the nucleolus (Fig. 9) which, after isolation by various procedures, have been shown to contain the modified long preribosomal RNA chains and, in addition, some proteins that migrate to cytoplasmic ribosomes and others that do not.

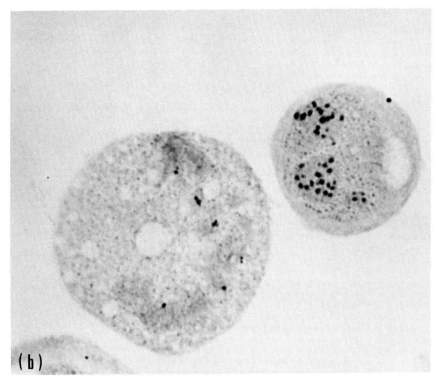

Fig. 24. *Continued*

Further maturation of nucleolar products is believed to occur in the nuclear ribonucleoprotein network (Busch and Smetana, 1970) which may provide the locus for joining additional ribosomal and polysomal proteins to these pre-ribosomal elements to complete the fully matured polysomes.

The fibrillar elements of the nucleolus (Fig. 9) apparently provide the matrix

TABLE VI

Specific Nucleolar Components

I. rDNA
II. U3 low molecular weight RNA
III. Specific elements
A. Fibrillar elements
B. Granular elements
C. Interelement "spaces"
IV. Proteins
A. C23
B. B23

composed of the rDNA, the RNA polymerase I, and juxtaposed enzymes which produce the earliest stages of synthesis of preribosomal RNA.

F. rDNA

Beginning with the demonstration of the nucleolar organizer region (NOR) by Heitz (1933) and the extended studies of McClintock (1934, 1961), further studies have been made on nucleolar DNA in a wide variety of species (Busch and Smetana, 1970). The "secondary constrictions" or NOR in chromosomes have been described earlier (Fig. 24). The presence in the nucleolus of several classes of DNA has been demonstrated by light and electron microscopic techniques and special stains (Fig. 24b). Some DNA regions can be "geographically" segregated into perinucleolar chromatin and intranucleolar chromatin. rDNA (Fig. 25) may also be subfractioned into condensed and dispersed nucleolar chromatin. In essence, the precise coding chromatin for the nucleolar rDNA has not yet been defined in these geographical entities.

Electron microscopic analysis has been made (Busch and Smetana, 1970) of DNA within the nucleoli after specific types of digestion. The "Miller" pictures (Fig. 26) using the spreading technique of Kleinschmidt (1968), have shown

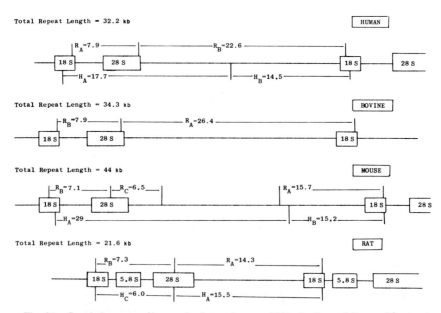

Fig. 25.   Restriction maps of human, bovine, and mouse rDNA. R_A, R_B, and R_C = subfragments produced by restriction endonuclease EcoRI; H_A, H_B, and H_C = subfragments produced by restriction endonuclease Hind III.

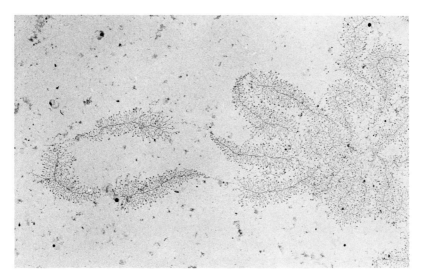

Fig. 26. ''Miller'' picture of ''Christmas trees'' of nucleolar rRNA readouts, synthesized pre-ribosomal RNP elements. (Courtesy of Dr. O. L. Miller.)

rRNA in the nucleolar cores of *Xenopus* and other species (Miller and Beatty, 1969). The results support the concept of tandem redundant rDNA genes transcribed simultaneously. Although these products have still not been related to chemical entities, the concept of progressive growth of chains fits well with very long final products of pre-RNA and the associated RNP.

With the development of improved hybridization techniques, attempts have been developed to establish specific information on localization of the rDNA genes. Studies in our laboratory (Sitz *et al.*, 1973) showed that the concentration of rDNA in the nucleolus of Novikoff hepatoma ascites cells is ten times that of the rDNA throughout the remainder of the nucleus. Accordingly, it appears that the nucleoli contain 90% or more of the total rDNA.

G. Products of Nucleolar RNA

The initial RNA product of the nucleolus is 45 S pre-RNA and oligomers of sedimentation coefficients up to 85 S. By a series of unique and specific endonucleolytic cleavages, these giant nucleolar RNAs are cleaved to three major ribosome species 28 S, 18 S, and 5.8 S rRNA (Busch and Smetana, 1970).

H. Nucleolar Proteins and Control of Nucleolar Function

Nucleolar proteins can be divided into (1) structural elements including (a) the histones, (b) special proteins of the preribosomal particles, (c) ribosomal proteins; (2) enzymes of RNA synthesis (RNA polymerase I) and processing (exonucleases and endonucleases); and (3) gene control proteins.

Gene control of nucleolar function may reside in specific elements that are either phosphoproteins (see below), or other specific types of nonhistone proteins. The participation of the nucleolus in important regulatory and phase-specific events indicates that its controls are more responsive than those for many mRNA species.

With the improved methods for isolation of rDNA and various binding proteins, it now becomes possible to achieve a more satisfactory approach to isolation and analysis of proteins involved in promotion or derepression of rDNA and $DNA_{r\text{-}prot}$. Such studies are of great importance in understanding the production of most cellular RNA and in understanding of specific controls on a major gene set.

At one time, the nucleolus was considered to be a simple structure with a small number of elements. The development of technology for determination of the numbers and types of those constituents has led to the view that the nucleolus contains approximately 200 species of proteins (Orrick *et al.*, 1973). Two-dimensional polyacrylamide gel electrophoresis (Fig. 27) has established that, in

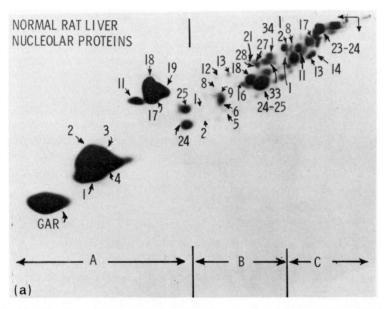

Fig. 27.   Two-dimensional gel electrophoretic patterns of normal and regenerating liver nucleolar proteins (Orrick *et al.*, 1973). Marked changes were found in the concentration of proteins A11, A24, C13, and C14 from the normal levels (a), 4 hour (b), 8 hour (c), 24 hour (d), and 48 hour (e) of regenerating liver. Regions A, B, and C represent the most rapid, intermediate and least rapid migrating protein spots in the two dimensions of the gel.

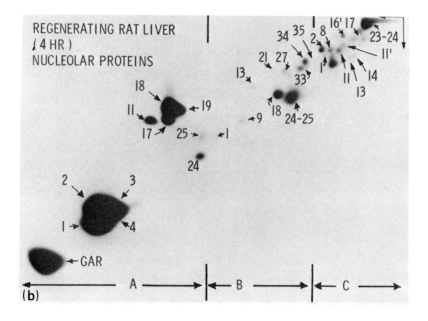

(b)

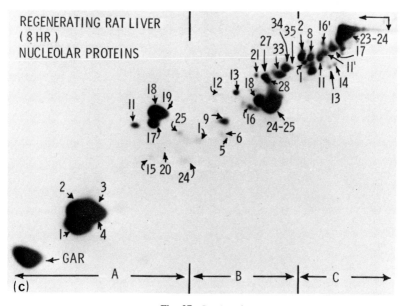

(c)

Fig. 27. *Continued*

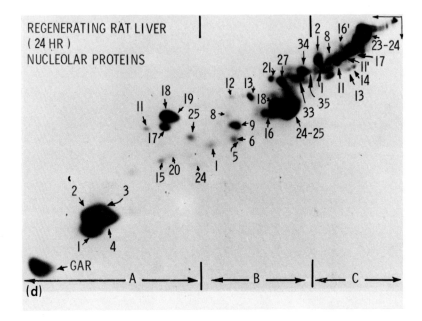

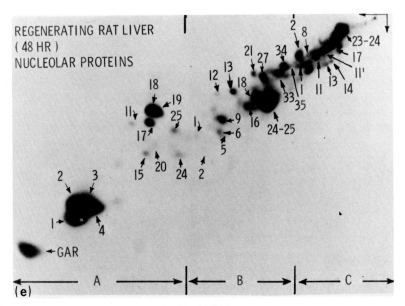

Fig. 27. *Continued*

addition to all the varieties of histones, approximately 90 nonhistone proteins are extractable from nucleoli with 0.4 N H_2SO_4. Another group of proteins is acid insoluble but is extractable under conditions that require solvents that dissociate hydrogen bonds and destroy hydrophobic molecular interactions. The RNA polymerase I that is uniquely localized to the nucleolus accounts for several polypeptides which are presumably enzyme subunits. There are also many proteins that are elements of the nucleolar ribonucleoproteins of the granular elements and the ribosomes.

Of the nuclear phosphoproteins (Stein *et al.*, 1972, 1975), one is specifically localized to the nucleolus, i.e., protein C23, a recently described nucleolus-specific phosphoprotein (Fig. 28) which apparently accounts for the bulk of ^{32}P incorporated into nucleolar proteins (Olson *et al.*, 1974, 1975). This protein may be related to silver staining of the B23, the NOR, and nucleolar granules (Smetana and Busch, 1979; Busch *et al.*, 1979).

Silver Stained Nucleolar Proteins

Recently, a rapid silver staining technique specific for nucleolar organizer regions (NOR), nucleoli, and "nucleolar satellites" was developed to provide cytochemical analysis of argyrophilic nucleolar structures and to analyze quantitative changes in highly argyrophilic nucleolar elements in hepatocytes and other cells (Smetana and Busch, 1979). Quantitative analysis of the numbers of the dense, highly argyrophilic granules in the nuclei and nucleoli of cells with varying nucleolar function and growth rate indicated that the largest numbers of grains (13 per nucleolus) were in the rapidly dividing tumor cells, and the smallest number were in mature lymphocytes (1.3 per nucleolus). In the normal liver there were 4.2 grains per nucleolus. This number increased to 7.8 and 13.7 in the regenerating liver 6 and 18 hours posthepatectomy (Busch *et al.*, 1979b).

In Novikoff hepatoma, KB, and HeLa cells, some of the arrays of nucleolar argyrophilic granules consisted on linearly arranged discrete granules, and others were in two to three rows each, containing three to five granules (Fig. 29a). Corresponding formations were not found in either the normal or regenerating liver nucleoli. The liver nucleoli contained an argyrophilic network in which the dark argyrophilic fibrils of the reticulum were observed. Interestingly, the nucleolar argyrophilic granules were readily identifiable in the separated nuclei of the tumor daughter cells in telophase, suggesting that the increased nucleolar activity of the G_1 phase begins in these cells even before cell division has been completed (Fig. 29b).

I. Morphological Correlates of Increased rRNA Production

The synthetic reactions of the nucleolus are catalyzed by RNA polymerase I, a specific polymerase localized to the nucleolus. The activity in synthesis of pre-

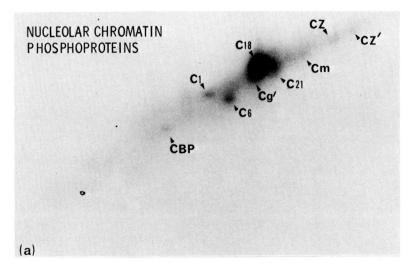

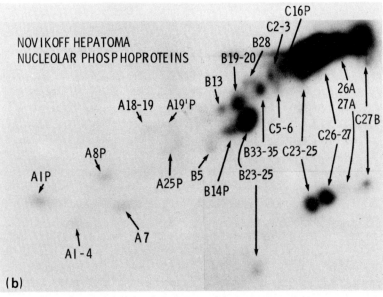

Fig. 28. Nucleolar phosphoproteins of Novikoff hepatoma ^{32}P-labeled nuclear chromatin preparations (a) showing the dense spot C18(23); (b) the nucleolar extract showing dense spots of proteins B23–B25 and C23–C27.

rRNA varies greatly with the state of the nucleolus and the cell. In a cell such as the circulating lymphocyte, there is a very small nucleolus, and the amount of rRNA produced is correspondingly very limited. The amount of granular elements produced by these nucleoli is very small, and the rate of ribosome replacement is correspondingly very limited (Busch and Smetana, 1970).

The nucleolus of the normal liver is also a rather small structure, i.e., it contains relatively large amounts of fibrillar elements and relatively small amounts of granular elements. In the normal liver, the rate of production of 45 S pre-rRNA is approximately 3–5 fg/min/nucleolus.

The nucleoli with the highest rates of production of ribosomes are the large nucleoli of rapidly growing tissues including malignant tumors, regenerating liver, "activated" lymphocytes, and nucleoli of some drug-treated cells. In the thioacetamide-treated cells, and in some malignant tumors, the rate of 45 S pre-rRNA biosynthesis is 40–45 fg/min/nucleolus (Busch and Smetana, 1970).

Nucleolar Antigens

Nucleoli of tumor cells have been shown to differ from those of normal cells by several techniques. Morphologically, nucleoli in most neoplastic cells are larger and more irregularly shaped than in normal cells, and such morphological differences have been diagnostically useful.

In previous work in this laboratory, nucleolar specific antibodies were produced in rabbits immunized with whole nucleoli. Antigens (such as NoAg-1) were found in the nucleolar chromatin of Novikoff hepatoma ascites cells but not in those of normal liver cells; the converse was also true (Busch and Busch, 1977) (Fig. 30).

In studies designed to purify nucleolar antigens, first by differential solubilization of nucleolar proteins, antigens soluble in the Zubay–Doty buffer (0.075 M NaCl and 0.025 M EDTA), 10 mM Tris-HCl, and 0.6 M NaCl were isolated from normal liver and Novikoff hepatoma nucleoli and compared by Ouchterlony double immunodiffusion and immunoelectrophoresis (Davis et al., 1978).

The various extracts differed both in the number of antigenic species precipitated and in density of immunoprecipin bands (Fig. 31). Four precipitin bands were found between the anti-liver nucleolar antiserum (AbLi) and liver nucleolar extracts (Table VII). Seven distinct antigenic species precipitated in extracts from Novikoff nucleoli by anti-tumor nucleolar antiserum (AbTu) (Table VII). Some of these, such as the middle precipitin band in the ribonucleoprotein (RNP) and chromation (Chr) fractions were found in more than one fraction.

Studies were done to determine whether antigens were mainly present in normal liver (Li), Novikoff hepatoma (Tu) nucleoli, or in extracts of fetal liver nuclei (Fe) (Table VII). As shown in Table VII, one antigen was present in the tumor only, and two were present in the tumor and fetal liver and may be referred to as oncofetal antigens.

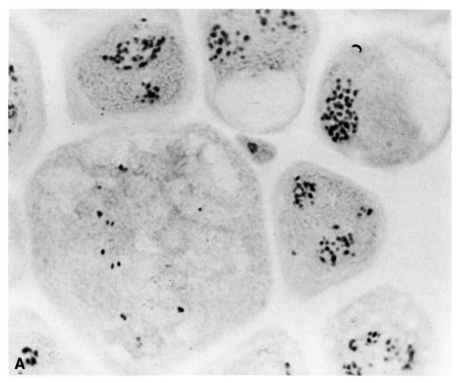

Fig. 29. (A) Silver stained Novikoff hepatoma cells showing a large cell containing doublets of NOR spots and interphase cells with three or more granules in a row in the nucleoli. (B) Two

Corresponding studies on immunofluorescent nucleolar antigens have now been performed (Davis *et al.*, 1979) with a variety of human tumor and non-tumor tissues, as shown in Tables VIII, IX, and X. With antisera to HeLa cell nucleoli, positive fluorescence was obtained in each of the tumors studied. On the other hand, the nontumor tissues, except for the slowly growing fetal WI-38 cell, did not exhibit positive immunofluorescence. This result is a potentially important indication of antigenic differences between nucleolar proteins of human cancer cells and other human tissues; the implications of this result may be useful for immunodiagnosis.

J. Coupled Synthesis of rRNA and mRNA$_{prot}$

In a variety of bacterial systems, evidence has been presented for coassociated ribosomal protein and ribosomal RNA synthesis (Jaskunas *et al.*, 1975; Lindahl

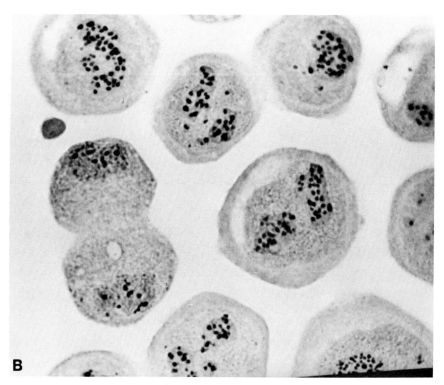

Novikoff hepatoma cells in telophase showing many granules in the nuclei and nucleoli. These formations suggest that the G$_1$ phase may begin in these cells before completion of mitosis.

et al., 1975; Watson *et al.,* 1975). This coupling has been based in part on gene proximity as well as the obvious need for correlated or simultaneous synthesis. In eukaryotic cells, the synthesis of rRNA and ribosomal proteins (r proteins) is only now coming under study with respect to its temporal similarity, i.e., the likelihood that the two are made together has now been supported by evidence for increases in both products during liver regeneration (Wu *et al.,* 1977).

Although the genes for rRNA are clustered and tandomly related, the r protein genes are not identified, and the suggestion has been made that the corresponding mRNAs are derived from a broad group of genes in various chromosomes. If this is the case, the "triggers" for their synthesis must be capable of affecting a very broad range of genes throughout the genome. Because of the numbers and types of genes that must be involved, the establishment of the mechanisms of these activations will require extensive study.

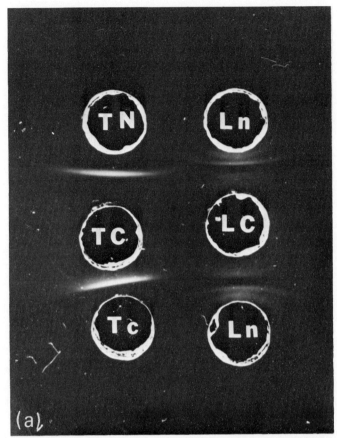

Fig. 30. (a) Immunoprecipitin bands showing that antibodies to tumor chromatin (TC), and liver chromatin (LC) formed specific immunoprecipitates with liver (Ln) and tumor (TN) nucleolar extracts. Only one dense band was found in the tumor where three (or four) were found for the liver. There was no cross-immunoreactivity in these preparations (Busch and Busch, 1977). (b) Immunofluorescence of cells reacted with preabsorbed antinucleolar antisera; preabsorbed antitumor nucleolar antiserum and Novikoff hepatoma cells (B1) or normal liver cells (B4), preabsorbed antiliver nucleolar antiserum with Novikoff hepatoma cells (B2) or normal liver cells (B3). × 1800. (Davis *et al.*, 1978.)

Fig. 31. Immunoelectrophoretic profile of liver, tumor, and fetal Zubay–Doty extracts and amniotic fluid. A precipitin arc in the extract from Novikoff nucleoli which is not detected in the other fractions is marked with an arrow. TuNo = Tumor nucleoli; LiNo = liver nucleoli; ZD = Zubay–Doty extract (0.075 *M* NaCl/0.025 *M* EDTA, pH 8); Amn. = amniotic fluid; FeNu = fetal nuclei. (Davis *et al.*, 1978.)

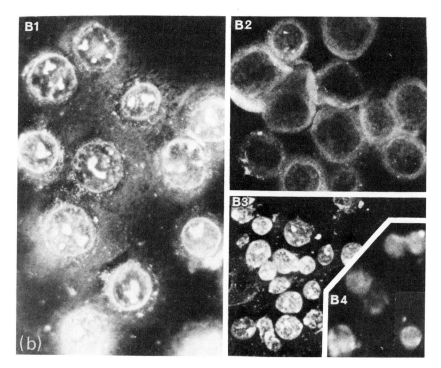

Fig. 30. *Continued*

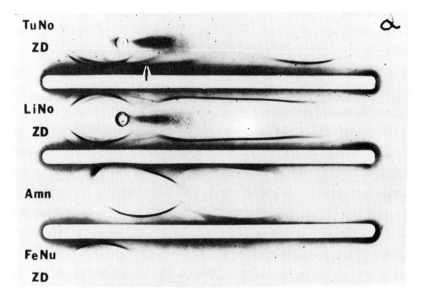

Fig. 31.

TABLE VII

Antigens Detected by Anti-Tumor Nucleolar Antiserum[a]

	Number of antigens found in extract[b]						
Extract	L only	T only	F only	L + T only	L + F only	T + F only	L + T + F
Zubay–Doty (NaCl/EDTA)	0	1	0	0	0	0	2
Tris	0	0	0	0	0	0	3
RNP	0	1	0	0	0	0	2
Chromatin	0	0	0	0	0	2	3
Residue	0	0	0	0	0	2	2

[a] Davis et al., 1978.
[b] L, liver; T, tumor; F, fetal.

K. Messenger RNA

In a sense, mRNA synthesis is the most specific function of the nucleus. The biosynthetic reactions involve complex events in enzymatic and structural chemistry. Through interaction of specific nonhistone proteins with the genome, specific mRNA species are produced and transported to the cytoplasm (Fig. 32).

Many individual mRNA species have been isolated including mRNA for hemoglobin, histones, globin, ovalbumin, and insulin. The polysomes which ultimately translate mRNA into proteins are associated with a host of initiation and elongation factors (Busch et al., 1976a).

L. Synthesis of mRNA

The processes involved in messenger RNA synthesis are apparently very similar to those for rRNA synthesis. The enzyme RNA polymerase II catalyzes the readout of mRNA as a consequence of availability of "open gene complexes." This enzyme, and its associated factors, link nucleoside triphosphates covalently into 3′,5′-phosphodiester bonds of mRNA. There are critical elements of the "initiation reactions" involved in starting these gene readouts as well as termination factors that are incompletely understood. Termination occurs when appropriate triplet "codons" are encountered by RNA polymerase II, but recognition proteins are apparently important to the termination process. Although mRNA is linearly synthesized in the nucleus, critical modification reactions are known to occur at each end of mRNA (Fig. 33). A large portion of the mRNA molecules become polyadenylated, i.e., an oligomer of approximately 200 adenylic residues is added to the 3′ end by poly(A) polymerase reactions (Busch et al., 1976a,b).

TABLE VIII

Bright Nucleolar Fluorescence in Human Malignant Tumor Specimens[a,b]

I. Carcinomas	II. Sarcomas
A. Lung	A. Chondrosarcoma (1)
1. Adenocarcinoma (3)	B. Fibrosarcoma (4)
2. Oat cell (4)	C. Giant cell tumor (1)
3. Squamous cell (22)	D. Granulocytic myoblastoma (2)
B. Gastrointestinal	E. Leiomyosarcoma (4)
1. Oral cavity (8)	F. Lymphoma (10)
2. Pharynx (4)	G. Meningiosarcoma (1)
3. Esophagus, squamous cell (5)	H. Myoblastoma (2)
4. Stomach, adenocarcinoma (5)	I. Osteogenic (6)
metastasis: liver	J. Pulmonary blastoma (1)
metastasis: lymph node	K. Reticulum cell sarcoma (1)
5. Colon, adenocarcinoma (9)	L. Synovial sarcoma (1)
metastasis: liver (2)	
transplantable carcinoma (GW-39)	III. Hematological Neoplasms
6. Liver, primary carcinoma (3)	A. Acute lymphocytic leukemia (2)
7. Pancreas (4)	B. Acute myelocytic leukemia (7)
C. Genitourinary	C. Acute monocytic leukemia (2)
1. Kidney (4)	D. Chronic myelocytic leukemia (5)
2. Prostate, adenocarcinoma (22)	E. Hodgkins disease (9)
3. Bladder (4)	F. Leukemia: CLL (12), hairy cell (1)
D. CNS	G. Mycosis fungoides
1. Glioblastoma (1)	H. Plasmacytomas (7)
2. Astrocytoma (5)	
E. Endocrine	
1. Breast (3)	
2. Cervix (4)	
3. Parathyroid (1)	
4. Thyroid (5)	
F. Skin	
1. Basal cell (8)	
2. Eccrine gland (1)	
3. Squamous cell (7)	
metastasis: lymph node	
4. Melanoma, malignant (4)	
cerebral metastasis (1)	
5. Sweat gland (3)	

[a] From Busch et al., 1979b.
[b] Numbers of specimens are in parentheses.

    Virtually all functional mRNA must contain "5′ cap" structures in order to be active in protein synthesis (Fig. 33). The 5′ cap is added by a series of reactions involving guanylyl transferases and methylating enzymes that form the $m^7G(5′)ppp(5′)Y^mpZ^mp$ "cap." The formation of this cap (Busch, 1976b) occurs mainly in the nucleus and partly in the cytoplasm. The 5′ cap serves as an

TABLE IX

Negative Nucleolar Fluorescence in Human Tissues[a]

I. Normal tissue
  A. Lung
  B. Gastrointestinal
    1. Stomach
    2. Intestine
        small, crypts of Lieberkuhn
        large
    3. Liver
    4. Pancreas
  C. Genital urinary
    1. Kidney
    2. Bladder
    3. Prostate
  D. Endocrine
    1. Thyroid
    2. Breast
    3. Placenta
  E. Skin
II. Hematologic
  A. Bone marrow
  B. Lymph nodes
    1. Lymphocytes
    2. Hyperplastic lymph nodes
  C. Benign growing tissues
    1. Thyroid, goiter
    2. Prostate, hyperplastic
III. Inflammatory diseases
  A. Chronic ulcerative colitis
  B. Glomerulonephritis
  C. Granuloma and fibrosis of lung
  D. Liver: cirrhosis, hepatitis
  E. Lupus profundus (mammary gland and skin)
  F. Pemphigus: bullous
  G. Ulcer, gastric

---

[a] From Busch et al., 1979b.

allosteric binding site for proteins involved in the initiation of protein synthesis, or for mRNA binding directly to special ribosomal proteins (Busch et al., 1975, 1976a). The specific enzyme, RNA polymerase II is involved in transcription of mRNA or DNA templates. It must be closely associated in these transcriptional events with the methylases, pyrophosphorylases, and poly(A) polymerases that are responsible for the synthesis of the completed mRNA. In addition, there are important initiation factors and termination factors that have been identified in

TABLE X

Negative Nucleolar Fluorescence in Benign Tumors[a]

Adrenal Cortex (2)
Angioimmunoblastic lymphadenopathy (2)
Apocrine (4)
Breast (7)
Chondroma (1)
Colon (6)
Fibroma (2)
Hamartoma (1)
Kidney (2)
Leiomyoma (2)
Meningioma (3)
Mixed tumors
Myoblastoma (2)
Oncocytoma (2)
Parathyroid (5)
Thyroid adenomas (3)

[a] From Busch *et al.*, 1979b.

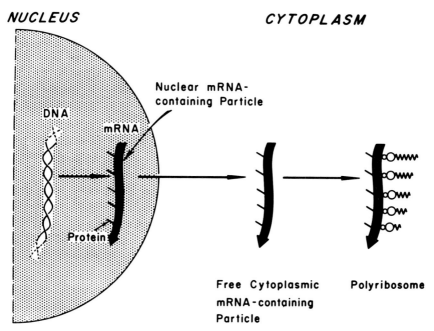

Fig. 32. Scheme of synthesis and transport of mRNA from the nucleus to the cytoplasm where it functions as part of the polyribosome complex. (Courtesy of Dr. Edgar C. Henshaw, Harvard University Medical School.)

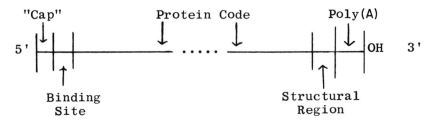

Fig. 33.   Topology of a typical messenger RNA molecule.

both bacterial and eukaryotic systems. For detailed studies on transcription of a specific mRNA, much more sharply defined systems must be developed.

M. Low Molecular Weight Nuclear RNA

Special interest from both structural and functional points of view has been recently directed to special low molecular weight nuclear (LMWN) RNA (Figs. 34 and 35) which differs markedly in structure from other types of cellular RNA (Busch *et al.*, 1971; Busch, 1976b; Hellung-Larsen, 1978). Studies on these molecules first revealed the remarkable "5' cap" of RNA species (Busch, 1976b). The 5' cap of these molecules is different from the 5' cap of mRNA by virtue of the presence of the base $m^{2,2,7}$-trimethylguanosine, rather than the m^7G of mRNA in the 5'-terminal nucleotide. The presence of this base apparently eliminates the possibility that translational systems in the cytoplasm can utilize these low molecular weight RNA species as mRNA.

Of the three major species of the LMWN RNA, one (U3 RNA) is specifically localized to the nucleolus. It does not appear to be present in any other site in the cell. Accordingly, it has been reasoned that this RNA may serve an important role in transcription of the rRNA from the rDNA templates. The number of U3 RNA molecules in the nucleolus is approximately 200,000 (0.3 attamoles or 0.2 pg/nucleolus), which is in large excess over the rDNA genes or the numbers of polymerase molecules. It is possible these are regulatory, since many kinds of control elements are present in large excess over the number of genes with which they interact, i.e., the estrogen receptors in the cell nucleus are in large excess (20,000- to 100,000-fold) over the number of gene sites available for specific readouts.

Among the suggestions for the function of the U3 RNA and other LMWN RNA are the following: (a) maintain "stable open gene complexes"; (b) critical components of the nucleolar fibrillar elements which are the presumed sites of transcription of the rDNA; and (c) form an RNP complex with subunits of RNA polymerases which transcribe the RNA. Little was known about the overall sequence of the U3 RNA because the methods used to label it *in vivo* had not

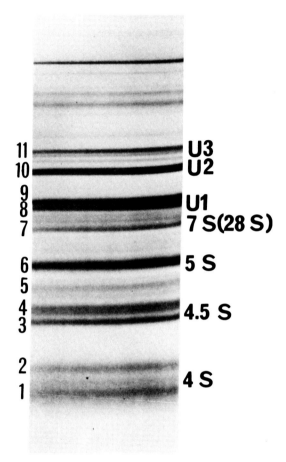

Fig. 34. Polyacrylamide gel (12%) electrophoresis of LMWN RNA from Novikoff hepatoma cell nuclei. Electrophoresis was carried out for 50 hours with a current of 40 mA at a voltage of 300 V in a buffer containing 0.02 M Tris-HCl (pH 7.2), 0.02 M NaCl, and 0.04 M EDTA. (Ro-Choi and Busch, 1973, 1974.)

yielded sufficient amounts of isotope for complete structural analysis. The structure of U3 RNA has recently been determined (Fig. 35).

IV. DISCUSSION

Thus far, no special properties of cancer cells have been detected that are not exhibited by nontumor cells at some point in ontogeny (Busch, 1976a). For example, growth is a property of all cells, invasiveness is a property of several

$pm_3^{2,2,7}G$
|
p
|

$\quad\quad\quad\quad\quad\quad 10 \quad\quad\quad\quad\quad\quad\quad\quad\quad\quad 20$
pAm-A-G-U-G-A-C-U-A-ψ-A-C-U-ψ-U-C-A-G-G-G-A-U-C-A-U-
$\quad\quad 30 \quad\quad\quad\quad\quad\quad\quad\quad 40 \quad\quad\quad\quad\quad\quad\quad\quad 50$
U-U-C-U-A-U-A-G-U-U-C-G-U-U-A-C-U-A-G-A-G-A-A-G-U-U-
$\quad\quad\quad\quad 60 \quad\quad\quad\quad\quad\quad\quad\quad\quad\quad 70$
U-C-U-C-U-G-A-C-U-G-U-G-U-A-G-A-G-C-C-C-A-C-G-A-A-A-
$\quad\quad 80 \quad\quad\quad\quad\quad\quad\quad\quad 90 \quad\quad\quad\quad\quad\quad\quad 100$
C-C-A-C-G-A-G-G-A-C-G-A-G-A-C-A-U-A-G-C-G-U-C-C-C-C-U-
$\quad\quad 110 \quad\quad\quad\quad\quad\quad\quad 120 \quad\quad\quad\quad\quad\quad\quad 130$
C-C-U-G-A-G-C-G-U-G-A-A-G-C-C-G-G-C-U-C-U-A-G-G-U-G-
$\quad\quad\quad\quad\quad 140 \quad\quad\quad\quad\quad\quad\quad\quad 150$
C-U-G-C-U-U-C-U-G-C-C-U-C-U-U-G-C-C-A-U-U-G-G-C-A-G-
$\quad\quad 160 \quad\quad\quad\quad\quad\quad\quad 170 \quad\quad\quad\quad\quad\quad\quad 180$
C-U-G-A-U-G-A-U-C-G-U-C-U-U-C-U-C-U-C-C-U-U-C-G-G-G-
$\quad\quad\quad\quad\quad 190 \quad\quad\quad\quad\quad\quad\quad\quad 200$
G-G-G-G-U-A-A-G-A-G-G-G-A-G-G-G-A-A-C-G-C-A-G-U-C-
210 $\quad\quad\quad\quad$ 216
U-G-A-G-U-G-G-A$_{OH}$

Fig. 35. Primary nucleotide sequence of U_3-B RNA. (From Reddy *et al.*, 1979.)

types of white cells and metastasis is a common embryonic phenomenon. Although production of abnormal chromosomes is an uncommon and pathological event in nontumor cells and generally leads to destruction of the affected cell, alterations in chromosome number such as polyploidy commonly occur in liver cells with maturation and aging.

As recently pointed out in studies from many laboratories, the "tumor antigens" of human cells and nonviral animal tumors frequently represent fetal gene readouts ranging from late fetal stages to as early as elements of sperm and ovum. Simply expressed, along with neoplastic transformation, there frequently is a fetal gene activation which is apparently quite random in terms of the "biological clock." Of course, it is by no means proven that such fetal gene readouts have any more to do with meaningful neoplastic processes than do the activation of genes for production of the many isozymes reported to exist in various tumors.

The concept that fetal genes are active in the process of neoplasia is an attractive one (Busch, 1976a). However, it is possible that substances responsible for the normal maturation processes at specific times of embryogenesis would function in tumor cells to reorder or eliminate the specific readouts related to the cancer process. The "fetal readouts" which may be responsible for "growth, invasiveness and metastasis" are likely to be timing errors of a dislocated genome for which proper timing may be restored by the substances normally involved in this "reordering" process.

Recently, a common nucleolar antigen has been found in a broad range of human malignant tumor specimens now numbering over 300 in the series of studies in our laboratory and related laboratories. It was indeed unexpected that a broad array of tumors would give a positive nucleolar fluorescence with antibodies to HeLa cell nuclear or nucleolar antigens. Further studies are required with improved analytical techniques to define the number and types of antigens in these preparations. In preliminary studies of the proteins of the 0.01 M Tris-HCl (pH 8) extract of nuclei by isoelectric focusing, there appeared to be only one major antigen band at pI 6.3. Preliminary analysis showed the antigen is a protein or contains protein elements, but the possibility has not been excluded that the antigen is a ribonucleoprotein or other type of complex protein. Further attempts are in progress to prepare sufficient quantities of the antigen(s) for analysis of their composition and properties. It remains to be determined whether the antigen represents a substance that is present in high concentrations in cancer cells and very low concentrations in noncancerous cells or is a fetal antigen as was found earlier in the comparative studies on nucleolar antigens of the rat Novikoff hepatoma and normal rat liver cells.

ACKNOWLEDGMENTS

These studies were supported by the Cancer Research Grant CA-10893, awarded by the National Cancer Institute, DHEW, the Bristol Fund, the Pauline Sterne Wolff Memorial Fund, and a generous gift from Mrs. Jack Hutchins.

REFERENCES

Barrett, T., and Gould, H. J. (1973). *Biochim. Biophys. Acta* **294**, 165.
Bouteille, M., Laval, M., and Dupuy-Coin, A. M. (1974). *In* "The Cell Nucleus" (H. Busch, ed.), Vol. I, pp. 3-71. Academic Press, New York.
Busch, G. I., Yeoman, L. C., Taylor, C. W., and Busch, H. (1974). *Physiol. Chem. Phys.* **6**, 1-10.
Busch, H. (1965). "Histones and Other Nuclear Proteins." Academic Press, New York.
Busch, H. (1974). *In* "The Molecular Biology of Cancer" (H. Busch, ed.), pp. 1-39. Academic Press, New York.
Busch, H. (1976a). *Cancer Res.* **36**, 4291-4294.
Busch, H. (1976b). *Perspect. Biol. Med.* **19**, 549-567.
Busch, H., ed. (1978a). "The Cell Nucleus," Vol. 4. Academic Press, New York.
Busch, H., ed. (1978b). "The Cell Nucleus," Vol. 5. Academic Press, New York.
Busch, H., ed. (1978c). "The Cell Nucleus," Vol. 6. Academic Press, New York.
Busch, H., and Smetana, K. (1970). "The Nucleolus." Academic Press, New York.
Busch, H., Ro-Choi, T. S., Prestayko, A. W., Shibata, H., Crooke, S. T., El-Khatib, S. M., Choi, Y. C., and Mauritzen, C. M. (1971). *Perspect. Biol. Med.* **15**, 117-139.

Busch. H., Ballal, N. R., Olson, M. O. J., and Yeoman, L. C. (1975). *Methods Cancer Res.* **11**, 43–121.

Busch, H., Choi, Y. C., Daskal, Y., Liarakos, C. D., Rao, M. R. S., Ro-Choi, T. S., and Wu, B. C. (1976a). *Methods Cancer Res.* **8**, 101–197.

Busch, H., Hirsch, F., Gupta, K. K., Rao, M., Spohn, W., and Wu, B. (1976b). *Prog. Nucleic Acids Res.* **19**, 39–61.

Busch, H., Daskal, Y., Györkey, F., and Smetana, K. (1979a). *Cancer Res.* **39**, 857–863.

Busch, H., Györkey, F., Busch, R. K., Davis, F. M., Györkey, P., and Smetana, K. (1979b). *Cancer Res.* **39**, 3024–3030.

Busch, R. K., and Busch, H. (1977). *Tumori* **63**, 347–357.

Chambon, P., Gissinger, F., Kedinger, C., Mandel, J. L., and Meilhac, M. (1974). *In* "The Cell Nucleus" (H. Busch, ed.), Vol. 3, pp. 270–308. Academic Press, New York.

Chytil, F., and Spelsberg, T. (1971). *Nature (London), New Biol.* **223**, 215.

Comings, D. E., and Harris, D. C. (1975). *Exp. Cell Res.* **96**, 161–179.

Comings, D. E., and Tack, L. O. (1973). *Exp. Cell Res.* **82**, 175–191.

Daskal, Y., Mace, M. L., Jr., Wray, W., and Busch, H. (1976). *Exp. Cell Res.* **100**, 204–212.

Davis, F. M., Busch, R. K., Yeoman, L. C., and Busch, H. (1978). *Cancer Res.* **38**, 1906–1915.

Davis, F. M., Györkey, F., Busch, R. K., and Busch, H. (1979). *Proc. Natl. Acad. Sci. U.S.A.* **76**, 892–896.

Douvas, A. S., Harrington, C. A., and Bonner, J. (1975). *Proc. Natl. Acad. Sci. U.S.A.* **72**, 3902–3906.

Elgin, S. C. R., and Weintraub, H. (1975). *Annu. Rev. Biochem.* **44**, 725–774.

Fidler, I. (1979). *Methods Cancer Res.* **15**, 399–439.

Fishman, W. H., and Busch, H., eds. (1979). "Oncodevelopmental Antigens in Methods in Cancer Research," Vol. 18. Academic Press, New York.

Fishman, W. H., and Sells, S. (1976). "Onco-Developmental Gene Expression." Academic Press, New York.

Franke, W. W., and Scheer, U. (1974). *In* "The Cell Nucleus" (H. Busch, ed.), Vol. I, pp. 220–347. Academic Press, New York.

Furth, J., and Kahn, M. C. (1937). *Am. J. Cancer* **31**, 276–282.

Gilmour, R. S., and Paul, J. (1970). *FEBS Lett.* **9**, 242.

Goldknopf, I. L., French, M. F., Musso, R., and Busch, H. (1977). *Proc. Natl. Acad. Sci. U.S.A.* **74**, 5492–5495.

Goodwin, G. H., Nicolas, R. H., and Johns, E. W. (1975). *Biochim. Biophys. Acta* **405**, 280–291.

Goodwin, G. H., Walker, J. M., and Johns, E. W. (1978). *In* "The Cell Nucleus" (Busch, H., ed.), Vol. 6, pp. 182–219. Academic Press, New York.

Gurdon, J. B. (1974). *In* "The Cell Nucleus" (H. Busch, ed.), Vol. 1, pp. 471–489. Academic Press, New York.

Heitz, E. (1933). *Z. Zellforsch. Mikrosk. Anat.* **19**, 720–742.

Hellung-Larsen, P. (1978). "Low Molecular Weight RNA Components in Eukaryotic Cells." FADL's Forlag, Copenhagen.

Hirsch, F. W., Nall, K. N., Busch, F. N., Morris, H. P., and Busch, H. (1978). *Cancer Res.* **38**, 1514–1522.

Hosokawa, K. (1950). *Gann* **41**, 236–237.

Illmensee, K., and Mintz, B. (1976). *Proc. Natl. Acad. Sci. U.S.A.* **73**, 549–553.

Ishibashi, K. (1950). *Gann* **41**, 1–14.

Jaskunas, S. R., Burgess, R., Lindahl, L., and Nomura, M. (1975). *Nature (London)* **257**, 458–462.

Jensen, E. V., and DeSombre, E. R. (1972). *Annu. Rev. Biochem.* **41**, 203–230.

Kadohama, N., and Turkington, R. W. (1973). *Cancer Res.* **33**, 1194.

Kamiyama, M., Dastugue, B., Defer, N., and Kruh, J. (1972). *Biochim. Biophys. Acta* **277**, 576.

Kleinschmidt, A. K. (1968). "Methods in Enzymology" (L. Grossman and K. Moldave, eds.), Vol. 12, Part B. pp. 361-377. Academic Press, New York.

Kostraba, N. C., and Wang, T. Y. (1972a). *Biochim. Biophys. Acta* **262**, 169.

Kostraba, N. C., and Wang, T. Y. (1972b). *Cancer Res.* **32**, 2348.

Kostraba, N. C., and Wang, T. Y. (1973). *Exp. Cell Res.* **80**, 291.

LeStourgeon, W. M., Forer, A., Yang, Y.-Z., Betram, J. S., and Rusch, H. P. (1975). *Biochim. Biophys. Acta* **379**, 529-552.

Levy, R., Levy, S., Rosenberg, S. A., and Simpson, R. T. (1973). *Biochemistry* **12**, 224.

Lindahl, L., Jaskunas, S. R., Dennis, P., and Nomura, M. (1975). *Proc. Natl. Acad. Sci. U.S.A.* **72**, 2743-2747.

McClintock, B. (1934). *Z. Zellforsch. Mikrosk. Anat.* **21**, 294-328.

McClintock, B. (1961). *Am. Nat.* **95**, 265-328.

Miller, O. L., Jr., and Beatty, B. R. (1969). *Science* **164**, 955-957.

Montgomery, T. H. (1898). *J. Morphol.* **15**, 265-564.

Olins, A. L., and Olins, D. E. (1974). *Science* **183**, 330-332.

Olson, M. O. J., Orrick, L. R., Jones, C., and Busch, H. (1974). *J. Biol. Chem.* **249**, 2823-2827.

Olson, M. O. J., Ezrailson, E. G., Guetzow, K., and Busch, H. (1975). *J. Molec. Biol.* **97**, 611-619.

Olson, M. O. J., Goldknopf, I. L., Guetzow, K. A., James, G. T., Hawkins, T. C., Mays-Rothberg, C. J., and Busch, H. (1976). *J. Biol. Chem.* **251**, 5901-5903.

O'Malley, B. W., and Means, A. R. (1974). *In* "The Cell Nucleus" (H. Busch, ed.), Vol. 3, pp. 380-416. Academic Press, New York.

O'Malley, B. W., and Schrader, W. T. (1976). *Sci. Am.* **231**, 32-43.

Orrick, L. R., Olson, M. O. J., and Busch, H. (1973). *Proc. Natl. Acad. Sci. U.S.A.* **70**, 1316-1320.

Pardon, J. F., and Richards, B. M. (1979). *In* "The Cell Nucleus" (H. Busch, ed.), Vol. 7, pp. 371-411. Academic Press, New York.

Paul, J., and Gilmour, R. S. (1966a). *J. Mol. Biol.* **16**, 242-244.

Paul, J., and Gilmour, R. S. (1966b). *Nature (London)* **210**, 992-993.

Paul, J., and Gilmour, R. S. (1968). *J. Mol. Biol.* **34**, 305-316.

Peterson, J. L., and McConkey, E. H. (1976a). *J. Biol. Chem.* **251**, 548-554.

Peterson, J. L., and McConkey, E. H. (1976b). *J. Biol. Chem.* **251**, 555-558.

Pogo, B. G. T., and Katz, J. R. (1974). *Cell Differ.* **2**, 119.

Reddy, R., Henning, D., and Busch, H. (1979). *J. Biol. Chem.* **254**, 11097-11105.

Richter, K. H., and Sekeris, C. E. (1972). *Arch. Biochem. Biophys.* **148**, 44.

Ro-Choi, T. S., and Busch, H. (1973). *In* "The Molecular Biology of Cancer" (H. Busch, ed.), pp. 241-276. Academic Press, New York.

Ro-Choi, T. S., and Busch, H. (1974). *In* "The Cell Nucleus" (H. Busch, ed.), Vol. 3, pp. 152-211. Academic Press, New York.

Roeder, R. G., and Rutter, W. J. (1969). *Nature (London)* **224**, 234-237.

Roeder, R. G., and Rutter, W. J. (1970). *Biochemistry* **9**, 2543-2553.

Rovera, G., and Baserga, R. (1971). *J. Cell Physiol.* **77**, 201.

Sandberg, A. A., and Sakurai, M. (1973). *In* "The Molecular Biology of Cancer" (H. Busch, ed.), pp. 81-106. Academic Press, New York.

Sato, S., and Sugimura, T. (1974). *Methods Cancer Res.* **12**, 259-315.

Sitz, T. O., Nazar, R. N., Spohn, W. H., and Busch, H. (1973). *Cancer Res.* **33**, 3312-3318.

Smetana, K., and Busch, H. (1979). *In* "Effects of Drugs in the Cell Nucleus" (H. Busch, S. Crooke, and Y. Daskal, eds.), pp. 89-105. Academic Press, New York.

Spelsberg, T. C., Steggles, A. W., and O'Malley, B. W. (1971). *Biochim. Biophys. Acta* **254**, 129.

Steele, W. J., and Busch, H. (1963). *Cancer Res.* **23**, 1153-1163.

Steggles, A. W., Spelsberg, T. C., and O'Malley, B. W. (1971). *Biochem. Biophys. Res. Commun.* **43**, 20.

Stein, G. S., and Kleinsmith, L. J., eds. (1975). "Chromosomal Proteins and Their Role in the Regulation of Gene Expression." Academic Press, New York.

Stein, G. S., Chaudhuri, S., and Baserga, R. (1972). *J. Biol. Chem.* **247**, 3918–3922.

Sugimura, T. (1976). "Control Mechanisms in Cancer." Raven Press, New York.

Takami, H., and Busch, H. (1979). *Cancer Res.* **39**, 507–518.

Teng, C. S., Teng, C. T., and Allfrey, V. G. (1971). *J. Biol. Chem.* **246**, 3597.

Vorbrodt, A. (1974). *In* "The Cell Nucleus" (H. Busch, ed.), Vol. 3, pp. 309–344. Academic Press, New York.

Watson, R. J., Parker, J., Fiil, N. P., Flaks, J. G., and Friesen, J. D. (1975). *Proc. Natl. Acad. Sci. U.S.A.* **72**, 2765–2769.

Weinhouse, S. (1972). *Cancer Res.* **32**, 2007–2016.

Wu, B. C., Rao, M. S., Gupta, K. K., Rothblum, L. I., Mamrack, P. C., and Busch, H. (1977). *Cell Biol. Int. Rep.* **1**, 31–44.

Yeoman, L. C., Taylor, C. W., and Busch, H. (1973a). *Biochem. Biophys. Res. Commun.* **51**, 956–966.

Yeoman, L. C., Taylor, C. W., Jordan, J. J., and Busch, H. (1973b). *Biochem. Biophys. Res. Commun.* **53**, 1067–1076.

Zardi, L., Lin, J.-C., and Baserga, R. (1973). *Nature (London), New Biol.* **245**, 211.

3

COMPARISON OF MALIGNANT AND NONMALIGNANT CELLS
James E. Strong

I. INTRODUCTION

In determining the molecular differences between neoplastic and normal cells, it is reasonable to begin our investigation by asking the question, what causes cancer? Most investigators would agree that the fundamental difference between normal and malignant cells is the loss of homeostatic control by the host over the tumor cells' growth. The degree of malignancy is generally correlated with a loss in cellular differentiation. The cancer cell may lose the specialized morphological and biochemical characteristics associated with the tissue of origin to become an efficient growth-oriented machine. Indeed, part of the problem associated with determining the relevant differences between cancer cells and normal cells is differentiating between characteristics associated with rapid cellular growth and those representative of the cancer phenotype. Expression of the cancer phenotype is probably controlled at the level of the cellular genome. Two mechanisms generally suggested for this process involve either genetic or epigenetic alterations. The first mechanism, genetic alteration, is supported by the observation that most carcinogenic chemicals are also mutagenic. In addition, oncogenic viruses are capable of integrating into host cellular DNA, thus ensuring genetic transmission of the cancer phenotype to daughter cells. A second mechanism, epigenetic alteration, is probably less obvious than the previous method. This mechanism suggests that no change in the genetic contribution need occur in malignant transformation. Rather, cancer is caused by activation of specific genetic sequences present in all normal cells. This theory is supported by evidence that under specific conditions, cancer cells may be made to appear and function the same as normal cells. Moreover, few, if any, new gene products are found in cancer cells that are not also present in normal cells, at some stage of development. These hypotheses are not mutually exclusive and both mechanisms probably coexist in cellular transformation and malignancy.

In this discussion, similarities and differences between cancer cells and normal cells will be presented that support either hypothesis. We will begin by examining the differentiation of neoplastic and normal cells, the fetal and embryonic characteristics of tumor cells, the metabolic alterations associated with malignancy, regulation of genetic information in cancer cells, and, finally, diseases associated with increased malignancy.

II. DIFFERENTIATION IN NEOPLASIA

During the development of a higher organism, billions of cells differentiate to form a great number of specific morphological, physiological, and biochemical cell types from a single activated egg. Available evidence indicates that this differential process does not involve a qualitative change in genetic information so that each differentiated cell has the potential for forming a new organism. Therefore, selective activation of gene functions must be controlled by epigenetic mechanisms. These mechanisms appear to be controlled largely by cytoplasmic factors which are capable of programming the nucleus to activate specific genetic expressions.

Since epigenetic mechanisms play an essential role in normal cellular differentiation, the question arises whether cancer cells might also be established and maintained through epigenetic mechanisms. This would require demonstration that all information necessary for the cancer phenotype can be present in normal cells and that the tumor cell phenotype is reversible.

The reversibility of the neoplastic state has been demonstrated in a number of different animal systems. One example is a highly malignant adenocarcinoma of the leopard frog caused by a herpes-type virus. Adenocarcinomas were induced in a triploid line of frogs so that a marker for the resultant cancer nuclei could be followed. The triploid nuclei were isolated from the cancer cells and injected into normal, enucleated frog eggs. The resultant triploid tadpoles were entirely normal. This experiment indicated that genetic information present in the cancer nucleus could be effectively manipulated by cytoplasmic factors to produce normal organisms (McKinnell et al., 1969).

Carcinogen-induced tumors in the European newt have also been shown to be reversible (Seilern-Aspang and Kratochwil, 1962). Carcinogenic hydrocarbons were injected to form tumors that infiltrated and metastasized killing over half of the treated newts. However, in many of the animals, spontaneous regression of the tumors occurred. The basis of the regression was not death of the tumor cells, but redifferentiation of those cells back to the nontumerous phenotype. Regression was most readily achieved in those animals undergoing regeneration of amputated tails.

Another example of reversibility of the neoplastic state occurs in teratocarcinoma of the mouse (Kleinsmith and Pierce, 1964). This teratocarcinoma consists of derivatives of the three embryonic germ layers and contains a wide variety of cell types interspersed with malignant cells. The multiple phenotypes appear to be formed from a common stem cell, since when malignant cells were injected into mice peritoneal cavaties, the resultant tumors were composed of the same differential cell types found in the original tumor. However, the differential cells had lost their tumorigenic capacity. These studies indicate embryonal cell carcinomas are multipotent stem cells capable of differentiating into a large number of nonmalignant phenotypes.

In humans, the best documented cases of tumor reversibility occurs in spontaneous remissions. In some instances, as illustrated in retinoblastomas, the regression may involve differentiation and maturation of malignant neuroblastoma cells into ganglionic cells which are nonmalignant (Dyke and Mulkey, 1967).

The findings that tumor cells may differentiate to become nonmalignant gives hope that new approaches to treatment might someday be based upon the control of genetic determinates. Indeed, one investigator has expressed the opinion that "oncogeny is blocked ontogeny" or cancer is caused when cells are arrested in the fetal–embryonic stages of development (Potter *et al.*, 1972). Understanding and control of differentiation, blocked in tumor cells, may someday allow manipulation of the neoplastic state.

III. FETAL–EMBRYONIC CHARACTERISTICS OF CANCER CELLS

In a comparison of normal and neoplastic tissue, one of the characteristics most persistently recognizable is the similarity between neoplastic and embryonic cells. Both cancer and embryonic cells may develop at a rapid rate, seemingly independent of host control mechanisms. Both cells also possess the ability to invade surrounding tissues and migrate to form new colonies. The loss of morphological differentiation observable in neoplastic cells may also be found in embryonic cells, especially at the early stages of development. Thus, it is not surprising that neoplastic cells possess many antigenic and biochemical similarities to fetal cells.

A. Biochemical Markers

1. Isozymes

The presence of multiple molecular forms or isozymes has been extensively documented in a number of enzyme systems. Some of these isozymes appear specific to the tissue of origin. There is much information available that indicates alterations occur in the isozymic patterns of neoplastic tissues. This is characterized by a progressive loss of specific tissue forms and their replacement by isozymic patterns often associated with fetal tissues. A listing of many fetal-like isozymes found in various tumors is shown in Table I.

Several specific examples of isozyme alteration associated with neoplastic development include glucose-ATP phosphotransferase (hexokinase), alkaline phosphatase, and pyruvate kinase. Glucose-ATP phosphotransferase has been found in four molecular forms. The fetal type isozyme pattern appears in most poorly differentiated hepatomas and in primary hepatomas induced by chemical carcinogens. However, highly differentiated hepatomas with very slow growth rates have an isozyme pattern similar to adult liver (Walker and Potter, 1972). A placental form of alkaline phosphatase, named Regan isozyme, was first discovered in a patient (Mr. Regan) with metastatic bronchogenic carcinoma (Fishman *et al.*, 1968). The Regan isozyme can be detected in greater than 10% of patients with a variety of tumors. Cultured human cancer cells (HeLa TCRC-1) also

TABLE I

Isozymes in Normal and Neoplastic Tissues[a]

Isozyme	Neoplastic tissue	Normal tissue
Thymidine kinase	Colon cancer	Placenta
	Hela cells	Human fetal cells
Pyruvate kinase	Hepatoma	Fetal tissue
Alcohol dehydrogenase	Hepatoma	Rat fetal liver
Aldolase C	Hepatoma	Rat fetal liver
	Human rhabdomyosarcoma	Rat fetal liver
	Yoshida ascites hepatoma	Rat fetal liver
	Zajdela ascites hepatoma	Rat fetal liver
Hexokinase	Uterine carcinomas	Fetal tissue
Uridine kinase	Novikoff ascites hepatoma	Fetal liver
Carbamylphosphate synthetase type II	Ehrlich ascites carcinomas Hepatomas	Fetal liver
Branched-chain amino acid transferases	Yoshida ascites hepatoma	Fetal liver
Alkaline phosphatase (Regan form)	Bronchogenic carcinoma Lung Gastrointestinal tract	Placenta
Alkaline phosphatase	Genital tract	Placenta
	Hepatocellular	Placenta
	Carcinomal of stomach	Placenta
Glutaminase	AH-130 hepatoma	Fetal liver
	Novikoff hepatoma	Fetal liver
	2C-18 hepatoma	Fetal liver
	Mammary carcinoma	Fetal liver

[a] From Stein *et al.* (1978).

possess the Regan isozyme. Growth of these cells in immunosuppressed rats resulted in reversion of the Regan isozyme to an adult type. However, returning these cells to tissue culture stimulated reappearance of the Regan isozyme (Singer and Fishman, 1974). Another example of isozymic similarities between tumor and fetal tissue occurs with pyruvate kinase. Pyruvate kinase can be resolved into three molecular forms: isozymes I, II, and III. Isozyme I predominates in adult liver whereas isozyme III activity is greatest in fetal liver. In transplantable hepatoma tumors, the ratio of isozyme III to I activity increases with loss of cellular differentiation (Farina *et al.*, 1974). A similar change from adult to fetal pyruvate kinase isozyme pattern occurred when rats were fed a hepatocarcinogen. The activity of isozyme I decreased 90% while a concomitant increase in isozyme III to greater than fivefold the initial value occurred 6 weeks after initiating the hepatocarcinogen diet (Walker and Potter, 1972).

2. Other Biochemical Similarities

In addition to isozymes, properties shared in common between embryonic and tumor cells (rapid cell growth, metastasis, and invasiveness) produce similar biochemical activities. The invasibility of tumor cells has been correlated with a specific protease, plasminogen activator, that is found in both embryonic and malignant cells (Sherman *et al.*, 1976). Tumor cells also resemble embryonic cells in their lack of ability to invade decidual tissue (Wilson, 1963). Cell surface properties are altered in malignantly transformed cells. Such changes are indicated by the ability of neoplastic cells to preferentially bind lectins, such as concanavalin A or wheat germ agglutinin (Inbar and Sacks, 1969). Embryonic cells are similarly agglutinated by concanavalin A and wheat germ agglutinin after proteolytic treatment to expose binding sites (Moscona, 1971).

Tumor cells produce a factor that stimulates vascularization to provide blood supply. A diffusible factor secreted by tumor cells which is mitogenic to vascular endothelium and stimulates capillary proliferation is known as tumor angiogenesis factor (TAF) (Folkman *et al.*, 1971). This angiogenesis factor is also found in the placenta (Folkman, 1972). Vascularization allows solid tumors to display their full potential for growth. Prior to vascularization, a solid tumor is limited in growth by diffusibility of nutrients into, and waste material out of, the tumor mass. However, stimulation of capillary development allows the tumor to escape these limitations and perhaps shed metastatic cells. Thus, investigation of "antiangiogenesis" factors offers a potential means for controlling tumor growth (Folkman, 1972).

An additional example of similarity between neoplasia and ontogenic development is found in the decondensation and reactivation of the normally condensed X chromosome (Teplitz *et al.*, 1972). This condition is usually found in human female cervical and gastric carcinomas and may represent a recurrence of a fetal condition, since both X chromosomes must be active during embryogenesis for normal fetal development (Lyon, 1961). Normal fetal development also requires an escape mechanism from antibody attack by the mother toward fetal antigens. Since this is a characteristic of tumor cells, a common escape mechanism has been suggested for both neoplastic and fetal cells (Coggin and Anderson, 1974).

B. Immunological Markers

1. α-Fetoprotein

This tumor-associated antigen can be detected by radioimmunoassay in greater than 70% of patients with hepatocellular carcinoma and greater than 60% of patients with teratocarcinomas (Goussev *et al.*, 1971). The presence of abnormal α-fetoprotein (α-FP) levels has also been observed in association with other pathological disorders, including alcoholic cirrhosis (Harai *et al.,* 1973). The principal source of α-FP during fetal development is the liver. The serum concentration drops rapidly at birth and after 1 month, α-FP is no longer detectable in the sera by immunodiffusion. However, radioimmunoassay indicates that the sera of healthy adults may contain between 5 and 20 ng/ml α-FP (Uriel, 1975). At present, α-FP does not appear pathognomic for neoplasia, although persistently high levels may be indicative of liver cancer. Determination of α-FP serum levels is of clinical usefulness, in periodically monitoring therapy or to detect residual and recurrent tumors.

2. Carcinoembryonic Antigen

Carcinoembryonic antigen (CEA) is a glycoprotein with a molecular weight of 200,000. CEA is generally associated with cell membranes in fetal and tumoral tissues of the digestive tract (Neville and Laurence, 1974). Normal adult plasma concentrations of CEA range from about 2.5 to 10.0 ng/ml. Raised levels of serum CEA have been reported in many patients with cancer of the gastrointestinal, genito-urinary, and pulmonary systems. Elevated levels have also been reported in patients with nonmalignant diseases (colitis, diverticulitis, alcoholic pancreatitis, and liver cirrhosis). Thus, CEA, like α-FP, is also of limited value in the differential diagnosis between neoplastic and non-neoplastic disease but is useful in clinical monitoring for therapeutic prognosis (Uriel, 1975).

3. Other Oncofetal Antigens

Studies have been conducted that indicate antigens arising in tumor cells following oncogenic viral infection may cross-react with fetal antigens. Infection of adult hamster cells with SV40 tumor virus results in induction of antigens that cross-react with hamster fetal cells (Baranska *et al.,* 1970). Several blood components normally found in fetal blood are also present during malignancy. These include α_2H-globulin, a ferroprotein normally occurring in fetal blood and found associated with childhood tumors (Buffe *et al.,* 1970). Another example of fetal blood components associated with malignancy is the appearance of fetal hemoglobin in leukemia and other hematological diseases (Miller, 1969).

Fetal antigens have been demonstrated on the surface of a variety of human solid tumors (Alexander, 1972; Avis *et al.,* 1973) and leukemia cells (Harris *et al.,* 1971). Sera from mice immunized with human leukemia blast cells reacted with fetal liver but not bone marrow or adult liver as determined by immunofluorescence (Granatek *et al.,* 1976). Although the function of many fetal antigens is unknown, some oncofetal antigens have been found that appear to perform similar functions in both neoplastic and fetal cells. An example of this may be the appearance of human chorionic gonadotropin (HCG) on the surface of human neoplastic cells. Immunochemical techniques were used to determine that in 25 of 28 human malignant tumor cells evaluated, there was present material antigenically similar to the β-chain of HCG (McManus *et al.*, 1976). Since it has been suggested that placental HCG may be involved in maternal immunological tolerance of the human fetus, a similar function has been proposed for the presence of HCG on the tumor cell surface (Adcock *et al.*, 1973). Although, initially fetal antigens were regarded as characteristic of the neoplastic state, recent studies indicate that normal adult cells may reexpress fetal antigens under circumstances unrelated to neoplasia but associated with cellular regeneration or rapid proliferation (Jerry *et al.*, 1976).

IV. METABOLIC ALTERATIONS IN NORMAL AND NEOPLASTIC CELLS

A. Molecular Correlation Concept

A metabolic imbalance associated with neoplasia was first described by Warburg (1931). He suggested that cancer was caused by an impaired respiratory mechanism with a resultant high rate of glycolysis. However, it has been demonstrated that in some tumors, the rate of respiration is normal and that some normal tissues have enhanced glycolytic activity. Subsequent to the Warburg hypothesis, the metabolic imbalance of cancer cells has been systematically examined by Weber who coined the phrase "molecular correlation concept" to describe the ordered pattern of enzymatic imbalance linked with malignancy (Weber, 1972). Weber suggested that the pattern of imbalance of key enzymes was biologically advantageous for cancer cell growth. This "metabolic imbalance" resulted in an enhanced activity of enzymes associated with nucleic acid and protein synthesis and a corresponding decrease in those enzymes constituting anabolic pathways. Conversely, enzymes associated with carbohydrate anabolism showed increased activity, while those contributing to carbohydrate synthesis, decreased.

In addition to quantitative changes in enzyme activities found in neoplastic cells, qualitative changes in isozyme patterns also help contribute to the metabolic imbalance. Within the glycolysis pathway, there is a change from the high K_m (dissociation constant), feedback-inhibited isozymes normally found in the liver for glucokinase and pyruvate kinase to the low K_m isozymes, for hexokinase and muscle-type pyruvate kinase. With the loss of glucokinase and liver-type pyruvate kinase, the sensitivity to control by phosphoenolpyruvate feedback inhibition is lost and the sensitivity to other inhibitors markedly decreased. Kinetic studies on the behavior of cyclic AMP phosphodiesterase activity also indicated a qualitative shift in this isozyme pattern in malignant transformation. The activity of a phosphodiesterase normally found in liver with a high K_m was replaced by a low K_m phosphodiesterase isozyme found in both slow and rapidly growing hepatomas. These findings are said by Weber to indicate that a selective gene activation of low K_m isozymes, unresponsive to normal control mechanisms, gives cancer cells a selective advantage for growth over normal cells.

Weber also suggests that the pattern of enzymatic activity for key enzymes involved in nucleic acid and carbohydrate metabolism indicates that neoplasia is not simply a regression to the fetal stage of differentiation. In a comparison of enzymatic activities found in hepatomas, regenerating liver, and fetal liver, numerous differences in the relative enzymatic rates were found. These differences were highly significant since tissue cells possessed similar rates of growth. Thus, these results indicated the presence of a specific molecular pattern, linked to the degree of malignant transformation, that was characteristic of cancer cells and not merely a return to the fetal state (Weber, 1977).

B. Other Metabolic Alterations

It has been reported that acute lymphocytic leukemic cells have lost the ability to synthesize asparagine (Capizzi et al., 1970). This difference between leukemia cells and normal cells has been the basis of chemotherapy with the enzyme L-asparaginase. The L-asparaginase depletes exogenous supplies of asparagine so that leukemic cells do not have plasma asparagine to utilize in protein synthesis. Thus the leukemic cells are selectively inhibited by L-asparaginase compared with normal blood cells that retain the ability to synthesize asparagine. Another metabolic difference associated with malignant cells was the enzyme 5′-nucleotidase. 5′-nucleotidase is either extremely low or absent in the cell membranes of chronic lymphocytic leukemia cells (Lopes et al., 1973).

V. ALTERATIONS IN CELL SURFACE

Membrane transport of glucose, amino acids, and certain cations is generally enhanced in malignantly transformed cells. One explanation is that increased membrane fluidity may contribute to the activity of membrane transport enzymes. The use of fluorescent polarization techniques (Shinitzky and Inbar, 1974) indicates that transformed lymphocytes have greater fluidity than normal lymphocytes. The binding of plant lectins to cell surfaces suggests that membrane fluidity is enhanced in transformed cells. A glycoprotein lectin from wheat seeds (wheat germ agglutinin) causes agglutination of cancer cells to a much greater degree than normal cells (Nicholson, 1974). However, normal and cancer cells appear to have the same number of binding sites for agglutinin attachment. That cancer cells agglutinate more effectively is thought to occur because the lectin binding sites freely diffuse in the tumor cell membrane to form dense patches of agglutinin receptors. These receptors allow effective cross-linking between cancer cells. However, normal cells do not apparently possess this diffusibility except during the mitotic stage of the cell cycle. During mitosis, normal cells agglutinate as effectively as cancer cells. The enhanced agglutinability of normal cells during mitosis has been correlated with loss of a fibrous protein beneath the cell membrane that may contribute to the rigidity of the normal cell surface at other stages of the cell cycle (Nicholson, 1974).

Various biochemical properties expressed on the surface of mammalian cells, distinguish cancer cells from normal cells (Emmelot, 1973). In rat hepatomas, there is a marked increase in cholesterol content of the plasma membrane. The RNA content also appears increased in the hepatoma plasma membrane. Cells transformed by temperature-sensitive oncogenic virus contain increased amounts of fucose-containing glycopeptide with an apparent higher molecular weight than those present in untransformed cells (Warren *et al.,* 1973). These cells showed characteristic glycopeptide patterns when grown at temperatures permissive for the tumor virus but were similar to nontransformed cells when grown at higher temperatures.

It seems likely that in normal cells, intercellular contact releases a chemical signal (probably cyclic AMP), leading to DNA synthesis inhibition and restriction of growth. The enzyme adenyl cyclase is firmly bound to the cell surface and may function as a "receptor complex" for contact inhibition by catalyzing the increased amounts of cyclic AMP synthesis found in normal contact inhibition (Weiss and Poste, 1976). However, in tumor cells, this mechanism does not appear functional. Tumor cells, in general, have lower levels of cyclic AMP, and the levels are not increased upon growth in high cell densities. Addition of cyclic AMP to either tumor or normal cells results in growth inhibition. Thus, one reason tumor cells may be resistant to contact inhibition is because they lack cell surface stimulation of adenyl cyclase catalyzed synthesis of cyclic AMP.

VI. REGULATION OF GENETIC EXPRESSION

Since regulation of genetic expression plays an important role in any phenotypic manifestation, comparison of the factors involved in this process between normal and neoplastic cells may aid in understanding (and possibly controlling) neoplasia.

A. Chromosomal Nucleoproteins

1. Histones

The histone fractions of chromosomal proteins probably are involved in nonspecific repression of genetic information and structural aspects of the

genome. Differences in histones and their posttranslational modifications between neoplastic cells and normal cells have not been established as specific
contributors to the neoplastic state. However, differences between cancer and
normal cells have been indicated, but it is difficult to interpret whether these may
be merely related to characteristics associated with rapidly growing cells. For
example, rapidly dividing tumors have a much higher level of phosphorylation of
histone F_1. However, phosphorylation of histone F_1 also increases during cell
proliferation in normal cells (Rovera, 1975). The DNA–histone ratios appear to
be consistent with normal controls in human leukemia and experimental rat
hepatomas, although some differences in this ratio have been found in
carcinogen-induced hepatomas (Gronow and Griffiths, 1974). Thus, the relationship between histones and neoplastic transformation is not apparent at this time.
However, the interactions between histones and nonhistone chromosomal proteins may play an important role in destabilizing the DNA–histone complex and
allow increased availability of genes transcribable for the cancer phenotype.

Differences in chromatin from normal and SV40 virus–transformed cells of the
same type have been detected by immunological techniques. Antisera made
using normal cell chromatin as antigen reacted weakly against transformed cell
chromatin. A similar result was obtained when the reverse experiment was performed. However, when the histone fractions were used as antigens, antisera
thus obtained reacted with histones extracted from either cell type. Nonhistone
chromosomal proteins used as antigens produced antisera that did not cross-react
with nonhistone chromosomal protein extracted from the heterologous cell type.
Thus, the specificity of antisera for nonhistone chromosomal proteins indicated
differences between immunoreactivity of normal and transformed cells chromatin resided with the nonhistone fraction (Zardi *et al.*, 1973).

2. *Nonhistone Chromosomal Proteins*

The nonhistone chromosomal proteins (NHCP) provide specific regulation of
genetic expression in mammalian cells. It is not surprising that alterations in
these proteins may be associated with malignant transformation; NHCP–DNA
ratios are significantly increased in hepatomas and human leukemias (Arnold *et
al.*, 1973). Both qualitative and quantitative differences have been found using
two-dimensional gel electrophoresis. By progressive extraction of nuclear fractions, many differences in NHCP in hepatoma and regenerating liver have been
found. Some proteins were present in hepatoma that were not found in liver, as
well as the converse (Wilson *et al.*, 1975; Yeoman *et al.*, 1974). Differences in
the NHCP of tumor and normal tissues have also been found in intestinal epithelial cells and human lymphocytes (Yeoman *et al.*, 1976a; Boffa and Allfrey,
1976). There may occasionally be similarity between NHCP of different tumors.
A nuclear antigen from Novikoff hepatoma cells cross-reacted with Walker 256
carcinosarcoma and fetal rat liver but not with normal or regenerating liver
chromatin (Yeoman *et al.*, 1976b). Antisera raised against NHCP–DNA com-

plexes from Novikoff hepatoma cross-reacted to a greater degree with NHCP–DNA complexes from Walker carcinosarcoma and AS30A hepatoma than normal rat liver NHCP–DNA complexes. Posttranslational modification differences also exist between NHCP of normal and transformed cells. Increased phosphorylation of NHCP of transformed cells may be as much as 10-fold greater than nontransformed cells of the same tissue. Enhanced phosphorylation may be significant in alteration of genetic regulation by NHCP. The regulation of NHCP phosphorylation may reside with the phosphorylating enzymes, since the protein kinases of neoplastic and normal tissues apparently differ (Thomson et al., 1975).

The presence of specific NHCP in the chromatin apparently controls the specificity of RNA transcription in both normal and neoplastic cells. When Walker 256 tumor nonhistone proteins were used to activate normal rat liver chromatin in experiments in which the chromatin was reconstituted in vitro, the RNA produced was similar to that produced by Walker 256 tumor chromatin (Kostraba and Wang, 1971, 1973). Although the results of reconstitution experiments should be interpreted cautiously, it seems clear that nonhistone chromasomal proteins are important in differences between normal and neoplastic cells.

B. Transcription

Investigations have been conducted into the differences between mRNA produced by tumor and normal cells. The enzyme reverse transcriptase can be used to synthesize cDNA from an RNA template. The cDNA (complimentary DNA) so produced has been used as a probe for hybridization with other mRNA. Using these techniques, approximately 45% of the mRNA in Novikoff hepatoma cells differed from that of normal liver and 35% differed from that of regenerating liver (Hirsch et al., 1977). The greatest quantitative differences appeared for the abundant mRNA species. The translational protein products of these different mRNAs from regenerating liver and tumor cells were also analyzed and suggested qualitative differences in the types of proteins synthesized.

Messenger RNA synthesized in mammalian cells generally has a finite lifteime for template activity in protein synthesis. The mRNA templates for the same protein appear to have different lifetimes in transformed cells than in normal cells (Shires et al., 1974). Though the mechanism for template stabilization is not completely understood, it may involve RNA association with membranes of the endoplasmic reticulum (Shires et al., 1974).

In mammalian cells, different RNA polymerases exist which are localized in the nucleus, mitochondria, and cytoplasm. New species of RNA polymerase have not been detected in tumor cells. However, considerable increase in activity of nuclear RNA polymerase appears to occur early in transformation to the malignant state (Mayer et al., 1976).

C. Translation

The mechanism of protein synthesis in normal and cancer cells does not appear to differ in any fundamental respect. However, variation in regulation of proteins synthesis may exist. Many investigators have reported differences in the specific aminoacyl-tRNAs of tumors and normal tissues. The existence of multiple forms of tRNA coding for the same amino acid indicate these molecules may play a role in translational regulation. The chromatographic profile from 20 aminoacyl-tRNAs of normal and leukemic lymphoblasts were compared, and there were small differences for leucyl-, seryl-, threonyl- and prolyl-tRNAs and pronounced differences between tyrosyl- and glutamyl-tRNA (Gallo and Pestka, 1970). A comparison between human myeloma cells and normal human lymphocytes also revealed differences in tRNA species (Fujioka and Gallo, 1971). Modifications in tRNA patterns are also common in virus-transformed cells. These alterations are probably the result of derepressed or modified host tRNA rather than viral genome product (Griffin, 1975).

VII. VIRUS-RELATED PROPERTIES OF NEOPLASTIC CELLS

The possibility that cancer can be caused by a human tumor virus has been the subject of intensive research. Despite this effort, no human tumor viruses have been definitely identified as causative agents in cancer. Although electron microscopy has revealed tumor virus-like particles in human cancer cells, it is uncertain whether these are causative agents of cancer or non-tumor-causing viruses associated with the malignant state. However, there is evidence that oncogenic virus-related proteins and nucleic acids are present in tumor cells. This evidence includes the following: (a) the presence of reverse transcriptase in human leukemia cells, (b) the appearance of structures with biophysical properties similar to RNA tumor viruses (oncornaviruses), (c) identification of oncornavirus specific nucleotide sequences, and (d) the presence of oncornavirus group-specific (gs) antigens in human leukemia (Gallo, 1976).

Shortly after the discovery of an enzyme that synthesized DNA from an RNA template (reverse transcriptase), this same enzyme was discovered in patients with acute leukemia (Gallo et al., 1970). The enzyme in leukemia had the known biochemical and biophysical properties of reverse transcriptases found in mammalian RNA tumor viruses (Gallo et al., 1973). The enzyme was also found in association with an RNA tumor virus-like particle, and it was antigenically similar to reverse transcriptase found in primate RNA tumor viruses (Baxt et al., 1973). The leukemia reverse transcriptase is highly specific for leukemic cells, since no enzyme with similar properties could be found in normal leukocytes, stimulated leukocytes, or human lymphoblast cell lines (Gallo, 1976). The particles containing reverse transcriptase in the cytoplasm of human leukemia cells also resembled RNA tumor viruses. The RNA present in these particles was the same size (70 S) as RNA in RNA tumor virus particles. Also, the density of these particles was similar to the density of RNA tumor viruses in other species. The presence of these particles and their associated reverse transcriptase may potentially aid in diagnosis of leukemia. Analysis of the reverse transcriptase associated with 70 S RNA in acute or chronic lymphoblastic and myelogenous leukemia cells revealed that more than 95% (22 of 23) of the patients had reverse transcriptase activity (Baxt et al., 1972). In contrast to these results, blood cells from 18 nonleukemic patients did not exhibit evidence of the specific 70 S RNA directed DNA polymerase activity. These findings are significant since half of the nonleukemic patients had elevated white blood cell counts caused by a variety of disorders, including polycythemia vera. Thus, tumor virus-like particles may be specific markers for human leukemia cells.

RNA tumor virus nucleotide sequences also appear unique to leukemia cells' genetic material. To investigate whether the DNA of malignant cells contain viral-related sequences that are not found in normal cells, DNA synthesized from the 70 S RNA by leukemia cell reverse transcriptase was used as a molecular probe. In these experiments, the tumor virus probe DNA was hybridized to normal and leukemic leukocyte DNA to look for unique sequences in the leukemia cell DNA that were not present in normal DNA. In eight patients studied, the DNA probe detected sequences in leukemia cell DNA that were not present in normal cells (Baxt and Spiegelman, 1972). Similar techniques demonstrated that Hodgkin's disease and Burkitt's lymphoma patients cells also had unique sequences (Kufe et al., 1973) not found in normal cells. The question was then asked whether the cancer patients' cells possessed unique DNA sequences through inherited or acquired alterations in cellular genetic material. To answer this question, studies were initiated on identical twins, only one of which had leukemia. The results obtained indicated that the leukemic twin's genome contained 70 S RNA particle-related sequences that could not be detected in the leukocytes of his healthy sibling (Buffe et al., 1970). Therefore, since identical twins differentiate from monozygotic origins, the unique DNA sequence of the leukemic individual had to be inserted following fertilization. This evidence supports the acquired rather than inherited mode of leukemia etiology.

VIII. DISEASES WITH ALTERED REPAIR THAT APPEAR ASSOCIATED WITH THE CANCER PHENOTYPE

Among the genetic traits that are associated with tumor development, cells with altered DNA repair mechanisms appear especially susceptible to neoplastic transformation. There are two main kinds of DNA repair processes in human cells: excision repair and postreplication repair. The excision repair process consists of several enzymatic activities that function to excise and patch regions of damaged DNA. These include an endonuclease to recognize the DNA damage and cause a single break near the damaged site, an exonuclease to remove a segment of DNA around the damaged site, a DNA polymerase to resynthesize DNA, and a ligase to join the newly synthesized DNA to the original strand. A second type of repair system, postreplication repair, involves a modification of normal replication by leaving gaps in newly synthesized DNA opposite damaged segments. Following DNA synthesis, the gaps are filled in by newly synthesized DNA and by recombination between parental and daughter strands.

A. Xeroderma Pigmentosum

The best established example of defective repair leading to malignancy is in xeroderma pigmentosum (XP). In most cases, XP is associated with defects in excision repair of damaged bases. The clinical manifestation of the disease is an extreme sensitivity to sunlight and a high incidence of skin cancer. Cells from XP patients exposed to UV light show enhanced lethality, chromosomal aberrations and mutations. The biochemical defect in excision repair defective XP cells is the UV endonuclease that initiates excision of DNA damage. However, a small group of XP patients have been found that are deficient in recombinational repair. Cells from these patients are unique in their sensitivity to caffeine, an agent known to inhibit recombinational repair (Cleaver and Bootsma, 1975).

B. Ataxia Telangiectasia

The clinical features of this disease are progressive cerebellar ataxia, telangiectasas of skin and conjunctiva, proneness to sinopulmonary infection, immunological deficiencies, and a tendency to develop lymphatic malignancy. The cellular characteristics include multiple chromosome aberrations and increased sensitivity to X rays. Cells apparently perform ultraviolet excision repair to a normal extent, and rejoin single-strand breaks made by X rays, but excise X-ray damaged bases slowly. Therefore, the defect may involve some stage in recognition and repair of X-ray damage (Paterson et al., 1976).

C. Blooms Syndrome

This disease is characterized by low birth weight, sensitivity to sunlight; characteristic facial features including prominent nose, hypoplastic molar areas, and retruded mandible; plus increased incidence of acute leukemia. Although there is a reduced rate of DNA chain elongation in these cells, the biochemical defect has yet to be identified (Hand and German, 1975).

D. Fanconi's Anemia

The prominent features of this disease are hypoplasia of all blood elements, pigmentary changes in the skin, malformation of the heart, and a tendency to develop acute leukemia and several solid tumors. Heterozygote carriers of this disease may also display an increased incidence of malignancy. Fanconi's anemia cellular characteristics include chromosomal aberrations. The biochemical defect associated with Fanconi's anemia is probably some stage in excision repair (Poon *et al.*, 1974).

E. Chronic Lymphocytic Leukemia

Unlike the previously mentioned alterations, chronic lymphocytic leukemia leukocytes appear to have an increased ability to excise UV damaged regions compared to normal cells (Huang *et al.*, 1972). Chronic lymphocytic leukemia lymphocytes also appear to have a DNA unwinding protein that is not found in normal lymphocytes (Huang *et al.*, 1975).

F. Progeria

This disease is characterized clinically by extreme premature senility and coronary artery disease. Patients' cells apparently display a normal sensitivity to ultraviolet light but enhanced susceptability to X rays (Epstein *et al.*, 1973). The defect may involve a reduced ability to rejoin X-ray induced DNA breaks (Regan and Setlow, 1974).

IX. DISCUSSION

A wide variety of biochemical differences have been observed which differentiate tumor cells from nonmalignant cells. Clearly, comparative studies have proved of value in furthering the understanding of the neoplastic process.

REFERENCES

Adcock, E. W., Teasdale, F., August, C. S., Cox, S., Meschia, G., Battaglia, F. C., and Naughton, M. A. (1973). *Science* **181**, 845–847.
Alexander, P. (1972). *Nature (London)* **235**, 137–140.
Arnold, E. A., Buksas, M. M., and Young, K. E. A. (1973). *Cancer Res.* **33**, 1169–1176.
Avis, P., Lewis, M. G., and Path, M. R. C. (1973). *J. Natl. Cancer Inst.* **51**, 1063–1065.
Baranska, W., Koldovsky, P., and Koprowski, H. (1970). *Proc. Natl. Acad. Sci. U.S.A.* **67**, 193–199.
Baxt, W. G., and Spiegelman, S. (1972). *Proc. Natl. Acad. Sci. U.S.A.* **69**, 3737–3741.

Baxt, W. G., Hehlmann, R., and Spiegelman, S. (1972). *Nature (London) New Biol.* **240**, 72-75.
Baxt, W. G., Yates, J. W., Wallace, H. J., Holland, J. F., and Spiegelman, S. (1973). *Proc. Natl. Acad. Sci. U.S.A.* **70**, 2629-2632.
Boffa, L. C., and Allfrey, V. G. (1976). *Cancer Res.* **36**, 2678-2865.
Buffe, D., Rimbout, C., Lemerle, J., Schweisguth, O., and Burtin, P. (1970). *Int. J. Cancer* **5**, 85-87.
Capizzi, R. L., Bertino, J. R., and Handschumacher, R. E. (1970). *Annu. Rev. Med.* **21**, 433-444.
Cleaver, J. E., and Bootsma, P. (1975). *Annu. Rev. Genet.* **9**, 19-38.
Coggin, J. H., and Anderson, N. G. (1974). *Adv. Cancer Res.* **19**, 105-165.
Dyke, P. C., and Mulkey, P. A. (1967). *Cancer* **20**, 1343-1349.
Emmelot, P. (1973). *Eur. J. Cancer* **9**, 319-333.
Epstein, J., Williams, J. R., and Little, J. B. (1973). *Proc. Natl. Acad. Sci. U.S.A.* **70**, 977-981.
Farina, F. A., Shatlon, J. B., Morris, H. P., and Weinhouse, S. (1974). *Cancer Res.* **34**, 1439-1446.
Fishman, W. H., Inglis, N. R., Stolbach, L. L., and Krant, M. J. (1968). *Cancer Res.* **28**, 150-154.
Folkman, J. (1972). *Ann. Surg.* **175**, 409-416.
Folkman, J., Merler, E., Abernathy, C., and William, G. (1971). *J. Exp. Med.* **133**, 275-288.
Fujioka, S., and Gallo, R. C. (1971). *Blood* **38**, 246-252.
Gallo, R. C. (1976). *In* "Molecular Base of Malignancy" (E. Deutsch, K. Moser, H. Rainer, and A. Stacker, eds.), pp. 171-177. Thieme, Stuttgart.
Gallo, R. C., and Pestka, S. (1970). *J. Mol. Biol.* **52**, 195-219.
Gallo, R. C., Yang, S. S., and Ting, R. C. (1970). *Nature (London)* **228**, 927-929.
Gallo, R. C., Miller, N. R., Saxinger, W. C., and Gillespie, D. (1973). *Proc. Natl. Acad. Sci. U.S.A.* **70**, 3219-3224.
Goussev, A. I., Englehardt, N. V., Massayeff, R., Camain, R., and Basteris, B. (1971). *Int. J. Cancer* **7**, 207-217.
Granatek, C. H., Hanna, M. G., Hersh, E. M., Gutterman, J. U., Mavligit, G. M., and Candler, E. L. (1976). *Cancer Res.* **36**, 3464-370.
Griffin, A. C. (1975). *In* "Cancer" (F. F. Becken, ed.), Vol. III, pp. 421-458. Plenum, New York.
Gronow, M., and Griffiths, G. (1974). *Exp. Pathol.* **9**, 73-78.
Hand, R., and German, J. (1975). *Proc. Natl. Acad. Sci. U.S.A.* **72**, 758-762.
Harai, M., Wishi, S., Watabe, M., and Tsukada, Y. (1973). GANN *Monogr.* **14**, 19-33.
Harris, R., Viza, D., Todd, R., Phillips, J., Sugar, R., Jennison, R. F., Marriott, G., and Gleeson, M. H. (1971). *Nature (London)* **233**, 556-557.
Hirsch, F. W., Nall, N. N., Hayes, L. C., Raju, K. S., Spohn, W. H., and Busch, H. (1977). *Cancer Res.* **37**, 3694-3700.
Huang, A. T., Kremer, W. B., Laszlo, J., and Setlow, R. B. (1972). *Nature (London)* **240**, 114-116.
Huang, A. T., Riddle, M. M., and Koons, L. S. (1975). *Cancer Res.* **35**, 981-986.
Inbar, M., and Sacks, L. (1969). *Nature (London)* **223**, 710-712.
Jerry, L. M., Lewis, M. G., Rowden, G., Sullivan, A. K., Ptizele, R., and Law, T. (1976). *Cancer Res.* **36**, 3446-3452.
Kleinsmith, L. J., and Pierce, G. B. (1964). *Cancer Res.* **24**, 1544-1551.
Kostraba, N. C., and Wang, T. Y. (1971). *Cancer Res.* **31**, 1663-1668.
Kostraba, N. C., and Wang, T. Y. (1973). *Exp. Cell Res.* **80**, 291-296.
Kufe, D. W., Peters, W. P., and Spiegelman, S. (1973). *Proc. Natl. Acad. Sci. U.S.A.* **70**, 3810-3814.
Lopes, J., Zucker-Franklin, O., and Silber, R. (1973). *J. Clin. Invest.* **52**, 1297-1300.
Lyon, M. F. (1961). *Nature (London)* **190**, 372-373.
McKinnell, R. G., Deggins, B. A., and Labar, D. D. (1969). *Science* **165**, 394.

McManus, L. M., Naughton, M. A., and Martinez-Hernandez, A. (1976). *Cancer Res.* **36,** 3476–3481.

Mayer, D., Eltze, M., Debuch, K. E., Jung, A., and Jackish, R. (1976). *In* "Molecular Base of Malignancy" (E. Deutsch, K. Moser, H. Rainer, and A. Stacker, eds.), pp. 60–66. Thieme, Stuttgart.

Miller, D. R. (1969). *Br. J. Haematol.* **17,** 103–112.

Moscona, A. A. (1971). *Science* **171,** 905–907.

Neville, A. M., and Laurence, D. J. R. (1974). *Int. J. Cancer* **14,** 1–18.

Nicholson, G. (1974). *Int. Rev. Cytol.* **39,** 90.

Paterson, M. D., Smith, B. P., Lohman, P. H. M., Anderson, A. K., and Fishman, L. (1976). *Nature (London)* **260,** 440–441.

Poon, P. K., O'Brien, R. L., and Parker, J. W. (1974). *Nature (London)* **250,** 223–225.

Potter, V. R., Walker, P. R., and Goodman, J. I. (1972). GANN *Monogr.* **13,** 121–134.

Regan, J. D., and Setlow, R. B. (1974). *Biochem. Biophys. Res. Commun.* **59,** 858–864.

Rovera, G. (1975). *In* "Cancer" (F. F. Becker, ed.), Vol. III, p. 405. Plenum, New York.

Seilern-Aspang, F., and Kratochwil, K. (1962). *J. Embryol. Exp. Morphol.* **10,** 337–356.

Sherman, M. L., Strickland, S., and Reich, E. (1976). *Cancer Res.* **36,** 4208–4216.

Shinitzky, M., and Inbar, M. (1974). *J. Mol. Biol.* **85,** 603–615.

Shires, T. K., Pitot, H. C., and Kauffman, F. A. (1974). *Biomembranes* **5,** 81–145.

Singer, R. M., and Fishman, W. H. (1974). *J. Cell Biol.* **60,** 777–780.

Stein, G. S., Stein, J. L., and Thomson, J. A. (1978). *Cancer Res.* **38,** 1181–1201.

Teplitz, R. L., Barr, K. J., and Laure, H. J. (1972). *In Vitro* **7,** 195–200.

Thomson, J. A., Chin, J. F., and Hnilica, L. S. (1975). *Biochim. Biophys. Acta* **407,** 114–119.

Uriel, J. (1975). *In* "Cancer" (F. F. Becker, ed.), Vol. III, pp. 21–54. Plenum, New York.

Walker, P. R., and Potter, V. R. (1972). *Adv. Enzyme Regul.* **10,** 339–364.

Warburg, O. (1931). "The Metabolism of Tumors." Constable Press, London.

Warren, L., Fuhrer, J. P., and Buck, C. A. (1973). *Fed. Proc., Fed. Am. Soc. Exp. Biol.* **32,** 80–85.

Weber, G. (1972). GANN *Monogr.* **13,** 47–77.

Weber, G. (1977). *N. Engl. J. Med.* **296,** 541–551.

Weiss, L., and Poste, G. (1976). *In* "Scientific Foundations of Oncology" (T. Symmington and R. L. Carter, eds.), p. 31. Yearbook Publ., Chicago, Illinois.

Wilson, B., Lee, M. A., Vidali, G., and Allfrey, V. G. (1975). *Cancer Res.* **35,** 2554–2558.

Wilson, I. B. (1963). *Proc. Zool. Soc. London* **141,** 137–151.

Yeoman, L. C., Taylor, C. W., and Busch, H. (1974). *Cancer Res.* **34,** 424–428.

Yeoman, L. C., Seeber, S., Taylor, C. W. Fernback, D. J., Faletta, J. M., Jordan, J. J., and Busch, H. (1976a). *Exp. Cell Res.* **100,** 47–55.

Yeoman, L. C., Jordan, J. J., Busch, R. K., Taylor, C. W., Savage, H. E., and Busch, H. (1976b). *Proc. Natl. Acad. Sci. U.S.A.* **73,** 3258–3262.

Zardi, L., Lin, J. C., and Baserga, R. (1973). *Nature (London) New Biol.* **245,** 211–213.

4

CELLULAR PHARMACOLOGY
Benjamin Drewinko

I. INTRODUCTION

New approaches to systemic treatment for unresectable neoplasias are continually being explored. These approaches include the search for new, more effective antitumor agents and the utilization of combinations of drugs and ionizing radiations. The magnitude of such search at the clinical level is hindered by the fact that it entails experimentation in human subjects with the consequent difficulties in standardization, reproducibility, and speed; its considerable expense; and the limitations in the number of compounds that can be evaluated. Cell cultures provide a rapid, efficient, and economic system for cytotoxicity screenings allowing elucidation of the mode of action of a drug in a controlled, systematic fashion with a high degree of resolution.

The main assumption for *in vitro* studies with chemotherapeutic agents is that the survival response of the cultured cells will reflect that of *in vivo* cells *once* the drug has reached the neoplastic elements (Drewinko, 1975). While no simple translation from *in vitro* to *in vivo* systems is possible, many responses of mammalian cells are reasonably similar to the two situations (Bhuyan, 1970; Madoc-Jones and Mauro, 1970; Rosenblum *et al.*, 1975; Kaneko and LePage, 1978). Therefore, cellular pharmacology has received considerable attention in the last decade, originated from the necessity of developing new and standardized techniques for drug evaluation (World Health Organization, 1966; Dawson, 1972).

One great advantage of *in vitro* systems is that they afford the possibility of studying neoplastic cells of human origin. Zubrod (1977) has proposed that the quickest route to more effective chemotherapy could reside in the efficient exploitation of known active drugs matched to the biological characteristics of the target cancer cells. This could be effectively done if more predictive screens for each type of neoplasm were developed. It is logical to assume that presently available established human cell lines could provide such superior screening systems. This point is particularly important since some agents shown to be active on L1210 leukemia, a routine *in vivo* screening system, failed to kill human neoplastic cells in clinical studies (Schepartz, 1971). In studies conducted in our laboratory, we have shown that anguidine and N-(Phosphonacetyl)-L-aspartate (PALA), drugs with considerable efficacy in murine colon carcinoma (Corbett *et al.*, 1976; Johnson *et al.*, 1976), failed to elicit lethal effects on cultured human colon carcinoma cells (Dosik *et al.*, 1978) predicting the subsequently observed poor clinical response to these agents.

Also, the selective action of a drug in terms of cell cycle specificity can be elucidated *in vitro*. This information may indicate the adequacy of a clinical trial. For example, it has been shown that camptothecin sodium, a drug considered inadequate in the treatment of gastrointestinal cancer, was largely ineffective in stages of the cell cycle other than S phase (Drewinko *et al.*, 1974); this provided at least one explanation for its failure in gastrointestinal tumors which present low fractions ($< 7\%$) of cells in S phase (Steel and Lamerton, 1969).

The methods used to assess cell lethality *in vitro* are of critical importance. Drug-induced cell killing is the result of an interplay between the type, extent, and duration of the damaging effect caused by a drug to critical biosynthetic pathways or subcellular structures, and the capacity of living elements to bypass or repair such damage. A lethally damaged cell may not only complete DNA synthesis but may even divide several times before the entire progeny perishes from the lethal damage inherited from their single ancestor (Whitmore and Till,

1964; Thompson and Suit, 1969; Peel and Cowen, 1972; Ehmann and Wheeler, 1978). Therefore, dye exclusion tests which measure cell membrane integrity, and tests which determine inhibition of DNA synthesis, under the assumption that a cell which completes DNA synthesis is viable, may grossly under- or overestimate the killing effectiveness of injurious agents (Bhuyan *et al.*, 1976; Roper and Drewinko, 1976). Hence, for proliferating populations, the lethal effects of an antitumor agent must be defined by its impairment of the reproductive integrity of the individual cells. *In vitro,* this impairment can be assessed by the inability of cells to proliferate indefinitely, forming colonies under the appropriate experimental conditions (Puck and Marcus, 1955). Applying this method to cell culture systems, dose–response effects can be analyzed quantitatively since the exact concentration of the drug bathing the cells and the duration of exposure is known, and these quantitative responses can be used to compare the efficacy of different agents on a given cell type or the activity of a specific drug on different cell classes.

II. THEORETICAL BACKGROUND

A. Fractional Kill

Cellular kill by many antineoplastic agents follows first order kinetics. Thus, the fraction of a cell population killed by a given dose of ionizing radiation or a cytotoxic agent tends to be constant. This implies that the proportion of cells rendered nonviable after exposure to such an injurious agent will be the same regardless of the initial cellular mass (i.e., 20 cells killed of 100 initial cells; 2×10^4 cells killed of 10^5 initial cells, and 2×10^7 of 10^8 initial cells, for a dose that kills 20% of the cells). This phenomenon of fractional cellular kill was originally observed and studied by early radiobiologists, and the principles and mathematical foundations for its analysis were laid down several decades ago (Atwood and Norman, 1949; Luria and Dulbecco, 1949; Lea, 1955; Barendsen *et al.*, 1960; Zimmer, 1961; Whitmore and Till, 1964; Fowler, 1966). With the advent of chemotherapeutic drugs for the treatment of neoplastic cells, a similar relation between drug dose and percent cell lethality was observed. This observation lead Skipper and collaborators (1964, 1965) to propose a fractional cell kill per drug dose theory which laid the foundation for escalating manipulations of drug dosage in the clinical management of tumors. This same principle is utilized in studies on the effects of drugs at the cellular level where escalating concentrations are used to measure the fractional cell kill as a function of the dose, thus originating the so-called cell survival curves. Frequently, the concentrations that the investigator must use *in vitro* are severalfold greater than those actually measured in plasma following injection of the drug being investigated, and the investigator must assume that the survival curves defined at higher concentrations will reflect the survival curve of cells at lower concentrations. This situation arises from the fact that the methods used to define the effect on cultured cells do not possess the sufficient resolution to permit definition of survival curves at low concentration increments.

B. Survival Analysis

For proliferating cell populations, the most important effect of an antitumor agent is impairment of the ability of a cell to originate a clone of similar cells under conditions in which untreated cells would do so. That is, cell survival must be equated to reproductive integrity, and, by inference, lethality is the loss of such function. An acceptable way to study drug-induced cell lethality is represented by survival analysis, which is the processing of experimental data based entirely on the individual members of the population to which the measured event (cellular death) has not occurred. Results are expressed in the form of survival curves representing the decreasing proportions of surviving clones as the concentration of drug augments. The shape of the survival curve is a function of the biological properties of the treated cells (i.e., membrane permeability, sensitive biosynthetic pathways or subcellular structures, rate of enzymatic transformation and degradation, and capacity to repair damaged subcellular structures) and the physiocochemical characteristics of the agents used (i.e., avidity and binding to target molecules, physicochemical stability, and active moieties). Thus, analysis of the shape of the elicited survival curve may provide vital information on the mechanisms leading to cell death which may contribute important knowledge for the design of improved therapeutic schemes. Unfortunately, the profusion of factors underlying the form of the survival curve and the limited knowledge about their interrelationship prevents a clear definition of the components involved in determining its shape.

One method, commonly used in radiobiology to analyze the shape of survival curves, is based on target theory, developed by Lea (1955) to interpret results of cell survival following treatment with ionizing radiations. Target theory assumes the intracellular existence of a number of distinct, discrete structures or entities engaged in some essential activity necessary to retain reproductive integrity. All or some of these "targets" have to be biologically inactivated before cell survival is abolished. A discrete quantized unit of the injurious agent is sufficient to cause one inactivation event per target. Quantities below this critical threshold will result in reversible damage, while those above this threshold will be superfluous. Similarly, a cell will lose its capacity for unlimited proliferation only if a given fixed number of targets are inactivated. A fraction of inactivated targets less than this critical total will not lead to reproductive death (sublethal damage), while the sum above this level results in "overkill."

Utilization of some concepts and the nomenclature of target theory can be a useful first approximation to the classification of cell–antitumor drug interactions. This approach has two distinct advantages: (a) It does not require *a priori* knowledge of drug effects at the molecular level or interpretation of the biochemical mechanisms leading to enhancement or decline of the cytotoxic effect, and (b) it provides a frame of reference to derive useful quantitative parameters for efficacy comparisons. For the analysis of drug-induced cytotoxicity, targets can be operationally defined as essential macromolecules or critical biosynthetic pathways, and the levels of damage (lethal and sublethal) envisioned as a reflection of the net intracellular concentration of drug molecules over fixed periods of time.

III. METHODOLOGY

Numerous investigators have implemented research programs to determine the effects of drugs on cultured cells (Barranco *et al.*, 1972, 1973a,b; Barranco and Novak, 1974; Bhuyan, 1970; Bhuyan and Fraser, 1974; Brachetti and Whitmore, 1969; Drewinko and Barlogie, 1976a,c; Drewinko and Gottlieb, 1973, 1975; Drewinko *et al.*, 1972, 1976c; Hirshaut *et al.*, 1969; Hryniuk *et al.*, 1969; Karon and Shirakawa, 1969; Kim *et al.*, 1968; Kim and Kim, 1972; Madoc-Jones and Mauro, 1974; Mauro and Madoc-Jones, 1970; Rosenkranz *et al.*, 1968; Thayer *et al.*, 1971; Wheeler *et al.*, 1975; Yataganas *et al.*, 1974). Although the species and histological types of cell origin may vary, the methodology used by most investigators to assess drug-induced cell lethality is basically similar. Techniques described below are those that have been used in our laboratory for the past 10 years.

A. Drugs

Drug solutions are always prepared in growth medium immediately before an experiment and the pH adjusted, if necessary, to 7.2. Water-soluble drugs are first diluted in saline solution. Lipid-soluble drugs (i.e., nitrosourea derivatives) are first diluted in pure ethanol or in 20% ethanol–80% propylene glycol. At the concentrations used, the solvent does not affect the viability of the treated cells.

B. Cell Survival

Stock cultures are harvested, aliquots of 5×10^5 cells are seeded in 60 mm plastic petri dishes, and incubated in fresh medium at 37°C in a 5% CO_2, in air, atmosphere (Fig. 1). After cells reach exponential growth, the medium is decanted and freshly prepared drug solutions in medium are added to the dishes.

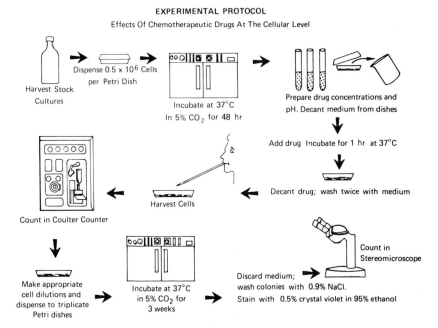

EXPERIMENTAL PROTOCOL
Effects Of Chemotherapeutic Drugs At The Cellular Level

Harvest Stock Cultures

Dispense 0.5 x 10^6 Cells per Petri Dish

Incubate at 37°C In 5% CO_2 for 48 hr

Prepare drug concentrations and pH. Decant medium from dishes

Add drug Incubate for 1 hr at 37°C

Decant drug; wash twice with medium

Harvest Cells

Count in Coulter Counter

Make appropriate cell dilutions and dispense to triplicate Petri dishes

Incubate at 37°C in 5% CO_2 for 3 weeks

Discard medium; wash colonies with 0.9% NaCl. Stain with 0.5% crystal violet in 95% ethanol

Count in Stereomicroscope

Fig. 1. Schema depicting sequential steps in the experimental protocol used to define drug-induced lethal effects at the cellular level. (From Drewinko, 1975.)

Following treatment for 1 hour at 37°C, the drug is decanted, cells are washed, harvested as a single cell suspension, and counted with an electronic particle counter (Coulter Counter Model ZBI, Coulter Electronics, Hialeah, Florida). Known aliquots are dispensed into 60 mm petri dishes so that 50–100 colonies appear after appropriate incubation intervals in a 5% CO_2, humidified atmosphere at 37°C (Fig. 2). The colonies are stained with 2% crystal violet in 95% ethanol and counted with a stereomicroscope. Viability is defined as the ability of single cells to give rise to a colony of $\geq$ 50 cells because it has been shown that when a treated cell undergoes five to six divisions at least one of the progeny elements will retain the capacity for unlimited proliferation (Whitmore and Till, 1964; Thompson and Suit, 1969). In every experiment, three replicate dishes for each dose point are inoculated, and the plating efficiency (PE) of at least six controls is assessed simultaneously. Plating efficiency is defined as the ratio of the number of colonies to the number of inoculated cells. Control cells are exposed to all mechanical manipulations undergone by the treated cells but do not receive drugs. Surviving fractions for each concentration point are calculated in reference to the control cultures by (PE treated cells)/(PE control).

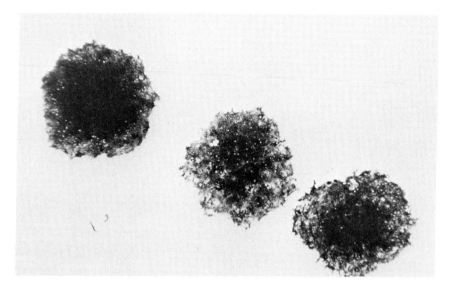

Fig. 2. Colonies obtained from a single cell suspension of human colon carcinoma cells (LoVo cells, Drewinko *et al.*, 1978a) incubated for 21 days.

IV. SURVIVAL PATTERNS

Survival curves of asynchronous exponentially growing cells treated for 1 hr with increasing concentrations of antitumor agents will correspond to one of five patterns (Fig. 3). For many agents the particular patterns will remain fixed, albeit with quantitative modifications depending on the cell type tested. However, for other agents the pattern elicited on a given cell type may not correspond to that observed for cells with different histological origins or obtained from a different species.

A. Type A: Simple Exponential

This survival curve is characterized by a logarithmic decrease in the number of surviving cells as a function of increasing drug concentrations. On a semilogarithmic plot the surviving fraction equals e^{-kD}, where D is the concentration and k is the constant numerical value of the slope. k can be depicted as $1/D_0$, where D_0 is numerically equal to the concentration that will reduce the surviving cells by 63%. In the context of target theory nomenclature, the D_0 represents the sensitivity of the critical cellular target (macromolecules, biosynthetic pathways, etc.) and can be used to compare the magnitude of the

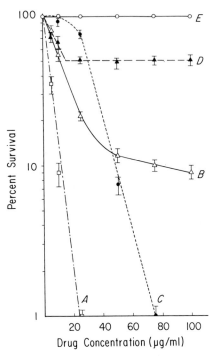

Fig. 3. The five patterns of cell survival curves following treatment with antitumor drugs *in vitro*. (A) Simple exponential. (B) Biphasic exponential. (C) Threshold exponential. (D) Exponential plateau. (E) Ineffectual. Data points depict actual results obtained for human lymphoma cells. (A) *cis*-Diamminedichloroplatinum (II); (B) bleomycin; (C) 1-(2-chloroethyl)-3-cyclohexyl-1-nitrosourea; (D) prednisolone; (E) arabinofuranosylcytosine. Points represent the average of at least two experiments with three replicates per dose point. Bars indicate the standard error. (From Drewinko *et al.*, 1979a.)

cytotoxic effect of different drugs on a given cell population or the sensitivity of different cell types to a single drug. It must be emphasized that the survival response to antitumor drugs depends not only on the concentration of the agent but also on the time interval of exposure (Drewinko, 1975; Drewinko and Gottlieb, 1975; Wheeler *et al.*, 1975). Hence, survival must be expressed not only as a function of dose (C) but also of time (t), or rather the product $C \times t$ (or some mathematical species thereof). This product has been termed the integral dose (Barranco *et al.*, 1975; Drewinko *et al.*, 1976c) or when defined more precisely, the exposure dose (Wheeler *et al.*, 1975). The equation can be approximated when the length of *in vitro* treatment is only 1 hr and, hence, the function is reduced to the numerical value of the concentration (i.e., $D_0 = ? \mu g/ml$, 1 hr). For varying exposure times, i.e., 30 min, 2 hr, 4 hr, etc., the D_0's cannot be compared unless the appropriate formulation for the time component is introduced (Wheeler *et al.*, 1975).

B. Type B: Biphasic Exponential

This curve is also characterized by a logarithmic decrease in survival as the drug concentration increases. However, it consists of two parts: an initially steep slope followed by a much shallower slope. By analogy with the preceding pattern this curve can be adequately described by the D_0 corresponding to each segment of the curve (sometimes achieved only by extrapolation) and by the concentration after which the killing rate changes (inflexion point). This inflexion point (I.P. = ? μg/ml, 1 hr) indicates the concentration which eradicates all of the more sensitive cells from the population. The shape of such curves can be explained by two separate mechanisms: (a) The drug may kill cells in a given stage of the cell cycle with an efficacy severalfold greater (first slope) than that exerted on cells in other stages (second slope); or (b) distinct cell populations, in terms of drug sensitivity, coexist within the seemingly homogeneous cell line and the biphasic curve results from differential killing of these two populations regardless of their position in the cycle. These two different possibilities can be distinguished in experiments that use synchronized cells; the biphasic curve should disappear if mode (a) is in operation.

C. Type C: Threshold Exponential

For certain agents, notably radiomimetic drugs, the survival response is characterized by the so-called threshold or type C curve (Gunter and Kohn, 1956) where at low concentrations no significant decrease of survival is observed, but higher concentrations produce an exponential killing effect. The linear exponential curve defined by the survival at high concentrations does not extrapolate to 1 (or 100% when the ordinate is expressed as percent survival) when the concentration is 0 and thus the curve is composed by a shoulder region and a linear part. In the context of target theory nomenclature, the shoulder reflects the capacity of the targets to absorb damage without expressing a cellular lethal effect or inactivation of an insufficient number of targets. This results from the capacity of cells to accumulate sublethal damage but does not imply cellular capacity to repair such damage (Drewinko *et al.*, 1976c, 1977). The extent of the shoulder can be quantified by extrapolating the linear part of the curve to the abscissa and defining the "quasithreshold" concentration (D_q) (Alper *et al.*, 1960) applying the same time-exposure factor considerations previously discussed for the D_0 (Wheeler *et al.*, 1975). Thus, Type C curves can be compared on the basis of their D_0 (1 hr) and their D_q (1 hr).

D. Type D: Exponential Plateau

This response is common for cell cycle stage-sensitive antitumor agents, usually antimetabolites. These drugs produce an initially exponential decrease in survival. Survival reaches a plateau when all sensitive cells are sterilized and subsequent increments in drug concentration fail to augment the killing effect. These curves can be characterized by the D_0 (1 hr) of the initial part of the curve (usually obtained by extrapolation), the I.P. between the exponential and plateau segments of the curve, and the percent survivors (P_s, 1 hr) attained at plateau. For certain drugs, P_s may be reached at levels above those calculated from proportions of cells in the sensitive stage. This suggests that not all of the cells in a given stage, purportedly sensitive to a given agent, are necessarily candidates for sterilization by this drug.

E. Type E: Ineffectual

No killing effects are elicited during 1 hr treatment even when high drug concentrations are employed. The definition of the experimentally upper limit of "high" drug concentration is by necessity arbitrary. In our studies, it is fixed at 5000 μg/ml (50 times the upper limit of the range 0.1–100 μg/ml at which most drugs express their lethal effects). No quantitative parameter can be used to describe type E survival curves. However, the magnitude of the resistance can be indicated by presenting the largest concentration that fails to elicit *in vitro* cell killing during 1 hr exposure ($C_{max} = ? \mu$l, 1 hr). This type of response is frequently seen for drugs that inhibit DNA synthesis and kill cells by the mechanism of "unbalanced growth" (Kim *et al.*, 1968; Lambert and Studzinsky, 1967). To achieve lethality by this mechanism, inhibition of DNA synthesis must be maintained for a period longer than the generation time (Brachetti and Whitmore, 1969), lest the cells resume their growth, synchronized but capable of unlimited proliferation. For drugs which bind irreversibly to their target enzymes, degrade slowly, and are exposed to cells which have a limited capacity to synthesize new enzymes, continuous DNA inhibition may be achieved even after brief exposure to the drug. If one or more of these conditions are not satisfied, lethality can only be obtained if the cells are continuously incubated with the antitumor agents.

Although the above described survival patterns characterize the lethal effects of most antitumor drugs and provide an operational framework to derive quantifiable parameters for comparing their efficacy, it would be premature to predict that they may have an immediate clinical application. Whether the proposed classification has relevance in the design of chemotherapeutic protocols must await appropriate clinical investigation, and be used in conjunction with other pertinent factors, such as pharmacokinetics and cell population growth kinetics. Yet, on a first approximation, the following guidelines may apply: (a) For type A survival curves, the drugs in the group appear potentially effective in reducing tumor burden singly and independently of scheduling. (b) Drugs in the type B survival curve group mimic, in part, the behavior of type A drugs. Yet, a considerable fraction of cells may be less sensitive to the agent and best results may be expected by utilizing these drugs in combination. (c) For drugs with type C survival responses, low concentrations may yield clinically irrelevant killing effects; superior results may be observed by rapid escalation of the employed dosages. (d) All drugs of the type D survival curve group are usually cell cycle stage sensitive. Hence, judicious scheduling or combination with other agents should provide the best results for these agents. (e) Drugs in group E are marginally effective in a "push" modality, and the best results can be anticipated by administration via continuous intravenous infusion.

V. NONEXPONENTIALLY GROWING CELLS

One of the major drawbacks of tissue culture experiments resides in the difficulty of extrapolating information obtained on exponentially growing cells to the expected responses of tumor cells *in vivo* where large fractions of the population may be in the quiescent state (G_0 cells). This is especially important in the case of solid tumors where the available information suggests a small proportion of proliferating cells (growth fraction) as reflected by the low labeling index values shown by these tumors (Steel and Lamerton, 1969). Recent investigations suggest the usefulness of utilizing stationary phase cultures as an adequate *in vitro* model of neoplasias with low growth fractions (Hahn et al., 1968; Hahn and Little, 1972; Barranco and Novak, 1974). Some investigators have studied the response of such culture systems to the lethal action of antitumor agents and reported considerable differences with respect to that obtained for exponentially growing cultures (Barranco and Novak, 1974; Hahn et al., 1974; Barranco et al., 1975). These differences might be significantly exploited at the clinical level (Twentyman, 1976). Stationary phase cultures are obtained by allowing cells to replicate without refeeding until such time when no net increment in cell numbers is demonstrated (Fig. 4). This can result from either cessation of multiplication (with elongation of cell cycle transit times) or from a balance between cell death and cell multiplication (i.e., the number of cells born per unit time equals the number of cells disintegrating per unit time). Several factors may be responsible for the stationary phase of growth of mammalian cells including cell-to-cell contact inhibition; exhaustion of metabolites and/or increased catabolites in the nutrient medium; and cellular synthesis of a molecular mediator (chalone) that inhibits cell proliferation by negative feedback. Recent studies have shown that stationary phase due to metabolic deprivation can be overcome by refeeding with fresh medium. Cells resume multiplication until they enter a second stage of growth inhibition induced by cell crowding. This situation cannot be reversed by refeeding and can be changed only if cells are subcultured at lower densities (Skehan and Friedman, 1976).

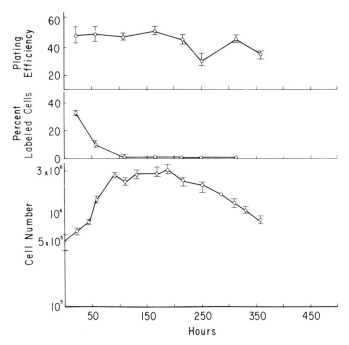

Fig. 4. Growth kinetics parameters of LoVo cells as a function of proliferation status. Upper panel, plating efficiency; middle panel, labeling index; lower panel, cell number. Plating efficiency was measured by the colony formation technique. Labeling index was assessed by autoradiography on cells pulse-labeled with [³H]TdR; cell number was determined with a Coulter counter. Bars represent standard errors. The growth curve enters a plateau just when the labeling index falls to zero, while the plating efficiency remains intact. After 4 days the cultures die as reflected by the declining slope of the cell counts. (From Drewinko *et al.*, 1979b.)

Another technique, recently proposed by Sutherland *et al.* (1971) suggests the use of multicellular spheroids as an alternative, useful *in vitro* model for noncycling cells. Multicellular spheroids are obtained from the continuous replication of cells maintained in suspension cultures (Fig. 5). If cells remain attached to each other after division, the group grows in a three-dimensional fashion. Cells positioned on the surface layers of the spheroids are in close contact with the nutrient medium and proliferate vigorously. The core of the spheroid conducts its gas and metabolite exchange with difficulty and, therefore, its cells either proliferate slowly, become quiescent, or die (Sutherland, 1974; Haji-Karim and Carlsson, 1978). Thus, the kinetic conditions of the spheroid mimic those described for *in vivo* solid tumors where cell proliferation is a function of the distance to vascular channels (Tannock, 1968). Under appropriate conditions, the different layers of the spheroid can be ''peeled'' in successive layers (Suther-

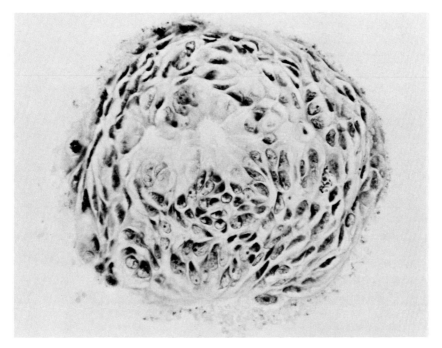

Fig. 5.   Multicellular spheroid obtained from a single cell suspension of colon carcinoma cells (line SW 403) 2 weeks after incubation.

land, 1974). Thus, drug treatment can be carried out on the entire spheroid, but cell survival can be analyzed for each layer, which possesses differential kinetic properties and presumably different survival responses. For cells that do not routinely remain attached, a useful alternative is represented by the soft agar cloning technique independently described by Yuhas *et al.* (1977) and by Haji-Karim and Carlsson (1978).

VI. CELL RECOVERY

One of the most important factors determining cell survival after drug treatment is the capacity of cells to repair drug-induced potentially lethal and sublethal damage. Potentially lethal damage is that which ordinarily causes cell death but may be prevented by posttreatment manipulations. The basic technique usually employed for studying recovery from potentially lethal damage is that described by Little (1971) which consists of maintaining the treated cells in spent medium for various time intervals before harvesting and replating for colony formation. Another method, described by Whitmore and Gulyas (1967), consists of maintaining the posttreated cells at suboptimal temperatures (4° or 22°C) for various time intervals before harvesting for colony formation. In both instances recovery is accomplished by preventing the cells from transiting through the cycle at their normal rate. Conceivably, the mechanisms leading to this type of repair require a long interval to dispose of the damaged "target" which becomes irreversible if cells reach mitosis before repair.

Sublethal damage results from insufficient injury to the structures or biochemical pathways responsible for maintaining integrity of the reproductive capacity. However, accumulation of sublethal damage will result in a lethal outcome. Repair of sublethal damage is usually investigated with the split-dose method described by Elkind and Sutton (1959) for cells treated with ionizing radiations. Cells receive the total dose of the injurious agent in two exposures of one-half the total dose separated in time. If recovery from sublethal damage exists, the time between exposures will be used to effect this repair, and the cells will respond to the second one-half dose as if they had never received previous treatment. Hence, the percent survival will be greater than that resulting from cells exposed to the total dose at one time (Fig. 6). However, repair of the injurious effect of chemotherapeutic agents cannot be determined accurately by the split-dose method used for radiation studies. This is due to the fact that lethal effects of

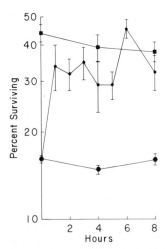

Fig. 6.   Survival of human lymphoma cells after split-dose treatment with *cis*-acid. Upper curve (squares) demonstrates the survival of cells exposed to 50 μg/ml for 15 min at the times indicated by the points. Lower curve (hexagons) indicates the survival of cells exposed to 100 μg/ml for 15 min at the times indicated by the points. The middle curve (circles) represents the survival of cells exposed to 50 μg/ml for 15 min at time 0, washed, reincubated with fresh medium, and exposed to an additional 50 μg/ml of *cis*-acid for 15 min at the times indicated by the points. (From Drewinko, *et al.*, 1977.)

drugs are not promptly dissipated because of the relatively prolonged chemical half-life of drugs inside cells. Yet, by investigating the cumulative effects of fractionated exposure, the clinical situation is imitated and a better understanding of the mechanisms of protracted treatment can be achieved.

VII. CELL CYCLE STAGE-DEPENDENT SURVIVAL

The position in the cell cycle occupied by a cell at the time it is exposed to an antitumor agent is an important determinant for survival. Some agents, notably inhibitors of DNA synthesis, will kill cells only in S phase (cell cycle stage-specific agents), while most antitumor drugs demonstrate significant differences in efficacy as a function of position in the cycle (cell cycle stage-sensitive agents). These cell cycle stage-dependent differences may have significant impact in the development of superior clinical chemotherapeutic regimens. The kinetics of *in vitro* cell killing may indicate dose and time manipulations of clinical scheduling for different combinations of drugs given simultaneously or in sequence. Thus, it may be possible to accumulate a large population of cells in a given stage of the cell cycle and utilize a second drug (or combination of drugs), the main killing effect of which occurs in that specific stage to sterilize the tumor efficiently. On the other hand, agents with widely different activities in distinct stages of the cycle could be combined in a paired delivery in order to attack all of the cells composing the tumor population. Therefore, *in vitro* studies on the modes of action of the various drugs, in conjunction with cytokinetic data, may provide a rational approach to combination therapy which could prove more effective than the largely empirical methods utilized to date. To conduct these sorts of studies, synchronized cells are exposed to the antitumor agents at regular intervals throughout their cell cycle transit (Fig. 7). A synchronized population of cells is that which consists of cells that pass through a specific point of the cell cycle at the same time. However, three considerations should be mentioned with respect to the technical limitations of obtaining synchronized populations that are imposed by currently available methods. (a) Synchronization does not imply the phasing of all cellular processes, but refers to the simultaneous manifestation of some distinct marker such as the synthesis of DNA or the mitotic apparatus. While the cell population may appear completely phased with respect to one biochemical process, other biochemical activities which should normally occur in subsequent stages may have already taken place during the interval required to obtain the synchronous population. (b) No technique provides more than partial synchrony. Although cells in one stage of the cycle may predominate, the population is spread at various points throughout that stage and even in other stages of the cycle. (c) Synchronization is an ephemeral event, since the cells have random rates of transit through the cycle stages; this decay in synchrony prevents clear-cut interpretation of results obtained after the release of the synchrony induction.

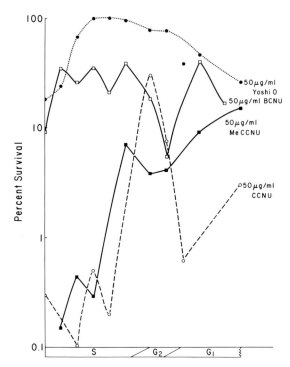

Fig. 7. Survival of human lymphoma cells exposed for 1 hr at 37°C to a single concentration of various alkylating antitumor agents at different periods of the cell cycle. (From Drewinko, 1975.)

In spite of these shortcomings considerable information has been accumulated on the cell cycle stage-dependent effects of a variety of antitumor agents (Bhuyan *et al.*, 1972; Madoc-Jones and Mauro, 1974). This information has been utilized by some clinical oncologists to develop "kinetic" chemotherapeutic regimes which have met with varying, mostly unsatisfactory, degrees of success in terms of improved clinical responses (Klein and Lennartz, 1974; Lampkin *et al.*, 1971; Livingston *et al.*, 1976). Yet, this implementation of the *in vitro* information may have been somewhat premature. A chemotherapeutic strategy based on a cell kinetics rationale requires accurate knowledge of the fraction of proliferating cells and the durations of the phases of the cell cycle, features that probably change during the natural history of disease (Skipper, 1971; Tannock and Frei, 1971; Drewinko and Alexanian, 1977). Such variations may require alterations in the scheduling tactics of drugs in accordance with the fluctuating growth kinetics properties of the neoplastic cells. Most "kinetic" protocols have thus far adhered to rigid schema of drug scheduling and were based on insufficient information on the growth kinetics properties of human tumors. Development of new and better techniques for studying these parameters and acquisition of a vast data bank on human tumor growth dynamics will probably alter this situation in the future. It is then when the full impact of the *in vitro* information on cell cycle stage-dependent drug effects may be finally attained.

VIII. CELL CYCLE PROGRESSION DELAY

At the cellular level, antitumor drugs exert both lethal and cytokinetic effects (Drewinko and Barlogie, 1976c; Barlogie and Drewinko, 1977a). The latter results in a delay or complete block of the normal transit of cells through the cycle which may or may not be reversible. Thus, an agent may temporarily decrease cell proliferation because of (a) actual cell kill, (b) cell cycle progression delay, (c) cell cycle stage block, and (d) more commonly, a combination of the above. While (b) and (c) contribute to the measured decrease in cell proliferation, they do not necessarily imply cell death, as the cells may resume normal growth once the agent is removed. Differential effects on killing and cell progression delay can be investigated by observing the transit of cells through the cell cycle during and after drug treatment; thus, evaluation of the kinetic response of tumor cells to cytostatic agents may provide useful knowledge for the design of chemotherapy protocols (Schabel, 1969; van Putten, 1974). For this purpose, many investigators utilize well-defined markers, such as the presence of mitotic figures and the incorporation of radiolabeled DNA precursors to define the distribution of cells in the mitotic cycle. However, these techniques only provide information on cells contained within two compartments of the cell cycle, S phase and mitosis. A more useful method is the determination of cellular DNA content as a function of cell cycle stage (Vendrely, 1971). The method is based on the analysis of DNA histograms representing the distribution of cells with various discrete DNA contents within a given population, thus allowing the direct measurement of cells in stages other than S phase (Fig. 8). However, because G_1 and G_0 and G_2 and M phase cells share the same DNA content, they cannot be distinguished from each other. The laborious and slow slide-oriented cytophotometric techniques used by early workers for this purpose can now be replaced by high-speed cytophotometry of cells in suspension (Kamentsky *et al.*, 1965; van Dilla *et al.*, 1969). Recently, several investigators (Tobey and Crissman, 1972; Yataganas and Clarkson, 1974; Krishan *et al.*, 1975; Tobey *et al.*, 1975) have used various staining techniques (Tobey and Crissman, 1972; Berkhan, 1975; Krishan *et al.*, 1975) and different flow systems to study drug-induced perturbation effects on cell cycle progression.

In our laboratory, drug-induced cell cycle progression delay is investigated by sequential DNA histograms obtained by flow cytometry (FCM) utilizing a Phywe ICP-11 pulse cytophotometer. Our technique provides rapid (< 20 min) and precise (coefficient of variation < 2%) determination of cell distribution in

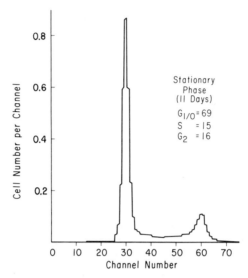

Fig. 8. DNA content histogram of human colon carcinoma cells stained with mithramycin–ethidium bromide and measured in a Phywe ICP 11 pulse cytophotometer; peak centered on channel 30 represents cells in G_1 and G_0; peak centered on channel G_0 represents G_2 + M cells. (From Drewinko *et al.*, 1978a.)

the various stages of the cell cycle (Barlogie *et al.*, 1976a,b; Drewinko *et al.*, 1978a); thus, we are capable of accurately monitoring the cell cycle transit of cells during and after the influence of antitumor drugs (Barlogie *et al.*, 1976c,d; Drewinko and Barlogie, 1976a,b,c; Barlogie and Drewinko, 1977b). In our studies, we have documented that all antitumor drugs induce a major delay in G_2 phase, the degree and reversibility of which depends on the concentration and length of incubation and on the particular drug studied. Each drug effects this block regardless of the stage of the cell cycle in which the cells are treated, even when exposed for brief periods. However, the stage of the cycle most sensitive to this effect varies for each drug. We also noted that, with the exception of adriamycin, there was no correlation between the magnitude and duration of the G_2 block and the degree of cytotoxicity and have concluded that cell killing and progression delay are the result of independent mechanisms (Barlogie *et al.*, 1976d; Drewinko and Barlogie, 1976c). While most agents induce the G_2 block during the life span of the treated cells, alkylating drugs exert this effect during the life span of the immediate progeny of the treated cells (Barlogie and Drewinko, 1978) (Figs. 9 and 10). Continuous implementation of such a program of investigation on drug-induced cell progression delay may uncover synchronizing agents useful in the management of cancer during certain phases of the disease, when a large fraction of neoplastic cells are proliferating. Although most of these agents also induce a considerable degree of irreversible G_2 block with subsequent

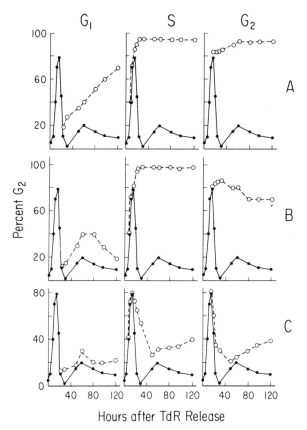

Fig. 9. Sequential fluctuations in the size of the G_2 compartment of human lymphoma cells treated in G_1, S, and G_2 phase for 1 hr at 37°C with anthracycline derivatives. (A) Adriamycin (0.5 μg/ml). (B) Adriamycin–DNA complex (0.5 μg/ml). (C) Rubidazone (1.0 μg/ml). Closed circles represent control cells. Open circles depict treated cells. (From Barlogie and Drewinko, 1978.)

cell death, cells able to escape this block will emerge partially synchronized. A fraction of these cells (or their progeny) will subsequently die from the inherited damage, but those cells which escape the G_2 block with intact reproductive capacities will be amenable to complete sterilization by the scheduling of a second phase-sensitive drug at full cytocidal dose employed after the adequate time interval.

For the clinical oncologist, FCM offers the possibility of rapidly monitoring kinetic effects of anticancer agents in patients with accessible tumor sites. This may allow for individual timing of combination chemotherapy schedules, according to the individual patient's tumor growth characteristics before and after drug perturbation. Thus, kinetic concepts can be used that utilize cell synchronization

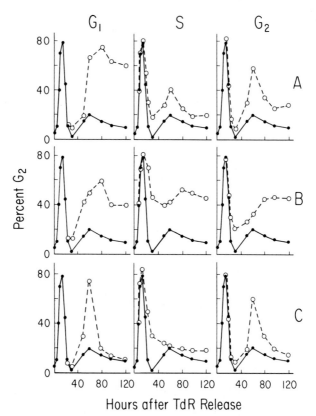

Fig. 10. Sequential fluctuations in the size of G_2 compartment of human lymphoma cells treated in G_1, S, and G_2 phase for 1 hr at 37°C with alkylating agents. (A) L-Phenylalanine mustard. (B) Peptichemio. (C) Yoshi compound 864. Closed circles represent control cells. Open circles depict treated cells. (From Barlogie and Drewinko, 1978.)

and/or recruitment of resting cells into the proliferative cycle, thereby increasing the therapeutic efficacy of antineoplastic treatment.

IX. COMBINATION CHEMOTHERAPY *IN VITRO*

The success of combination chemotherapy has been repeatedly proved in a variety of human malignancies (Henderson and Samaha, 1969; Alexanian *et al.*, 1972; Frei, 1972). Oncologists are presently searching for new and more effective combinations to control the growth of every neoplasm. Yet, the search for such effective drug combinations has been mostly empirical, although rational bases have been proposed to facilitate rapid and economic developments in this field (Sartorelli, 1969; Skipper *et al.,* 1970; DeVita and Schein, 1973; Goldin, 1973; Bono, 1974). Effective combinations, in terms of therapeutic gain, can emerge from three possible circumstances: (a) adequate manipulation of growth kinetics properties; (b) selective use of drugs that elicit less than additive toxic effects while providing at least additive therapeutic effects, and (c) biological synergism. A fourth category exists in which miscellaneous pharmacological properties are exploited, such as the "rescue" effect elicited by citrovorum factor after methotrexate (MTX) therapy (Bertino *et al.,* 1971) or the enhancement of efficacy of certain chemotherapeutic drugs by other agents not effective by themselves (Elion *et al.,* 1963; Neil *et al.,* 1970; Cohen and Carbone, 1972). The rationale of using growth kinetics parameters to obtain a therapeutic gain is based on (a) the simultaneous or sequential treatment with drugs that exert maximum lethal effects in different stages of the cell cycle or (b) the pairing of drugs, one of which blocks the progression of cells through the cycle eliciting at least partial synchronization of cells in one stage of the cycle with subsequent treatment with a second drug which exerts its maximum lethal effect in that stage. The practical application of this approach to human oncology is restricted by the fact that it requires precise knowledge of cell cycle parameters, a knowledge which presently is not available for most human tumors. Selective use of drugs with different toxicities has been the most frequently used clinical method in the design of multiple drug combinations entailing, by necessity, human experimentation. However, animal model systems can be used as effective screening systems to predict potentiation of toxic effects (Skipper, 1974). Unfortunately, in most clinical situations subadditive effects are elicited by drug combinations. The third approach, namely, the search for biologic synergism, is perhaps the most satisfying one for basic researchers. It pairs drugs having different modes of activity in combinations which enhance their mutual effects at the cellular level, and such investigations can be efficiently and economically carried out *in vitro* (Bono, 1974; Grunwald *et al.,* 1978). Biologic synergism of drug effects may occur through one of three possible mechanisms (Sartorelli, 1969): (a) sequential inhibition upon different enzymes in a limited portion of a multienzyme sequence, (b) concurrent inhibition on alternate metabolic pathways available for the synthesis of an essential metabolite, and (c) complementary inhibition whereby drugs that cause damage to macromolecules are combined with drugs that inhibit the formation of precursor molecules necessary for the repair of such damage. Therefore, the selection of drug pairs for combination chemotherapy studies requires precise knowledge of the lethal mode of action of each drug. However, this information is not available for most drugs, and various possible models of cell killing are proposed. Even in cases such as MTX where the main molecular effect of a drug is known, it is not clear whether this effect is lethal (Borsa, 1971). Furthermore, clinically effective synergistic pairs, such as vincristine and prednisolone and melphalan and prednisolone (Alexanian *et al.,*

1972), and synergistic pairs noted in experimental animal systems, such as cyclophosphamide and *cis*-platinum, and MeCCNU and CCNU, (Goldin, 1973), have emerged which are not discovered on the basis of the above limited rationale.

It is difficult to visualize and interpret the interaction at the cellular level of a pair of drugs which do not potentiate each other by any of the above-mentioned mechanisms. Utilizing the colony-forming method, apparent, but not necessarily true, subadditive or antagonistic effects may be elicited. In fact, due to random interaction of drugs with cells, such subadditive or antagonistic results should be the rule rather than the exception. Additive results would indicate some inter-dependence of both drugs, while synergistic results would suggest biologic potentiation. Consider the possible situations depicted in Fig. 11, intended to demonstrate the various ways in which two drugs may interact with cells. Drugs A and B, when used alone, kill a given fraction of cells, while a smaller fraction of cells may be damaged sublethally. Cells will die when sufficient damaging events are accumulated. Combination treatment (C) may produce "overkill" by interacting at random with cells already lethally damaged by either drug A or B.

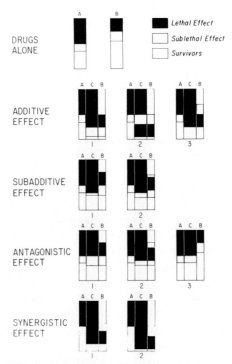

Fig. 11. Schema depicting possible results of the interaction of two antitumor agents at the cellular level. (From Drewinko *et al.*, 1976a.)

True additive effects, defined as the summation of the killing of each drug alone will result if drug B is able to bypass cells lethally damaged by drug A and (1) affects only viable cells and/or cells sublethally damaged by drug A, (2) affects only viable cells and sublethal damage is not additive, or (3) both A and B affect viable cells and cells sublethally damaged by the other drug.

Subadditive effects will be noted by (1) quantitative modifications of the former model or (2) "overkill" by drug B on cells already damaged by drug A and partial accumulation of sublethal damage induced independently by both drugs. This latter situation, although not strictly a biochemical synergism, may be considered a biological potentiation. Yet, cell survival experiments will fail to denote such a synergistic effect.

Apparent, but not true, antagonistic effects may result from (1) drugs A and B affect cells already damaged by each other and the sublethal damage induced independently by each drug is not cumulative enough to render cells nonviable. (2) Both drugs affect most cells damaged by each other, sublethal damage is not cumulative, and only a small fraction of viable cells is additionally affected. In this situation, it is only a matter of quantitative results in deciding whether the observed response is antagonistic or subadditive. (3) Lethal and sublethal damage effected by drug B occurs only on cells already lethally damaged by drug A.

Synergistic effects will be noted only when the sublethal damage induced by both drugs operates additively, quantitative differences observed for situations depicted by models 1 and 2 in Fig. 11.

Only true synergistic effects, with killing greater than that predicted from an additive effect, or true antagonistic effects, with killing less than that expected from that of any drug alone, can be readily recognized from survival data. Any degree of killing between that resulting from the most efficient drug in the pair and that equal to a predicted additive effect, may mask biological antagonistic or synergistic effects. For these reasons in our studies we arbitrarily define true synergistic effects as those quantitatively greater by more than threefold from the predicted additive effect. Deviations from additive effects smaller than threefold are called supra- or subadditive; true antagonistic effects are defined by cellular killing less than that obtained by the most powerful drug of the pair alone.

Even though it is impossible to study every possible pair combination (Lloyd, 1974), during the past several years we have investigated the combined effects of many drugs in an attempt to detect additive and synergistic pairs. A drug is paired with other chemotherapeutic agents in order to observe whether the first drug can increase the killing effect of the second agent. Significant deviations from the additive response and their magnitude are defined as follows: For each dose point of the drug tested in combination, an additive response (percent of expected survival) is defined by the geometric sum of the survival resulting from treatment with each drug alone. An additive response for the tested drug is defined by a score obtained from the arithmetic sum of the results at each dose point. The variance of this score is determined by the technique of propagation of error (Kendall and Stuart, 1963). Deviations from the additive effect are considered significant when they exceeded $1.96 \times (\text{variance})^{\frac{1}{2}}$ (Remington and Schork, 1970). The overall significance of the deviation is accepted when the results are recomputed after eliminating the dose point with the greatest deviation. This procedure is instituted to avoid bias in the overall estimation introduced by a single dose point. In order to quantify deviations from additive effects, we devised a performance index. This performance index is obtained by averaging the sum of ratios of observed and expected survivals for each data point. To

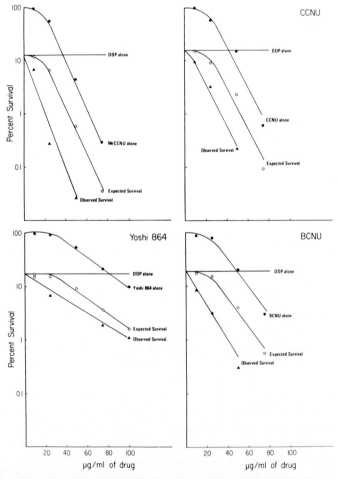

Fig. 12. Survival curves demonstrating synergistic killing effects of *cis-* diaminedichlroplatinum (DDP) (10 μg/ml) used in simultaneous pair combination treatment with increasing concentrations of alkylating agents and nitrosourea derivatives. (From Drewinko *et al.,* 1976b.)

calculate the ratios of synergistic drugs, the expected response is used as the numerator. The observed response is used as the denominator in antagonistic situations. This is done in order to obtain values greater than 1 so that the efficiency of antagonistic and synergistic drugs can be compared.

Our studies have disclosed several unsuspected synergistic drug pairs for potential clinical application (Drewinko *et al.*, 1976a,b, 1978b) and have also opened new important avenues of research. For instance a combination which is biologically synergistic may be considered a new "drug," with properties that may differ from those of each of its components. Hence, for any such combination discovered, cell cycle stage-sensitivity studies should be carried out to observe whether (a) the potentiation effect results from a simple additive effect of the killing by individual agents at the same stages of the cycle where they were shown effective when administered in single fashion, (b) one agent potentiates the stage-sensitivity effect of the other drug, or (c) the pair has acquired new cell age-dependent characteristics with a stage-sensitivity pattern not previously shown by each member of the pair. Additionally, we documented the fact that the major effect of *cis*-diaminedichloroplatinum in combination with agents that display a type C response pattern was to reduce or totally obliterate the shoulder region of the survival curve (Fig. 12) (Drewinko *et al.*, 1976b). Thus, this drug may represent a unique agent to investigate the mechanisms that permit cells to absorb drug-induced damage without expressing a lethal effect.

X. DISCUSSION

Tissue culture experimentation constitutes a fundamental stage in the orderly development of an antitumor agent for clinical application. This experimental system permits adequate and multiphasic investigation of the biological properties of many antitumor drugs within reasonable time spans and acceptable economic limits. Some of the inherent problems of this sort of investigation, namely, the inadequacy of exponentially growing cells to reflect the entire *in vivo* tumor mass, are being actively addressed with the development of stationary phase and multicellular spheroid cultures. Although a given cell line may not be representative of all human tumors (not even of a specific tissue type), further establishment of new lines will provide panels of cell types that may adequately cover a sufficient range of behavioral responses for predicting clinical results in most patients. Thus, the future role of tissue culture will be increasingly expanded until its full impact in antitumor agent development is finally achieved.

ACKNOWLEDGMENT

This work was supported by Grants CA-14528, CA-16763, and CA-23272 and by Contract CM-43801 from the National Cancer Institute, United States Department of Health, Education and Welfare.

REFERENCES

Alexanian, R., Bonnet, J., Gehan, E., Haut, A., Hewlett, J., Lane, M., Monto, R., and Wilson, H. (1972). *Cancer* **30**, 382–389.

Alper, T., Gillies, N. E., and Elkind, M. M. (1960). *Nature (London)* **186**, 1062–1063.

Atwood, K. C., and Norman, A. (1949). *Proc. Natl. Acad. Sci. U.S.A.* **35**, 696–709.

Barendsen, G. W., Beusker, T. L. J., Vergroesen, A. J., and Budke, L. (1960). *Radiat. Res.* **13**, 841–849.

Barlogie, B., and Drewinko, B. (1977a). *In* "Growth Kinetics and Biochemical Regulation of Normal and Malignant Cells" (B. Drewinko and R. M. Humphrey, eds.), pp. 315–328. Williams & Wilkins, Baltimore, Maryland.

Barlogie, B., and Drewinko, B. (1977b). *Cancer Treat. Rep.* **61**, 425–436.

Barlogie, B., and Drewinko, B. (1978). *Eur. J. Cancer* **14**, 741–745.

Barlogie, B., Drewinko, B., Büchner, T., Göhde, W., Schumann, J., Hauss, W. H., and Freireich, E. J. (1976a). *Cancer Res.* **36**, 1176–1181.

Barlogie, B., Drewinko, B., Schumann, J., Büchner, T., Göhde, W., Hart, J. S., and Johnston, D. A. (1976b). *In* "Pulse Cytophotometry" (W. Göhde, J. Schumann, and T. Büchner, eds.), pp. 125–136. European Press, Ghent, Belgium.

Barlogie, B., Drewinko, B., Schumann, J., and Freireich, E. J. (1976c). *Cancer Res.* **36**, 1182–1187.

Barlogie, B., Drewinko, B., Johnston, D. A., and Freireich, E. J. (1976d). *Cancer Res.* **36**, 1975–1979.

Barranco, S. C., and Novak, J. K. (1974). *Cancer Res.* **34**, 1616–1618.

Barranco, S. C., Ho, D. H., Drewinko, B., Romsdahl, M. M., and Humphrey, R. M. (1972). *Cancer Res.* **32**, 2733–2736.

Barranco, S. C., Romsdahl, M. M., Drewinko, B., and Humphrey, R. M. (1973a). *Mutat. Res.* **19**, 277–280.

Barranco, S. C., Gerner, E. W., Burk, K. H., and Humphrey, R. M. (1973). *Cancer Res.* **33**, 11–16.

Barranco, S. C., Novak, J. K., and Humphrey, R. M. (1975). *Cancer Res.* **35**, 1194.

Berkhan, E. (1975). *In* "Impulscytophotometrie" (M. Andreeff, ed.), pp. 11–13. Springer-Verlag, Berlin and New York.

Bertino, J. R., Levitt, M., McCullough, J. L., and Chabner, B. (1971). *Ann. N.Y. Acad. Sci.* **186**, 486–495.

Bhuyan, B. K. (1970). *Cancer Res.* **30**, 2017–2023.

Bhuyan, B. K., and Fraser, T. J. (1974). *Cancer Res.* **34**, 778–782.

Bhuyan, B. K., Scheidt, L. G., and Fraser, T. J. (1972). *Cancer Res.* **32**, 398–407.

Bhuyan, B. K., Loughman, B. E., Fraser, T. J., and Day, K. J. (1976). *Exp. Cell Res.* **97**, 275–280.

Bono, V. H. (1974). *Cancer Chemother. Rep., Part 2* **4**, 131–136.

Borsa, J. (1971). *Ann. N.Y. Acad. Sci.* **186**, 359–362.

Brachetti, S., and Whitmore, G. F. (1969). *Cell Tissue Kinet.* **2**, 193–211.

Cohen, M. H., and Carbone, P. P. (1972). *J. Natl. Cancer Inst.* **48**, 921–926.

Corbett, T. H., Griswald, D. P., Roberts, B. J., Peckham, J. C., and Schabel, F. M. (1976). *Cancer* **40**, 2660–2680.

Dawson, M. (1972). "Cellular Pharmacology." Thomas, Springfield, Illinois.

DeVita, V. T., and Schein, P. S. (1973). *N. Engl. J. Med.* **288**, 998–1006.

Dosik, G. M., Barlogie, B., Johnston, D. A., Murphrey, W. K., and Drewinko, B. (1978). *Cancer Res.* **38**, 3304–3309.

Drewinko, B. (1975). *In* "Cancer Chemotherapy. Fundamental Concepts and Recent Advances," p. 63. Yearbook Publ., Chicago, Illinois.

Drewinko, B., and Alexanian, R. (1977). *J. Natl. Cancer Inst.* **58**, 1247–1253.

Drewinko, B., and Barlogie, B. (1976a). *Cancer Treat. Rep.* **60**, 1295–1306.

Drewinko, B., and Barlogie, B. (1976b). *Cancer Treat. Rep.* **60**, 1637–1645.

Drewinko, B., and Barlogie, B. (1976c). *Cancer Chemother. Rep.* **60**, 1707–1717.

Drewinko, B., and Gottlieb, J. A. (1973). *Cancer Res.* **33**, 1141–1145.

Drewinko, B., and Gottlieb, J. A. (1975). *Cancer Chemother. Rep.* **59**, 665–673.

Drewinko, B., Ho, D. H., and Barranco, S. C. (1972). *Cancer Res.* **32**, 2737–2742.

Drewinko, B., Freireich, E. J., and Gottlieb, J. A. (1974). *Cancer Res.* **34**, 747–750.

Drewinko, B., Loo, T. L., Brown, B., Gottlieb, J. A., and Freireich, E. J. (1976a). *Cancer Biochem. Biophys.* **1**, 187.

Drewinko, B., Green, C., and Loo, T. L. (1976b). *Cancer Treat. Rep.* **60**, 1619–1625.

Drewinko, B., Loo, T. L., and Gottlieb, J. A. (1976c). *Cancer Res.* **36**, 511–515.

Drewinko, B., Green, C., and Loo, T. L. (1977). *Cancer Treat. Rep.* **61**, 1513–1518.

Drewinko, B., Yang, L. Y., Barlogie, B., Romsdahl, M. M., Meistrich, M., Malahy, M. A., and Giovanella, B. (1978a). *J. Natl. Cancer Inst.* **61**, 75–84.

Drewinko, B., Loo, T. L., and Freireich, E. J. (1978b). *Cancer Treat. Rep.* **63**, 373–375.

Drewinko, B., Roper, P. R., and Barlogie, B. (1979a). *Eur J. Cancer* **15**, 93–99.

Drewinko, B., Barlogie, B., and Freireich, E. J. (1979b). *Cancer Res.* **39**, 2630–2636.

Ehmann, U. K., and Wheeler, K. T. (1978). *Proc. Am. Assoc. Cancer Res.* **19**, 18.

Elion, G. B., Callahan, S., Nathan, H., Bieber, S., Rumdles, R. W., and Hitchings, G. H. (1963). *Biochem. Pharmacol.* **12**, 85–93.

Elkind, M. M., and Sutton, H. (1959). *Nature (London)* **184**, 1293–1295.

Fowler, J. F. (1966). *Curr. Top. Radiat. Res.* **2**, 303–364.

Frei, E. (1972). *Cancer Res.* **32**, 2593–2607.

Goldin, A. (1973). *Cancer Chemother. Rep., Part 3* **4**, 189–198.

Grunwald, H. W., Rosner, F., and Hirshaut, Y. (1978). *Am. J. Hematol.* **4**, 35.

Gunter, S. E., and Kohn, H. I. (1956). *J. Bacteriol.* **72**, 422–428.

Hahn, G. M., and Little, J. B. (1972). *Curr. Top. Radiat. Res.* **8**, 39–83.

Hahn, G. M., Stewart, J. R., Yang, S. J., and Parker, V. (1968). *Exp. Cell Res.* **49**, 285–292.

Hahn, G. M., Gordon, L. F., and Kurkjian, S. D. (1974). *Cancer Res.* **34**, 2373–2377.

Haji-Karim, M., and Carlsson, J. (1978). *Cancer Res.* **38**, 1457–1464.

Henderson, E. H., and Samaha, R. J. (1969). *Cancer Res.* **29**, 2272–2280.

Hirshaut, Y., Weiss, G. H., and Perry, S. (1969). *Cancer Res.* **29**, 1732–1740.

Hryniuk, W. M., Fischer, G. A., and Bertino, J. R. (1969). *Mol. Pharmacol.* **5**, 557–564.

Johnson, R. K., Inouye, T., Goldin, A., and Stark, G. R. (1976). *Cancer Res.* **36**, 2720–2725.

Kamentsky, L. A., Melamed, M. R., and Derman, H. (1965). *Science* **150**, 630–631.

Kaneko, T., and LePage, G. A. (1978). *Cancer Res.* **38**, 2084–2090.

Karon, M., and Shirakawa, S. (1969). *Cancer Res.* **29**, 687–696.

Kendall, M. G., and Stuart, A. (1963). "The Advanced Theory of Statistics," Vol. 1, Sect. 10.6; Vol. 2, Chapters 17 and 18. Hafner, New York.

Kim, J. H., Perez, A. G., and Djordjevic, B. (1968). *Cancer Res.* **28**, 2443–2447.

Kim, S. H., and Kim, J. H. (1972). *Cancer Res.* **32**, 323–325.

Klein, H. O., and Lennartz, K. J. (1974). *Semin. Hematol.* **11**, 203–227.

Krishan, A., Paika, K., and Frei, E. (1975). *J. Cell Biol.* **66**, 521–530.

Lambert, W. C., and Studzinsky, G. (1967). *Cancer Res.* **27**, 2364–2369.

Lampkin, B. C., Nagao, T., and Mauer, A. M. (1971). *J. Clin. Invest.* **50**, 2204–2214.

Lea, D. E. (1955). "Action of Radiation of Living Cells." Cambridge Univ. Press, London and New York.

Little, J. B. (1971). *Int. J. Radiat. Biol.* **20**, 87–92.

Livingston, R. B., Fels, W. H., Einhorn, L. H., Burgess, M. A., Freireich, E. J., Gottlieb, J. A., and Farber, M. O. (1976). *Cancer* **37**, 1237–1242.

Lloyd, H. H. (1974). *Cancer Chemother. Rep., Part 2* **4**, 157–165.

Luria, S. E., and Dulbecco, R. (1949). *Genetics* **34**, 93–125.

Madoc-Jones, H., and Mauro, F. (1970). *J. Natl. Cancer Inst.* **45**, 1131–1143.

Madoc-Jones, H., and Mauro, F. (1974). *In* "Handbook of Experimental Pharmacology. Antineoplastic and Immunosuppressive Agents" (A. C. Sartorelli and D. G. Johns, eds.) Part 1, pp. 629–691. Springer-Verlag, Berlin and New York.

Mauro, F., and Madoc-Jones, H. (1970). *Cancer Res.* **30**, 1397–1408.

Neil, G. L., Moxley, T. E., and Manak, R. C. (1970). *Cancer Res.* **30**, 2166–2172.

Peel, S., and Cowen, D. M. (1972). *Br. J. Cancer* **26**, 304–314.

Puck, T. T., and Marcus, P. I. (1955). *Proc. Natl. Acad. Sci. U.S.A.* **41**, 432–437.

Remington, R. D., and Schork, M. A. (1970). "Statistics With Applications to the Biological and Health Sciences." Prentice-Hall, Englewood Cliffs, New Jersey.

Roper, P., and Drewinko, B. (1976). *Cancer Res.* **36**, 2182–2188.

Rosenblum, M. L., Wheeler, K. T., Wilson, C. B., Barker, M., and Kuebel, K. D. (1975). *Cancer Res.* **35**, 1387–1391.

Rosenkranz, H. S., Jacobs, S. H., and Carr, H. J. (1968). *Biochim. Biophys. Acta* **161**, 428–441.

Sartorelli, A. C. (1969). *Cancer Res.* **29**, 2292–2299.

Schabel, F. M. (1969). *Cancer Res.* **29**, 2384–2389.

Schepartz, S. A. (1971). *Cancer Chemother. Rep.* **3**, 3–8.

Skehan, P., and Friedman, S. J. (1976). *Exp. Cell Res.* **101**, 315–322.

Skipper, H. E. (1971). *Cancer* **28**, 1479–1499.

Skipper, H. E. (1974). *Cancer Chemother. Rep., Part 2* **4**, 137–145.

Skipper, H. E., Schabel, F. M., and Wilcox, W. S. (1964). *Cancer Chemother. Rep.* **35**, 1–111.

Skipper, H. E., Schabel, F. M., and Wilcox, W. S. (1965). *Cancer Chemother. Rep.* **45**, 5–28.

Skipper, H. E., Schabel, F. M., Mellet, L. B., Montgomery, J. A., Wilkoff, L. J., Lloyd, H. H., and Brockman, R. W. (1970). *Cancer Chemother. Rep.* **54**, 431–450.

Steel, G. G., and Lamerton, L. F. (1969). *Natl. Cancer Inst., Monogr.* **30**, 29–50.

Sutherland, R. M. (1974). *Cancer Res.* **34**, 3501–3503.

Sutherland, R. M., McCredie, J. A., and Inch, W. R. (1971). *J. Natl. Cancer Inst.* **46**, 113–117.

Tannock, I. F. (1968). *Br. J. Cancer* **22**, 258–273.

Tannock, I. F., and Frei, E. (1971). *Natl. Cancer Inst., Monogr.* **34**, 19–24.

Thayer, P. S., Himmelfarb, P., and Watts, G. L. (1971). *Cancer Chemother. Rep.* **2**, 1–25.

Thompson, L. H., and Suit, H. D. (1969). *Int. J. Radiat. Biol.* **13**, 391–397.

Tobey, R. A., and Crissman, H. A. (1972). *Cancer Res.* **32**, 2726–2732.

Tobey, R. A., Oka, M. S., and Crissman, H. A. (1975). *Eur. J. Cancer* **11**, 433–441.

Twentyman, P. R. (1976). *Cancer Treat. Rep.* **60**, 1719–1722.

van Dilla, M. A., Trujillo, T. T., Mullaney, P. F., and Coulter, J. R. (1969). *Science* **163**, 1213–1214.

van Putten, L. M. (1974). *Cell Tissue Kinet.* **7**, 493–504.

Vendrely, C. (1971). *In* "The Cell Cycle and Cancer" (R. Baserga, ed.), pp. 227–268. Dekker, New York.

Wheeler, K. T., Tel, N., Williams, M. R., Sheppard, S., Levin, V. A., and Kabra, P. M. (1975). *Cancer Res.* **35**, 1464–1469.

Whitmore, G. F., and Gulyas, S. (1967). *Natl. Cancer Inst., Monogr.* **24**, 141–156.

Whitmore, G. F., and Till, J. E. (1964). *Annu. Rev. Nucl. Sci.* **14**, 347–374.

World Health Organization (1966). *W.H.O., Tech. Rep. Ser.* **341.**

Yataganas, X., and Clarkson, B. D. (1974). *J. Histochem. Cytochem.* **22**, 651–659.

Yataganas, X., Strife, A., Perez, A., and Clarkson, B. D. (1974). *Cancer Res.* **34**, 2795–2806.

Yuhas, J. M., Li, A. P., Martinez, A. O., and Ladman, A. J. (1977). *Cancer Res.* **37**, 3639–3643.

Zimmer, K. G. (1961). "Studies on Quantitative Radiation Biology." Hafner, New York.

Zubrod, C. G. (1977). *Proc. 1977 Workshop Natl. Large Bowel Cancer Proj., 1977* p. 103.

5

CELL CYCLE: DRUG EFFECTS AND CLINICAL APPLICATIONS

S. C. Barranco

I. INTRODUCTION

Most solid tumors are composed of populations of dividing and nondividing cells (Mendelsohn, 1962). At least part of the tumor's response to chemotherapy will depend upon the differential sensitivities expressed by the cells in these two populations.

The cell cycle was described originally by Howard and Pelc (1953), and is composed of four major compartments, including mitosis (M), a pre-DNA synthesis phase (G_1), the DNA synthesis phase (S), and a post-DNA synthesis phase (G_2). Cells in an exponential growth state have rather fixed time parameters for each of these phases (Fig. 1) and are most sensitive to anticancer drugs. Under a variety of conditions cell populations may cease dividing or divide very slowly and conceptually can be described as having entered either an extended G_1 or G_2 period, or comprise a compartment of noncycling cells (G_0) which may reenter the cycle on demand (Fig. 1). The portion of tumor cells in the cell cycle is described as being in the growth fraction (Mendelsohn, 1962), i.e., when all of the tumor cells are dividing, the growth fraction is 100%; and for example, when 20% of the cells are in G_0, the growth fraction is only 80%.

The G_0 cells are usually less sensitive to anticancer drug therapy because many of the chemotherapeutic agents are antimetabolites which interfere with specific

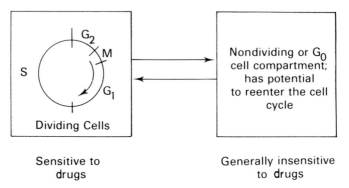

Fig. 1. An idealized view of the mammalian cell cycle showing the G_0 or nondividing cell compartment.

biochemical events occurring only during the cell cycle (such as DNA synthesis). It has also been shown in animal tumor models that the size of the G_0 population increases as the tumor becomes larger and as the distance between cells and capillaries increases (Tannock, 1968). This is generally taken to mean that less oxygen and nutrients can diffuse to these G_0 cells; therefore, anticancer drugs may have difficulty in reaching these G_0 areas within the tumor, and this would also result in reduced cytotoxicity.

In addition to the differential sensitivity expressed by dividing and nondividing cells in the tumor, the effects of a drug may be modulated by a large number of other factors such as those shown in Fig. 2: (1) membrane permeability, (2) the modification of the chemical to active or inactive form, (3) the transport of the chemical to an active site, (4) the interaction of the chemical with primary target molecules, (5) the subsequent molecular response, and (6) the ability of the cell to repair molecular damage and recover the capacity to divide. The effects of some of these factors can be demonstrated and are dealt with in other chapters of this series; however, many have not been dealt with at this time and, therefore, constitute a fertile ground for continued research. From the model, we further suggest that these factors, which have a direct or indirect influence on the cell's response, are controlled both qualitatively and quantitatively by the specific biochemical events being carried out in the cell at that time. This view of cell cycle modulated response to any agent would then lead to the inevitable conclusion that, in order to understand the mechanism of action of a perturbing agent, we will have to know a great deal more about specific events occurring during the cell cycle and their subsequent influence on the modifying factors shown here.

The purpose of this chapter will be to describe the effects of some anticancer drugs on cell survival and kinetics, and to suggest the clinical relevance of the data.

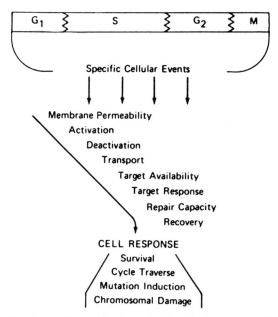

Fig. 2.   A general model for the modulation of cell response to drugs.

II. DRUG EFFECTS ON DIVIDING AND NONDIVIDING CELLS

Puck and Marcus (1956) developed the now classical quantitative colony formation method for determining the effect of radiation on single mammalian cells *in vitro*. The criterion of survival is based on the ability of a cell to divide at least five to six times when plated into an appropriate growth medium. The method (Fig. 3) is straightforward, and is adaptable to most mammalian cell lines and yields precise data on the killing efficiency of radiation and chemicals.

By using this colony formation assay *in vitro* it is possible to determine the drug effects on dividing and nondividing cells. Dividing cells were treated when they were in exponential growth. Nondividing or plateau phase cell cultures were produced *in vitro* by plating cells that were initially in exponential growth into medium and allowing them to progress into a plateau stage without refeeding the cultures. By starving these cultures a nondividing state, similar to G_0 *in vivo,* is produced, and treatment with drugs at this time allows the determination of cytotoxic effects of drugs on nondividing cell populations (Barranco *et al.,* 1973a).

The survival responses of dividing and nondividing cells following treatment with hydroxyurea (HU) are shown in Fig. 4. In exponential cells, survival decreases gradually at doses through 760 μg/ml for 1 hr. The survival fraction then

PLATING TECHNIQUE

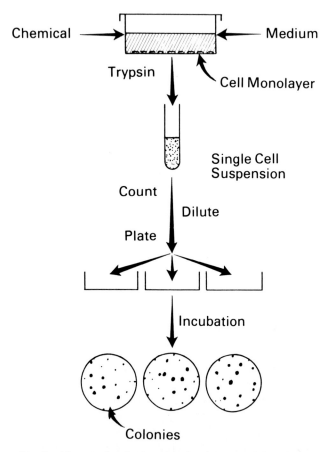

Fig. 3. The procedure for the colony forming assay of drug damage.

plateaus at 0.40, with no additional killing at doses as high as 7600 μg/ml. Since HU has been shown to be a drug which specifically kills cells during the DNA synthesis phase (Sinclair, 1967), and since approximately 60% of the exponentially growing CHO cells are in S phase (under the growth conditions of our laboratory), these data suggest that all S phase cells were killed. No plateau phase cells were killed by any of the doses used, since these cells were not in the cell cycle (Barranco and Novak, 1974). The data in Fig. 4 suggest, therefore, that drugs such as HU or cytosine arabinoside (another drug which kills cells best in S phase, Barranco and Novak, 1974) would not be effective agents to use in tumors whose growth fractions are small.

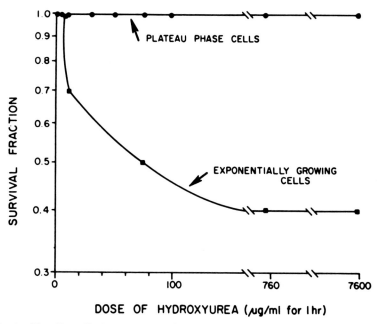

Fig. 4. The effect of hydroxyurea at varying concentrations on survival of dividing or nondividing CHO cells. (From Barranco and Novak, 1974.)

The effects of Bleomycin (Bleo) on survival are shown in Fig. 5. Bleo has been shown to inhibit DNA synthesis (Kunimoto, *et al.,* 1967) and to cause DNA strand scission (Susuki *et al.,* 1969). The survival responses vary considerably, depending on whether the cells are dividing, nondividing, or synchronized into G_1 phase of the cell cycle at the time of treatment. The survival curves are biphasic suggesting that there are sensitive and less sensitive cells in the treated populations. Nondividing plateau phase cells are ten times more sensitive (at the 100 μg/ml dose) than are dividing cells, and they are thirty times more sensitive than G_1 phase cells (Fig. 5). Similar results have been reported in other *in vitro* systems. More importantly, Hahn *et al.* (1973) have shown that nondividing EMT6 tumor cells *in vivo* are also more sensitive to Bleo. These data suggest, therefore, that the drug does diffuse to the G_0 areas of this tumor and may be a good agent to use in other tumors with low growth fractions.

Another example of how the survival characteristics of a cell population change as the growth fraction changes is shown in Fig. 6. Known numbers of dividing and nondividing CHO cells were mixed together and then treated immediately with the anticancer nitrosourea compound MeCCNU (1-*trans*-(2-chloroethyl)-3-(4-methylcyclohexyl)-1-nitrosourea). It can be seen that the sensitivity of the population increased as the number of cells in the growth

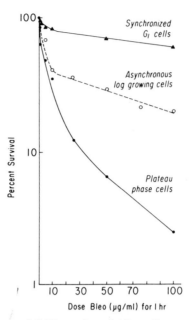

Fig. 5. Survival responses of dividing and nondividing cells treated for 1 hr with Bleomycin. (From Barranco *et al.*, 1973b.)

fraction decreased (Barranco, *et al.*, 1978b). Hahn *et al.* (1973) have also demonstrated this phenomenon *in vivo* in the EMT6 tumor system. Once again there is a possibility that considerable killing in G_0 tumor populations in human tumors may be observed following treatment with such compounds. In Table I a list of some of the anticancer drugs known to kill nondividing cells best includes Bleo, the nitrosoureas MeCCNU, CCNU [1-(2-chloroethyl)-3-cyclohexyl-1-nitrosourea], and BCNU [1, 3-bis(2-chloroethyl)-1-nitrosourea], and galactitol. Although adriamycin, actinomycin D, and diglycoaldehyde kill dividing cells better, they kill a significant fraction of nondividing cells and may also be useful in tumors having low growth fractions. However, HU and Cytosine Arabinoside (ara C) kill only dividing cells and would be much less effective against tumors having large populations of nondividing cells.

As was discussed earlier, the response to drug treatment depends somewhat on the biochemical events occurring in a particular cell at the time of treatment. Thus, it may be assumed that cells would respond differently if treated in various phases of the cell cycle. Cells were synchronized by either physical or chemical means into the various phases of the cell cycle (Barranco *et al.*, 1973c) and then treated with an anticancer drug to determine the differential cell cycle stage sensitivity. In Fig. 7 the Bleo dose response survival curves are shown. Mitotic

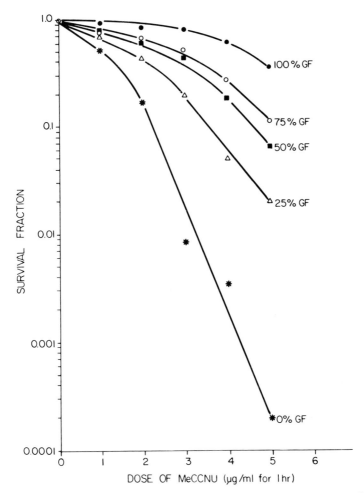

Fig. 6. The change in survival responses to MeCCNU in populations whose growth fractions (GF) vary from 0 to 100%. (From Barranco *et al.*, 1978b.)

cells are most sensitive, with greater than 97% of the cells being killed by doses of 50 μg/ml or greater. This sensitivity of mitotic cells correlates well with the report that mitotic cell DNA exhibits the greatest amount of Bleo-induced strand breaks (Clarkson *et al.*, 1976), and with another report that showed that mitotic cells were unable to recover from Bleo-induced damage (Barranco and Bolton, 1977). The survival curves in Fig. 7 also show that G_2 phase cells are very sensitive to Bleo; however, S phase cells are much less sensitive, and G_1 cells exhibit the least sensitivity.

TABLE I

A Selected List of Anticancer Drugs Whose
Effects May Depend upon the Growth
Fractions of the Tumors Treated

Most effective on nondividing cells
  Bleomycin
  MeCCNU
  CCNU
  BCNU
  1,2:5,6-Dianhydrogalactitol
Most effective on dividing cells
  Adriamycin
  Act D
  Diglycoaldehyde
Kills only dividing cells
  Hydroxyurea
  Ara C

III. DRUG EFFECTS ON CELL PROGRESSION KINETICS

Each chemical, based on its mode of action may block cells at specific positions in the cell cycle. Thus, a chemical which inhibits DNA synthesis will either prevent cells from initiating DNA replication so that they remain in late G_1 phase or reduce the rate of replication so that they remain in S phase. Therefore, once a chemical is applied to an *in vitro* or *in vivo* cell population, the kinetics of cellular progression will be altered and impose on the remaining viable population a completely changed pattern of drug response. From this fact, it follows that the action of a second agent must be influenced in some way by the first, the action of a third agent influenced by a summation of the first and second, and so on.

In Fig. 8, the kinetics effects of the anticancer agent, diglycoaldehyde (DGA), are shown. This drug is an inhibitor of ribonucleotide reductase (Cory *et al.*, 1976) and has been shown to *kill cells most effectively in S phase,* and while cells in G_0, M, G_1 and G_2 are relatively resistant (Bhuyan and Fraser, 1974; Barranco *et al.*, 1978a).

Mitotic cells treated with 500 μg/ml DGA progressed at control rates into G_1 phase. It can be seen in Fig. 8A that the fraction of cells in mitosis decreased from 93% to almost 0% within 1.5 hr in both the treated and control populations, indicating normal progression into G_1 phase.

Cells treated for 1 hr (see arrows, Fig. 8B) during early G_1 phase were delayed for approximately 2 hr, but then progressed at a slightly reduced rate into S phase. Cells in G_1 phase are not replicating DNA and, therefore, will not incor-

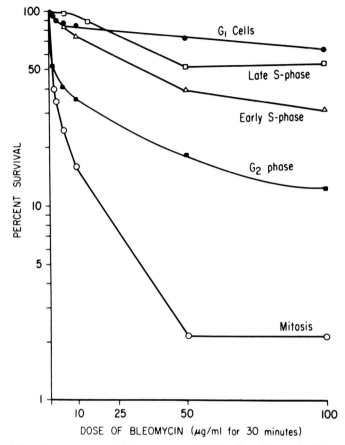

Fig. 7. The cell cycle stage sensitivity responses of CHO cells to Bleomycin. (From Barranco and Humphrey, 1971.)

porate DNA precursors. As G_1 cells progress into S phase they incorporate
[3]H-thymidine, and this assay can be used to measure cell progression. The
fraction of ^{3}H-thymidine labeled cells (*LI*) was essentially 0% at 0–2 hr after
plating mitotic cells, indicating that the cells were in G_1 at the time of treatment.
As the G_1 cells in the control populations progressed into S phase, the *LI*
increased. The rise in the *LI* of the treated population was delayed until the fourth
hour and then increased at a rate slower than that for controls, thus demonstrating
the effect of DGA on G_1 progression kinetics.

The *LI* in the synchronized control S phase populations in Fig. 8C was 92% by
the second hour after the end of synchrony and decreased when the majority of
cells began progressing out of S phase and into G_2. The *LI* decreased to 30% by

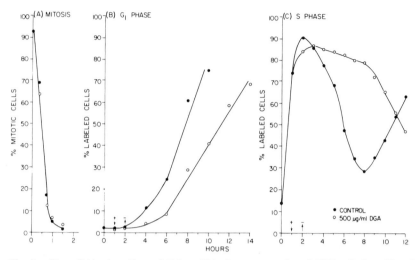

Fig. 8. The cell kinetics effects of diglycoaldehyde on progression of CHO cells from M to G_1 (A), from G_1 to S (B), or from S to G_2 (C). +, start drug treatment; −, stop drug treatment. (From Barranco *et al.*, 1978a.)

the eighth hour and rose again as some cells reentered the subsequent S phase. Cells treated for 1 hr in early S phase with 500 μg/ml DGA were delayed almost 5 hr longer in S phase before progressing into G_2 (Fig. 8c). At doses below 500 μg/ml, there were no effects on cell progression from G_1 to S, or from S to G_2 phases of the cell cycle. A dose-dependent effect on DGA on G_2 progression into M was also observed.

By employing such techniques as those used in the experiments shown in Fig. 8, the effects on cell kinetics of other drugs can also be studied. Presented in Table II is a selected group of anticancer agents showing where in the cell cycle they induce a kinetics block. The group headed by the nitrosourea compounds BCNU, CCNU, and MeCCNU stop cell progression in all stages of the cell cycle. Adriamycin and diglycoaldehyde block cell progression in all phases except mitosis.

The position of the kinetics blockade may or may not have any relationship to the killing effectiveness of a chemical. For example, the alkaloids, colchicine, vinblastine, and vincristine, are very effective specific inhibitors of mitosis for all mammalian cells. However, it has been reported (Mauro and Madoc-Jones, 1970) that in HeLa cells these alkaloids are most effective in killing S phase cells. Some relationship exists for Bleo in which the block is in G_2 and one of the most sensitive phases to killing is G_2 (Barranco and Humphrey, 1971). Hydroxyurea serves as an example, illustrating a very close relationship between blockage and cell killing efficiency. Hydroxyurea kills cells specifically in S

TABLE II

Location of Drug-induced Cell Kinetics Blocks by a Variety of Anticancer Drugs[a]

Drug	G_1	S	G_2	M
BCNU	+	+	+	+
CCNU	+	+	+	+
MeCCNU	+	+	+	+
Adriamycin	+	+	+	−
Diglycoaldehyde	+	+	+	−
Hydroxyurea	+	+	−	−
Galactitol	−	+	+	−
Bleomycin	−	−	+	−
Colcemide	−	−	−	+
Vincristine	−	−	−	+
Vinblastine	−	−	−	+

[a] +, indicates block; −, no block.

phase, blocks further progression out of S phase, and prevents cells in G_1 phase from entering into S phase. Those cells arrested in G_1 are not killed unless they remained blocked for a time approximately equal to one cell cycle time (Sinclair, 1967).

IV. DISCUSSION

The anticancer drugs in current use all produce some form of cytotoxicity to tumor cells as well as to the normal cells in the body. Perhaps the greatest toxic side effects are observed in cell renewal systems such as skin, bone marrow, and small intestine. It is extremely important, therefore, that toxicity be one of the major parameters considered when choosing drugs for chemotherapy. The pharmacological aspects of the drug must also be considered, i.e., the route of administration, the circulation half-life of the drug, and whether it gets to the tumor. Once these parameters (and others) are considered, one is faced with developing an effective drug schedule that will result in eradication of the tumor cells.

Because of a better knowledge of drug effects on the cell cycle obtained through experiments, such as those described in this chapter, it may now be possible to manipulate a patient's tumor kinetics in a way that would optimize treatment scheduling. For example, most large solid tumors contain only small fractions of cells in the growth fraction (Tannock, 1968). As we have seen in Fig. 4 and Table I, the cell cycle active anticancer drugs, specific for dividing cells will usually be only minimally effective. Likewise the effectiveness of cell cycle phase-specific anticancer drugs will be determined by the "size" of a particularly sensitive population in the cell cycle. Therefore, a tumor with only 8 to 10% of its cells in S phase will not be very sensitive to S phase agents, such as hydroxyurea or ara C. However, if the fraction of cells in S phase could be enriched, the tumor might become more sensitive to S phase-specific anticancer drugs. The rationale of this combination schedule is that the first drug may be used to enrich a fraction of cells into the phase of the cell cycle where a second drug kills them most effectively. Such enrichment may be achieved through the use of drug treatments which induce partial synchronization in the cell population. As was noted in Fig. 10, Bleo blocks cells only in G_2 phase, near the $S-G_2$ boundary. The blockade is reversible, depending on the dose given (Barranco and Humphrey, 1971). Continuous infusion of Bleo has been used *in vivo* in human tumors to enrich the fraction of cells in the $S-G_2$ area of the cell cycle (Barranco *et al.*, 1973b). The cells subsequently overcome the kinetics block and progress through the cell cycle, ultimately causing a severalfold enrichment in the fraction of cells in S phase. Treatment at that time with an S phase anticancer drug is several times more effective than when either drug is used alone (Costanzi *et al.*, 1976; Barranco *et al.*, 1973b).

Another example of a kinetics directed protocol is the combination of vincristine and Bleo. As was noted in Table II, vincristine blocks cells in mitosis and Bleo kills cells best in mitosis (Fig. 7). Therefore, if vincristine were to be administered first to enrich the fraction of cells in mitosis, and if Bleo was given some time later, when the mitotic index was increased severalfold, then, the effects of Bleo would be greatly enhanced. This schedule is, in fact, being used currently as a very effective chemotherapy protocol in the treatment of solid tumors (Livingston *et al.*, 1973; Spigel *et al.*, 1974).

Other examples can be given, but it should be clear that the characterizations of drug effects on survival and cell kinetics are valuable parameters to consider when planning chemotherapy protocols. That, coupled with a better knowledge of the tumor population kinetics should make it possible to design more effective tumor treatments.

ACKNOWLEDGMENTS

The author wishes to thank Mrs. R. Kenworthy for her help in preparing this manuscript. Work supported by National Institutes of Health Grants DHEW-5R01-CA-15397(06), DHEW-1R01-CA-23145(01), and DHEW-1P01-CA-23114(01).

REFERENCES

Barranco, S. C., and Bolton, W. E. (1977). *Cancer Res.* **37,** 2589–2591.
Barranco, S. C., and Humphrey, R. M. (1971). *Cancer Res.* **31,** 1218–1223.

Barranco, S. C., and Novak, J. K. (1974). *Cancer Res.* **34**, 1616-1618.

Barranco, S. C., Gerner, E. W., Burk, K. H., and Humphrey, R. M. (1973a). *Cancer Res.* **33**, 11-16.

Barranco, S. C., Novak, J. K., and Humphrey, R. M. (1973b). *Cancer Res.* **33**, 691-694.

Barranco, S. C., Luce, J. K., Romsdahl, M. M., and Humphrey, R. M. (1973c). *Cancer Res.* **33**, 882-887.

Barranco, S. C., Fluornoy, D. R., Bolton, W. E., and Oka, M. A. (1978a). *J. Natl. Cancer Inst.* **61**, 1307-1310.

Barranco, S. C., Bolton, W. E., and Novak, J. K. (1979). *Cell Tissue Kinet.* **12**, 11-16.

Bhuyan, B. K., and Fraser, T. J. (1974). *Cancer Chemother. Rep.* **58**, 149-155.

Clarkson, J. M., and Humphrey, R. M. (1976). *Cancer Res.* **36**, 2345-2349.

Cory, J. G., Mansel, M. M., and Whitford, T. W., Jr. (1976). *Cancer Res.* **36**, 3166-3170.

Costanzi, J. J., Loukas, D., Gagliano, R. G., Griffiths, C., and Barranco, S. C. (1976). *Cancer* **38**, 1503-1506.

Hahn, G. M., Ray, G. R., Gordon, L. F., and Kallman, R. F. (1973). *J. Natl. Cancer Inst.* **50**, 529-533.

Howard, A., and Pelc, S. R. (1953). *Heredity* **6**, 261-273.

Kunimoto, T., Hori, M., and Umezawa, H. (1967). *J. Antibiot., Ser. A.* **20**, 277-281.

Livingston, R. B., Bodey, G. P., Gottlieb, J. A., and Frei, E., III (1973). *Cancer Chemother. Rep.* **57**, 219-224.

Mauro, F., and Madoc-Jones, H. (1970). *Cancer Res.* **30**, 1397-1408.

Mendelsohn, M. L. (1962). *J. Natl. Cancer Inst.* **28**, 1015-1029.

Puck, T. T., and Marcus, P. I. (1956). *J. Exp. Med.* **103**, 653-666.

Sinclair, W. K. (1967). *Cancer Res.* **27**, 297-308.

Spigel, S. C., and Coltman, C. A., Jr. (1974). *Cancer Chemother. Rep.* **58**, 213-216.

Susuki, H., Nagai, K., Yamaki, H., Tanaka, N., and Umezawa, H. (1969). *J. Antibiot., Ser. A* **22**, 446-448.

Tannock, I. F. (1968). *Br. J. Cancer* **22**, 258-273.

6

MORPHOLOGICAL CORRELATES OF NEOPLASIA*

Yerach Daskal, Phyllis Gyorkey, and Ferenc Gyorkey

I. INTRODUCTION

The early hypothesis that the basis for malignancy resides within the cancer cell emanated from morphological observations which were followed by experimentation. According to Oberling and Bernhard (1961), the "arch cancer cell" is not identical in the different types of neoplasms, and the diversity of the cancer cells, morphologically, is as great as the various tumors themselves. Greenstein (1954) observed that there is only one kind of normal tissue, but there may be a number of different neoplasms which arise from this normal tissue.

With the advent of electron microscopy, vast information has been accumulated on the structure of various cell constituents; however, the search is still in progress to define the universal characteristic feature that will unequivocally delineate the normal cell from its neoplastic counterpart.

*In memory of a dear colleague Dr. Ramah Lapushin who lost her greatest battle.

CANCER AND CHEMOTHERAPY, VOL. I

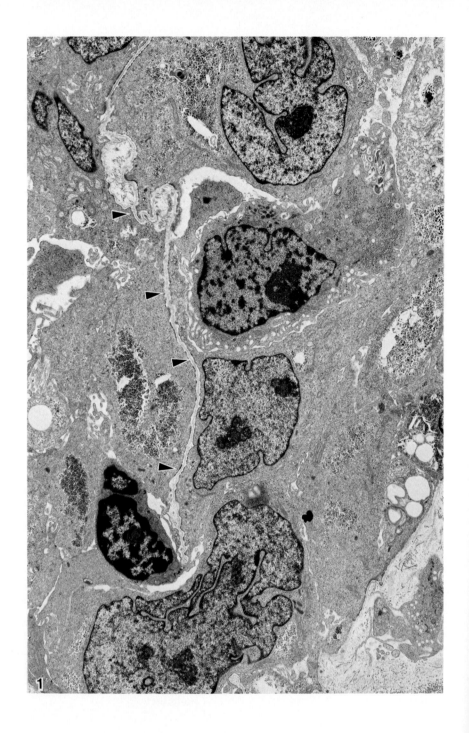

The reliable hallmarks of neoplasia are cellular pleomorphism, cell division, anaplasia, invasion, and metastasis into the surrounding tissues, vessels, and regional and distant lymph nodes. Anaplasia, or lack of differentiation, refers to the loss of cellular specialization or structural organization of tumor cells as compared to the tissue or cells of origin (Fig. 1). Moreover, the anaplastic process manifests itself not only in the light microscopy of the tumor cell but also at the subcellular level, such as in the structural organization of the cell nucleus and its organelles. At all levels, electron microscopy has provided meaningful data for the cytological classification of tumors. For example, in leiomyosarcoma, myofilaments in the cytoplasm of the cells in question are observed, thereby properly identifying and classifying such a tumor.

Malignant (metastatic) amelanotic melanomas can be diagnosed with the electron microscopy by the presence of promelanosomes and melanosomes in the cytoplasm of the tumor cells which are unobservable by light microscopic study. However, it is important to realize that cellular anaplasia is a wide and gradual change of structure and function of the neoplastic cell compared to its normal counterpart cell. With respect to tumor invasiveness, it seems that certain normal tissue components, such as the capsules of organs (kidney, liver), are more resistant to tumor invasion than others. Arterial walls or fibrous tissue, for example, may act as physical barriers for tumor metastasis as well. Whether factors such as the pressure exerted by the growing tumor mass confined within a limited space (Young, 1959) or the lack of contact inhibition of tumor cells proposed by Abercombie (1961) are mechanisms related to tumor invasiveness is not clearly defined. However, observations that tumor cells may infiltrate defined spaces, follow a preselected route, or even migrate along certain gradients where some form of cellular damage has occurred, have been reported (Babai and Tremblay, 1972). Figure 2 shows the penetration of a tumor cell (thyroid carcinoma) through a well-defined, but disrupted, basement membrane into the interstitium, possibly penetrating the lymphatics or the vascular system with metastases to distant sites by the same mechanism. Penetration through the disrupted basement membrane was perhaps due to a focal lesion induced by unknown factors, with possible mediation by the tumor cells themselves. Permeation into the vascular system represents a more advanced stage of neoplastic process (invasiveness) (Fig. 3). The tumor cells seem to penetrate into the vascular lumen through a gap between the endothelial cells, resulting in tumor dissemination in the various sites of the body via the vascular system.

Despite the high level of resolution of the electron microscope, important

---

Fig. 1. Metastatic renal cell carcinoma (human) showing pleomorphic nature of tumor cells. A basement membrane (arrowheads) undulates between the tumor cells. All four cells in the field differ by their nuclear configuration, chromatin condensation patterns, and the state of nucleolar activity. × 4750.

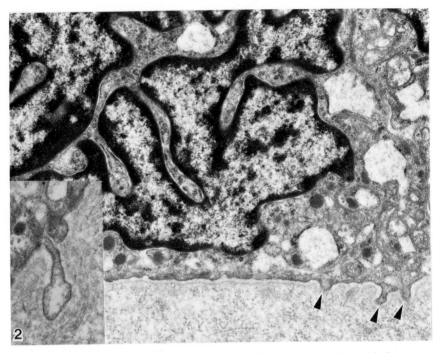

Fig. 2.   Well-differentiated follicular cell carcinoma of the thyroid gland (human) in the process of penetration of the cell through a gap in the basement membrane. × 18,000. Inset, × 38,000.

limitations must be borne in mind when the degree of differentiation of a tumor is to be determined, namely, what is the proper selection of the control or "normal" counterpart to a tumor cell. For example, experimentally induced tumors in animals may bear little resemblance to human neoplasms. On the other hand, the study of normal adult human tissues may be less relevant than the study of embryonic tissues, which because of the presence of varying degrees of cell differentiation may actually provide important morphological data that correlate to cellular anaplasia.

Since no one unique structural characteristic can be shown to describe the basic hallmark of neoplasia, several criteria for the definition of malignancy must be considered which may afford the recognition of a neoplastic process and provide some dimensions to the enormous range of the structural variations that are manifested by tumor cells (Luse, 1961).

Fig. 3.   Malignant melanoma metastatic to the brain (human). The tumor cell process extends into the blood vessel through the endothelial gap. Note the change in the structure of the cell extension ("pseudopod") in contact with the endothelium. At higher magnifications (b), fine filaments (contractile elements) are in the pseudopod. L, luminal space. (a) × 10,000. (b) × 36,000.

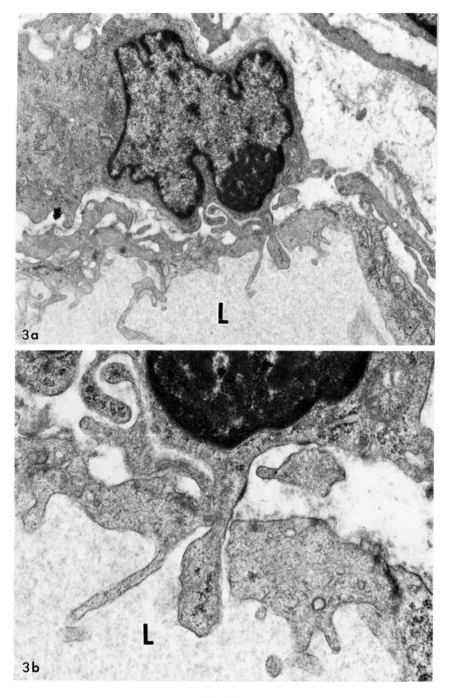

Fig. 3.

II. THE INTERPHASE NUCLEUS OF THE CANCER CELL

A. Shape, Size, and Chromatin Distribution

In general, the nucleus of the cancer cell is enlarged and often presents irregular contours (Fig. 4). The increase in the nuclear–cytoplasmic ratio (N/C) may be one of the more distinctive features of malignancy (Oberling and Bernhard, 1961). The change in nuclear contours is an important diagnostic marker for neoplasia and is a true manifestation of nuclear pleomorphism of the cancer cell. Deep clefts or invaginations are found in many tumors (Fig. 4) [hepatocellular carcinoma (Fig. 5a), carcinoma of the prostrate and kidney (Fig. 1), poorly differentiated neoplasms as well as in specialized cells, such as the Reed-Sternberg cell in Hodgkin's disease (Fig. 6a), and the Sezary cell that may be related to chronic lymphocytic leukemia (Fig. 6b)]. These lobulated nuclei are commonly referred to as "monstrous." Although the nuclear–cytoplasmic ratio increases in tumor cells, the nuclear lobulations seem to compensate for this deficiency by essentially increasing the nuclear cytoplasmic exchange surfaces (Ghadially, 1975).

Very frequently, nuclei that are "monstrous" also contain highly condensed chromatin clumps distributed within these nuclei, predominantly around the nuclear perimeter following the nuclear membrane (Figs. 1–5). These chromatin clumps, known as heterochromatin, are considered to represent inactive portions of the chromatin component of the cell (Frenster, 1974) that can be converted into euchromatin upon gene activation. Therefore, the relative amounts of heterochromatin within the tumor cell nucleus may reflect the overall synthetic activity of the cell rather than its synthetic capacity. In other instances, rapidly growing tumors, such as adenocarcinoma of the pancreas (Fig. 7), possess a highly contorted nucleus and contain little, if any, heterochromatic clumps. The increase in nuclear volume of tumor cells need not always be associated with irregularly shaped nuclear contours. Poorly differentiated tumors are frequently observed to have well expanded spherical nuclei with smooth contours characteristic of nuclei of embryonic cells (Fig. 7). The highly convoluted nuclear membranes in tumor cells may be the reason for the detection of the various nuclear inclusions that will be discussed below.

Although it is clear that the nuclear envelope may play an important role in the function of the normal and the tumor cell, it is not clear whether it has a defined role in the neoplastic process. Furthermore, it is not entirely understood what properties of the nuclear membranes are related to the formation of the bizarre nuclear profiles in tumor cells. No clear evidence is available at present (Franke and Scheer, 1974) as to the quantitative distribution of the number of nuclear pores per unit area in tumor cells versus normal cells.

The presence of "monstrous" nuclei in cells alone does not necessarily imply that the cell is malignant. The nuclear polymorphism of the tumor cells must be

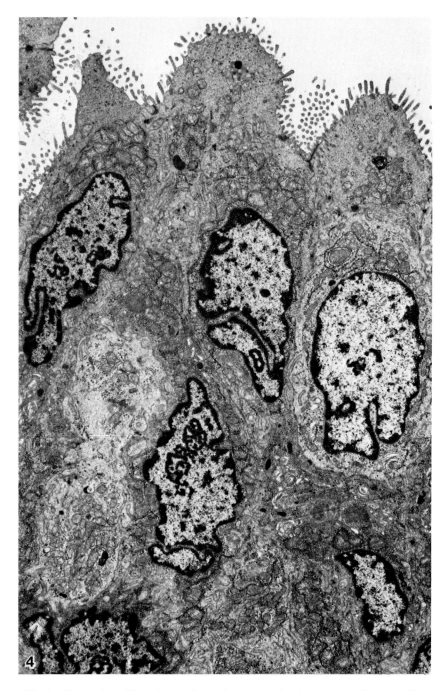

Fig. 4. Pancreatic papillary adenocarcinoma (human) showing the ''monstrous'' tumor cell nuclei. Note the filamentous nucleoli indicative of active synthesis. × 7500.

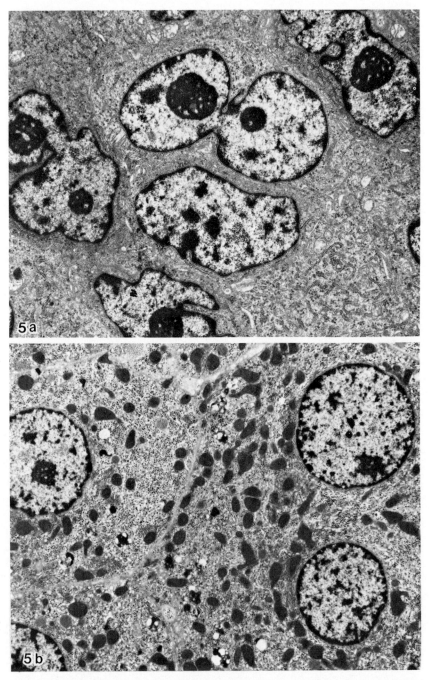

Fig. 5. Comparison between the nucleus of liver cell carcinoma (a) and normal liver (human) (b). There is a net increase in nuclear volume in carcinoma. Note the undulations in nuclear membranes and the increase in nucleolar volume (nucleolar hypertrophy) in the tumor cells. × 8500.

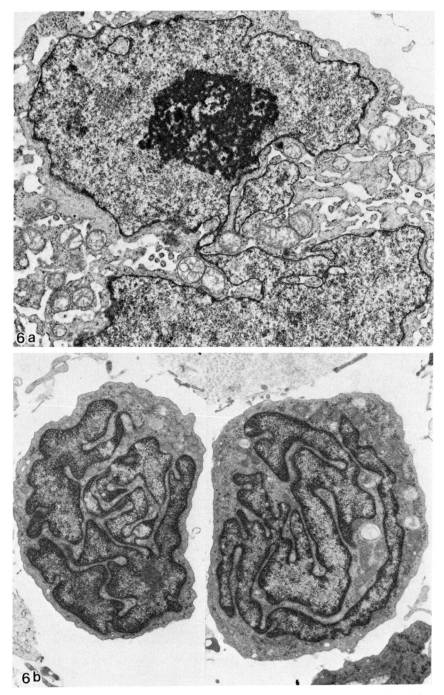

Fig. 6. The lobulated nuclei of the Reed–Sternberg cell of Hodgkin's disease (a) and that of the Sezary cell (b) are unique diagnostic markers. Note the active compact nucleolus of the Reed–Sternberg cell and the inactive ring-shape one in the Sezary cell. (a) × 6000. (b) × 12,000.

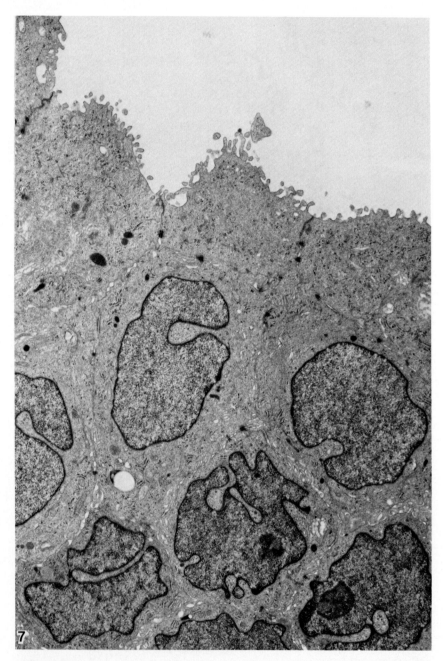

Fig. 7. Pancreatic adenocarcinoma in an abdominal mass (human). Nuclear pleomorphism of the neoplastic cells is apparent in the lobulated nuclei but without aggregates of heterochromatin (compare with Fig. 4). × 8000.

considered within the context of other data obtained prior to the final diagnostic determination.

B. Nucleolar Index and Morphology in Tumor Cells

Nucleolar hypertrophy and pleomorphisms are well known characteristics of tumor cells which were observed and reported by cytologists for more than 100 years (Pianese, 1896). As early as 1934, McCarthy and his associates established the statistical validity in correlating nucleolar hypertrophy and variability with neoplasia (McCarthy and Haumeder, 1934).

Historically, an increase in nucleolar size in excess of 5 μm has been regarded as a reliable marker for malignant cells (Busch and Smetana, 1973). In general, a nucleolar–nuclear ratio exceeding 0.25 is a strong indication for the presence of a tumor. Furthermore, the increase in nucleolar volume can be correlated readily with the increase in the grade of malignancy (Ferreira, 1941).

The nucleolus is the site where transcription and initial packaging of the preribosomal particles occur (Perry, 1966; Penman et al., 1967; Warner et al., 1966; Busch and Smetana, 1970). Three main structural components can be observed in the nucleolus: the granular component representing the partially assembled preribosomal particles (Figs. 8, 9b and d, and 11a–g), the fibrillar component that represents the transcriptional locus of the rRNA genes (Figs. 8a and 9a–d and 9f), and the nucleolus organizer (NOR), component (Figs. 8, 9, and 11b), similar in appearance to the fibrillar component but of lesser electron density (Bernhard and Granboulan, 1963; Busch and Smetana, 1970; Goessens, 1976; Daskal et al., 1976).

Nucleoli of tumor cells may vary in size and range from 0.5 to 3 μm in diameter. All nucleoli consist of the three main components previously described. However they may or may not be surrounded by a "shell" of nucleolus-associated chromatin penetrating the nucleolar body proper (Fig. 8a). The variation in nucleolar shape is due to the variation in the relative distribution pattern of nucleolar components (Fig. 10a–d).

Frequently, fast-growing tumors possess large filamentous nucleoli with elaborated intertwining of the fibrillar and granular components (nucleolonemas) (Figs. 1,4,10, and 11). Similar nucleoli may be observed in seminomas, uterine tumors, and a variety of fast-growing carcinomas (Figs. 10 and 11).

Nucleolar compaction may be related to a diminution in growth rates of the cells (Figs. 8c and 11). The total cessation of nucleolar RNA synthesis is manifested in the form of a highly compact spherical nucleolus in which the segregation of all elements occurs (Fig. 10). The biochemical events represented in the various segregation patterns of nucleoli of tumor cells are unknown at present. The inhibition of nucleolar synthetic activity may occur spontaneously (Fig. 9b–d).

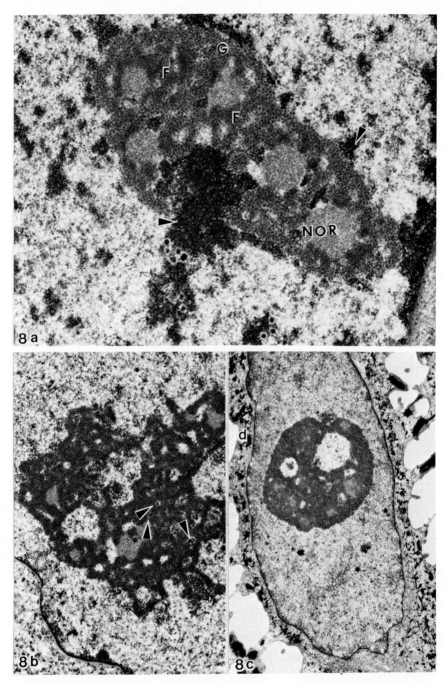

Fig. 8. The nucleolus of an asbestos-induced malignant mesothelioma of the lung (a). The perinucleolar chromatin (arrowheads) is penetrating into the nucleolar body. NOR, nucleolus organizer components; G, granular component; F, fibrillar component. The nucleolus of a well-

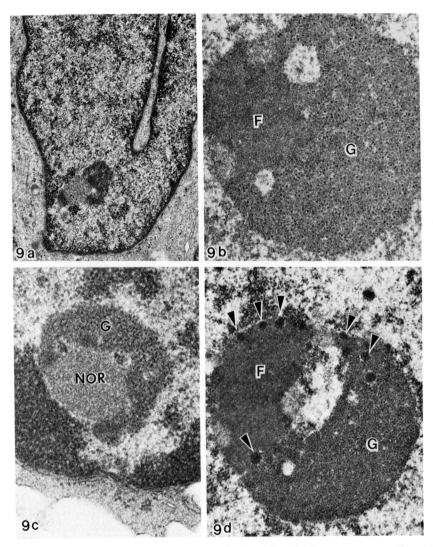

Fig. 9. The phenomenon of nucleolar segregation in tumor cells. Spontaneous segregation of nucleolar components in a well-differentiated human pancreatic adenocarcinoma (a). Segregation may be induced in tumor cells *in vitro* by various intercallating antitumor drugs (adriamycins, actinomycin D, and mitomycin C). During segregation, the nucleolus may (b) or may not produce microspherules (d) (arrowheads). In many hematologic neoplasms, naturally segregated nucleoli centered around the nucleolus organizer components (NOR) are frequently observed (c). Fr, fibrillar component; Gr, granular component. (a) × 7000. (b) × 26,000. (c) × 22,000.

differentiated squamous cell carcinoma of the tongue (b) contains microspherules (arrowheads). The nucleolus spreads out over a considerable area of the nucleus. Another squamous cell carcinoma of the larynx (c) contains a large spherical and compact nucleolus with large vacuoles, indicative of a temporary cessation in metabolic activity. (a) × 33,000. (b) and (c) × 9000.

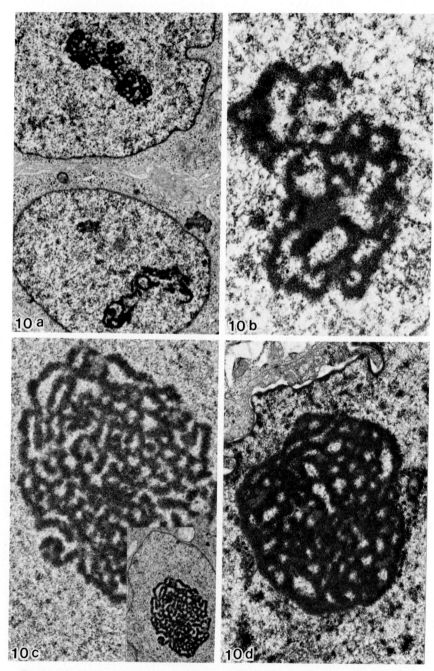

Fig. 10. Nucleolar pleomorphism in tumor cells. Ribbonlike nucleoli from a seminoma (human). The fibrillar component forms the backbone of these nucleoli [(a) and (b)]. The paucity of granular elements in these nucleoli is indicative of the high rate of rRNA synthesis without the accumulation of preribosomal particles in nucleolar body. The nucleolus of a rapidly growing rectal adenocarcinoma [(c) and inset]; the reticular nucleolus occupies a large portion of the nucleus (inset). Gradual compaction of the nucleolus in a fibrous histiocytoma (d) is indicative of a reduction in nucleolar activity. (a) × 5500. (b) × 18,000. (c) × 14,000; inset, × 5,000. (d) × 18,000.

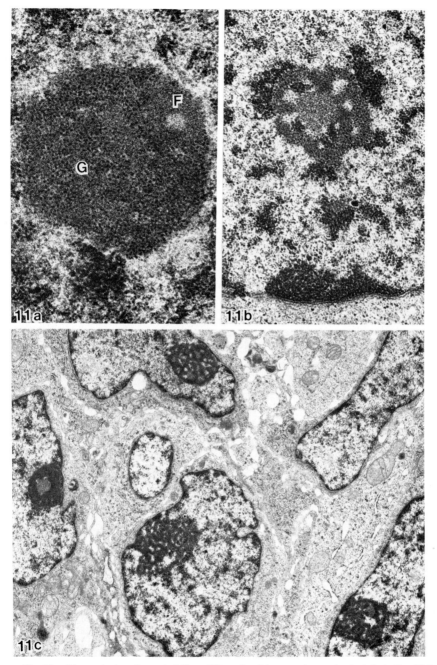

Fig. 11. The nucleolus of a metastatic undifferentiated lung carcinoma (metastatic to the skin) showing an intermediate stage in nucleolar inactivation (a). On the other hand, a nucleolus of a hairy cell leukemia (b) shows initial phases of activation by progressing to a reticular confrontation from a "ring-shaped" form. Nucleolar "margination" has been frequently reported to occur in tumor cells (c). Consideration must be given to the effects of cellular pressure in a rapidly growing tumor (e.g., plane of sectioning) on nucleolar orientation in the nucleus. (a) × 38,000. (b) × 20,000. (c) × 9000. F, fibrillar component; G, granular component.

An intermediate stage in nucleolar inactivation is the "ring-shape" nucleolus (Smetana *et al.*, 1970) frequently observed in hematological neoplasms and routinely in normal lymphoid tissues (Figs. 6b, 9c, and 11b). Various nucleolar inclusions have been reported in tumor cells (Busch and Smetana, 1973), such as microspherules (Figs. 8b and 9d) (Unuma and Busch, 1967) and nucleolar dense granules (Busch and Smetana, 1970). These may be induced in normal cells by various infectious agents, drugs, or environmental conditions; however, it appears that, quantitatively, there may be a preponderance of these in tumor cells.

Nucleolar invagination (Fig. 11c) is considered to be present in higher frequency in tumor cells. However, the displacement of the nucleolus within the nucleus may be the result of directional pressure exerted by the growing tumor cells, as well as selective orientation of the cells during sectioning. To date, there is no evidence to indicate that the position of the nucleolus within the nucleoplasm is fixed and that the nucleoli are essentially stationary (Daskal *et al.*, 1978).

Based on these observations and other similar data obtained from nucleolar profiles, it may be concluded that the morphology of the nucleolus of the cancer cells, although representative of the state of rRNA metabolism of the cell, and thus its growth rate, does not exhibit any unique specific or tumor related ultrastructural alterations. The observed variations in nucleolar pleomorphism should be considered within the context of other parameters that may be suggestive of tumor growth.

C. Extranuclear Organelles

1. Perichromatin Granules (PCG)

These nuclear granules, 300–400 Å in diameter, are a universal component of the cell nucleus. First described by Watson in 1968, their function, precise structure, biogenesis, and overall composition are still unknown (Daskal *et al.*, 1978). The perichromatin granules (PCG) can be identified readily by the clear surrounding halo (Fig. 12a–c) and their localization in the midst of heterochromatin clumps. It has been calculated that the average cell nucleus contains about 2000–2500 PCGs. These granules are found in tumor cells as well. More-

---

Fig. 12. Perichromatinic granules (PCGs) in the cell nucleus of cycloheximide treated rat liver cell (a), fibrous histiocytoma (b), and malignant mesothelioma (c). The PCGs are 300–400 Å in diameter and are recognized by the surrounding halo. Although present in all normal cells as well, the clustering of these granules is frequently observed in either drug-treated or in tumor cells. Similarly, interchromatinic granules (ICGs) (d) may occupy large areas of tumor cell nuclei. At higher magnifications (d, inset), the fine interconnecting filaments of the ICGs can be observed in this bronchioloalveolar carcinoma. Arrowheads, the boundaries of the ICG complex. (a) × 60,000. (b) × 25,000. (c) × 33,000. (d) × 50,000; inset, × 70,000.

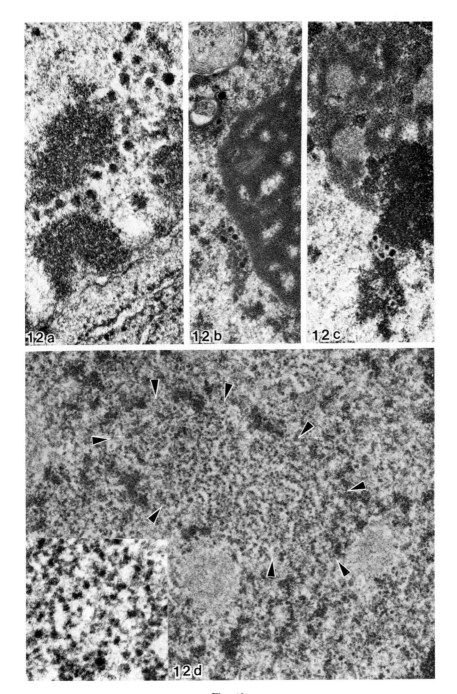

Fig. 12.

over, it appears that in tumors that contain nuclei with hypercondensed chromatin, the number of perichromatin granules grouped in clusters is increased over that of the normal cell (Fig. 12) (Daskal *et al.*, 1975). The increase in the number of perichromatin granules in certain tumors (Ghadially, 1975; Murad and Scarpelli, 1967) is related to the transcriptional activity of these tumors which is reflected in the increased or decreased numbers of perichromatin granules causal to the neoplastic process. Inactivation of nuclear transcription with mitomycin C, cycloheximide (Daskal *et al.*, 1975; Daskal and Crooke, 1979), lasiocarpine and aflatoxin (Monneron and Bernhard, 1969) α-amanitin (Petrov and Sekeris, 1971), riboflavin deficiency (Norton *et al.*, 1977) and supranormal temperatures (Heine *et al.*, 1971) will also cause an increase in the number of perichromatin granules in the cell nucleus.

2. *Interchromatinic Granules (ICG)*

First described by Swift in 1959 (Fig. 12d), the ICGs are compact granules organized in spherical patches throughout the cell nucleus. The individual ICGs are about 200–25 Å in diameter, interconnected by filamentous elements (Fig. 12d), and apparently contain ribonucleoproteins (Busch and Smetana, 1973). Their number seems also to increase in tumor cells where interchromatinic complexes may occupy large regions of the cell nucleus (Fig. 12d). The dimensions of the individual ICG patches may be as large as 2–3 μm in diameter. Although no statistical data are available to determine the frequency distribution of the ICGs, it has been reported that these granules are consistently enlarged and increased in hepatocarcinomas (Reddy and Svoboda, 1968). The ease of identification of the interchromatinic granules in tumor cells may be related to the particular states of chromatin condensation in the nucleoplasm (Fig. 12). However, no direct correlation exists between the increase in ICGs and the neoplastic process. Frequently, the interchromatinic granules appear as coiled structures, where the individual granule may be interconnected by fine filaments (Fig. 12d, inset).

3. *Nuclear Bodies*

These nuclear organelles are about 0.2–2.5 μm in diameter, and can be detected only by electron microscopy (Fig. 13). First described by De-The *et al.* (1960) the presence of these organelles in the normal cell nucleus is still in dispute, with others claiming that nuclear bodies are evidence for a pathological

---

Fig. 13. Nuclear bodies of tumor cells (bronchioalveolar carcinoma). The three most common varieties of nuclear bodies encountered in tumor cells are (a) the simple nuclear body (SNB), (b) the beaded nuclear body (BNB), and (c–e) the granular nuclear body (GNB). The granular elements in the GNB appear similar to the nucleolar granular components, suggesting a possible origin to these bodies. (a) and (b) $\times$ 50,000. (c) and (d) $\times$ 37,000. (e) $\times$ 47,000.

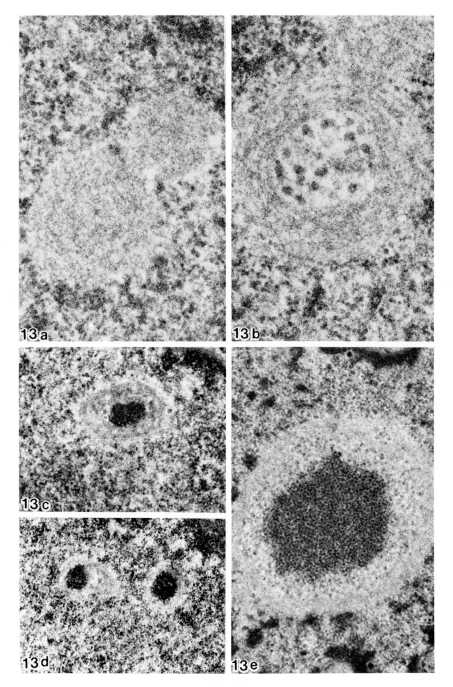

Fig. 13.

state of the cell nucleus. Buttner and Horstmann (1967) have concluded that nuclear bodies (sphareides) should be considered as a functional differentiation of the nucleoplasm of normal cells. Bouteille *et al.* (1974) suggested that the nuclear bodies are pathological manifestations of possible viral etiology. Nuclear bodies appear in three structural variants: the simple nuclear body (SNB), the beaded nuclear body (BNB), and granular nuclear body (GNB) (Fig. 13).

The simple nuclear body (Fig. 13a) may consist of concentric membranelike structure often found in the vicinity of nucleoli. The beaded nuclear body is a mixture of the concentric lamellae and granules of low electron density approximately 200–300 Å in diameter (Fig. 13b).

Finally, the granular nuclear body (Fig. 13c–e) consists mainly of granules 200–300 Å in diameter and similar to those observed in the granular portion of the nucleolus. It is interesting that a significant increase in the number of these bodies is found in bronchioalveolar carcinomas of the lung (Fig. 13c and d). Recently, similar increases in the number of these bodies was reported in a large number of carcinomas of the tongue studied in Japan (Yasuzumi *et al.*, 1976). An increase in the number of nuclear bodies in alveolar epithelial cells has been observed after the administration of bleomycin or busulfan as well (Daskal *et al.*, 1976; F. Gyorkey, unpublished observation).

4. Nuclear Lamellar Inclusions

In addition to the tortuous undulation in the nuclear membrane observed previously (Figs. 4 and 6), tumor cell nuclei frequently contain tubular inclusions (Fig. 14d–f) of a large variety of forms and configurations as well as size. It is not uncommon for bronchioalveolar carcinomas to contain nuclei and for more than 40–50% of their total volume is occupied by such nuclear inclusions. Serial sections have confirmed the nuclear origin of these structures, having been observed occasionally in normal tissues also, such as endometrium or other metabolically active cells (Fig. 14e and f). Whether the presence of these membranous structures is another mechanism for the increase of the nuclear–cytoplasmic exchange, in addition to the increase in nuclear identations of tumor cells, is unknown (Ghadially, 1975).

Fig. 14. A variety of nuclear inclusions detected in tumor cells. The nuclear rodlets (a) may be composed of subunits and quite similar to nuclear paracrystalline inclusions (b). Bizarre invagination of the nuclear membrane is quite common in tumor cells (c). These structures may be related to the generally increased undulations of the tumor cell nucleus. Various granular or particulate inclusions reminiscent of perichromatinic granules or even viral inclusions may be observed (d). Nuclear lamellar inclusions may occupy up to 70% of the total nuclear volume. These inclusions [(e) and (f)] are not associated with heterchromatin, but are derived from inner nuclear membrane and may be induced also by antitumor drugs, such as bleomycin or busulfan. (a) and (b) × 72,000. (c) × 60,000. (d) × 65,000. (e) × 14,500. (f) × 38,000.

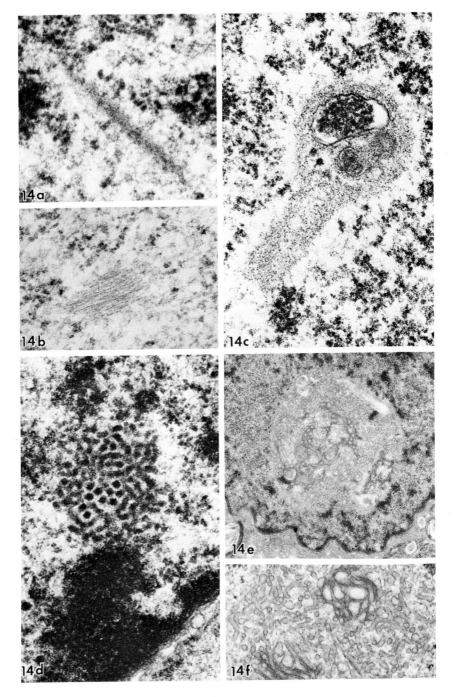

Fig. 14.

5. Miscellaneous Inclusions (Nuclear Rodlets, Fibrillar, and Granular Inclusions

This terminology has been applied to denote the presence of unusual structures in the cell nucleus (Fig. 14a and d).

Nuclear rodlets and fibrillar and granular inclusions are found rarely in normal tissues, but more frequently in pathological conditions, such as carcinoma of the prostate and Sezary syndrome. This does not eliminate the possibility that the nuclear rodlet (Fig. 14a and b) and other inclusions (Fig. 14d) may represent normal cell constituents. Their presence in higher frequencies in neoplastic cells may be either suggestive of aborted structural elements or another manifestation of the tendency of the tumor cell toward variation and anaplasia rather than to constancy and uniformity.

Although numerous observations of viral inclusions in tumor cell nuclei have been reported, a viral etiology to human neoplasma has not been established to date. Therefore, when viral particles are observed in tumor cell nuclei, consideration must be given to the case history of the specimen in question in order to determine possible origins of nuclear viral particles.

III. THE CYTOPLASM OF THE CANCER CELL

In addition to fundamental and so-called universal ultrastructural components, the normal cell cytoplasm contains structures that are unique to a cell type which has differentiated in a particular direction. Such specialized structures are, for example, the lamellar (surfactant containing) inclusions of type II alveolar cells, myofilaments in skeletal muscle cells, or procollagen fibrils in fibroblasts. Thus, with reference to the determination of the anaplastic character of the malignant cell, both the differentiated and elemental cytoplasmic components should be considered.

After 40 years of serial transplantation; the persistance of promelanosomes, with their characteristic ultrastructure, not only in highly malignant human melanoma cells (Fig. 15a) but also demonstrate *in vitro* the anaplastic character of malignant cells. On the other hand, loss of melanin granules occurs as in amelanotic melanomas and may be found both in human and experimental tumors. The characteristic ultrastructural features of the promelanosomes and melanosomes are identical in the malignant melanoma and normal melanocytes

---

Fig. 15.   Cytoplasmic structures useful for the identification of the cell of origin of tumor cell. In the case of a leiomyosarcoma (a), the presence of abortive structures similar to sarcomeres allowed the identification of this tumor. In the case of a malignant melonoma (b)–(d), the presence of mature melanin granules in the cytoplasm (c) or premelanosomes (d) with their characteristic crystalline organization revealed the nature of the tumor cell. (a) × 28,000. (b) × 9000. (c) and (d) × 45,000.

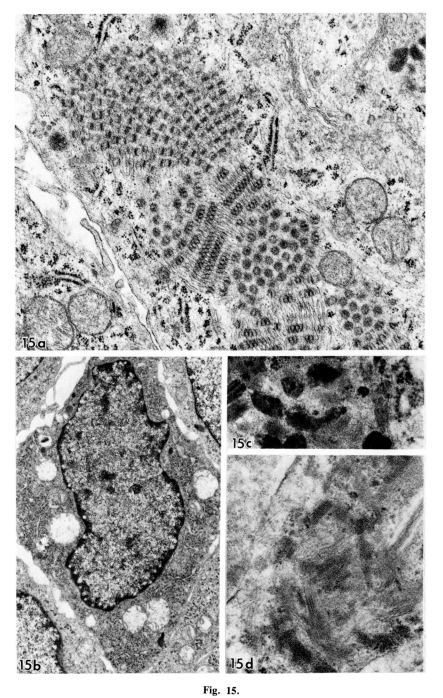

Fig. 15.

(Fig. 15b). Other examples in which neoplastic cells seem to retain some ultra-structural characteristics and can thus be classified as ''more differentiated'' tumors, are the sarcomas.

Bundlelike complexes reminiscent of bundles of myofilaments can be detected in the cytoplasm of myosarcomas (Fig. 15a). Similar ultrastructural elements of normal cells can be demonstrated by the presence of granules in adenocarcinoma of the pancreas and by the presence of prostate secretory granules in prostatic carcinomas.

The diagnostic importance of such ultrastructural features is self-evident. It allows the proper histological classification of tumors. But equally important is the developing concept that tumor cells have conserved some aspects of their genetic programming while other aspects were lost and replaced, yielding a structural–functional reorganization, manifested in the form of an anaplastic process.

Of the other cytoplasmic organelles, such as lysosomes, mitochondria, endo-

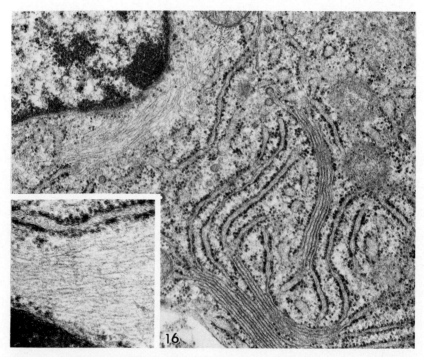

Fig. 16.   Electron microscopy revealed the characteristic organization of the endoplasmic re-ticulum (ER) in the cells. Based on the abnormal 70 Å filaments in the cytoplasm (inset), the ER, and the nuclear configuration, it was concluded that this cell retained the structures of plasma cell (myeloma). × 32,500. Inset, × 70,000.

plasmic reticulum (ER), or Golgi apparatus, no fundamental ultrastructural differences have been detected between normal and in tumor cells, although quantitative differences have been reported. For a complete in-depth analysis of this topic, the review of Oberling and Bernhard (1961) should be consulted.

Abnormal mitochondrial inclusions, such as paracrystalline structures, may be detected in tumor cells, but these are found in a variety of hepatic disorders as well and do not seem to be related to the malignant state. The amount of well-developed rough endoplasmic reticulum appears to be related to the synthetic potential of the cell as well as the retention of some of its differentiated function. Plasma cell ER organization, for example, is an ultrastructural marker characteristic of the cell. In the case of a plasmacytoma, some of this ER organization seems to be retained (Fig. 16). However, the anaplastic process also manifests itself in this case in the form of large bundles of fine fibrils, usually not found in this form in normal plasma cells (Fig. 16, inset).

IV. TUMOR CELL PERIPHERIES AND THE CYTOSKELETON

As discussed previously, the hallmarks of neoplasia are cellular anaplasia, invasiveness and metastasis. The invasive properties of the malignant cells have been attributed in part to their reduced adhesiveness, which, in turn, facilitates the separation of tumor cells from other cells and affords their migration or translocation to distant sites (see review by Carter, 1976). Abercombie and Ambros (1962) have suggested that the mobile potential of malignant cells may be related to their invasive properties.

The intercellular mechanical attachment of cells is mediated by the desmosomal complex or the macula adherens and the zonula adherens. The tight junction (zonula occludens) and the gap junction (the nexus) function in the prevention of intercellular diffusion of materials and electrical coupling as well as passages for small molecules, respectively. However, the ultrastructure of cell junctions in normal cells is identical to those of differentiated malignant ones. At times, fewer desmosomes have been observed in squamous cell carcinomas. Moreover, some reports claim that tumors also have gap junctions, thus, contributing support for the hypothesis of reduced cell adhesion in malignant cell growth. On the other hand, these findings may be attributed to abnormal cell-to-cell recognition patterns and the loss of contact inhibition, thereby resulting in the formation of multiple cell layers and aggregates seen in carcinomas. In summary, no significant qualitative (structural) differences in tumors of epithelial cell origin and normal intercellular junctions can be detected by electron microscopy. The presence of desmosomal complex and tonofibrils are also useful in the classification of poorly differentiated tumors, such as squamous cell carcinomas and sarcomas (Györkey *et al.*, 1975).

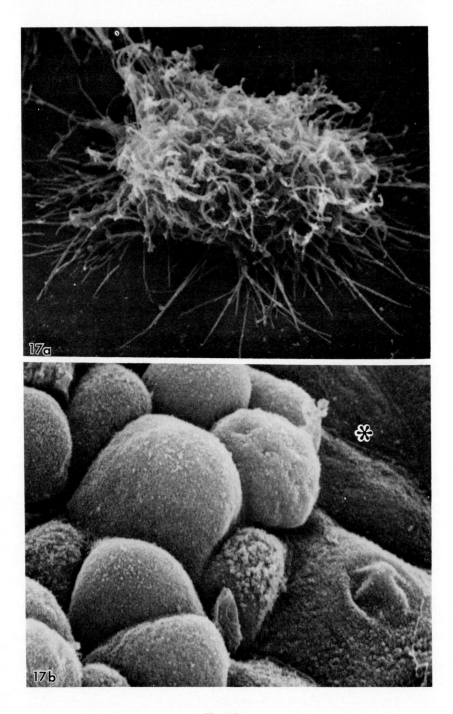

Fig. 17.

In addition to the lateral specializations of the plasma membrane in the form of the various junctions, the cytoplasm also contains a complex and delicate network of microfilaments and microtubules. These contractile components are especially abundant in epithelial cells, and essentially constitute the cytoskeletal structure of the cell (Porter, 1966). It is the cytoskeletal complex that confers the shape to growing cells (Fig. 17a). Cytoskeletal elements seem also to be involved in the mobility and activity of cell surface receptors (Edelman, 1976). Examination of tumor cells grown *in vitro* and *in vivo* by scanning electron microscopy (Fig. 17a and b) demonstrates the highly complex cell-to-cell interaction as well as the interaction of cells with substrate (for a review, see Wetzel, 1976). It seems that cell substrate interactions are not universal and depend largely on the nature of the substrate, culture conditions, age of tumors, transformation, and etiology (Wetzel, 1976).

Changes in cell substrate interactions and the transition from a flattened to a rounded configuration (Hale *et al.*, 1975) have been attributed to alterations in the architecture, and organization of the cytoskeletal components and can be directly correlated with the various processes that are responsible for the transformation of the normal cell to a malignant cell either *in vitro* or *in vivo*.

Recently, several laboratories have reported that unique morphological differences in the organization of the cytoskeletal elements exist between normal and transformed cells (Fonte and Porter, 1975; Brinkley *et al.*, 1975; Edelman and Yahara, 1976; Pollack *et al.*, 1975; also a recent review by Brinkley *et al.*, 1978). Malech and Lentz (1974) and McNutt *et al.*, (1973) have studied the distribution of microfilaments in carcinogen-treated epithelial cells in mice, detecting microfilaments in the transformed cells but not in the normal cells. Immunological studies on the distribution of contractile proteins in human cancers have been reported by Gabbiani *et al.* (1976). Basal and squamous cell carcinomas contained actin, actinin, myosin, and tropomyosin. Normal tissues did not. Furthermore, electron microscopic studies of the identical tissues have confirmed that the immunological findings were indeed related to the presence of microfilaments of two classes; 40–80 Å filaments were reported to be present in carcinomas (Schenk, 1974). Thus, it was proposed that the presence and the amount of contractile proteins in malignant cells may be of diagnostic importance (Schenk, 1974) and may be directly related to the invasive potential of tumors

---

Fig. 17. Scanning electron micrograph of a Novikoff hepatoma cell grown on a glass substrate. Note the intricate fillopodial extensions and the change in their structure as they contact the solid substrate. *In vivo* (b) a N-[4-(5-nitro-2-furyl)-2-thiazdyl] formamide (FANFT) induced urinary bladder transitional cell carcinoma grows in a papillary pattern. The tumor cells that extrude into the luminal space have much more complex intercellular interactions than the normal epithelial cells seen in the background (asterisk). (a) × 4800. (b) × 2700.

(Fig. 16). Using monovalent antibodies against either tubulin or actin (e.g., against microtubules and microfilaments, respectively), Miller *et al.* (1977), Fuller and Brinkley (1976), and others have elegantly shown that normal cells of established cultured lines *in vitro* contain a highly organized and complex cytoskeleton (Fig. 18). However, upon transformation of the cells by either chemical or viral means, the cytoskeletal structures of cells *in vitro* are not as elaborate and are frequently absent. Similar experiments carried out on primary cell lines of animal or human origin, as well as primary cultures of malignant cells, yielded negative results with respect to differences in the cytoskeleton organization.

It appears that some differences in the microfilaments of established cell lines could be detected, but no differences were found in the distribution patterns of the microtubules of these cells (Asch *et al.*, 1978). Further studies are needed to determine the significance of these results with respect to the cancer problem in general and human neoplasia in particular.

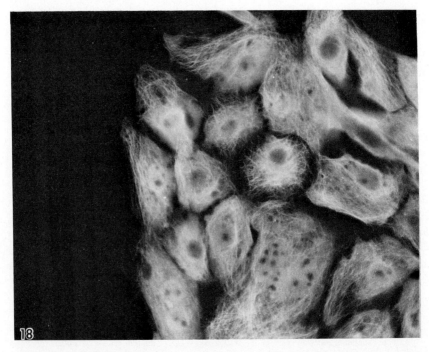

Fig. 18. 3T3 cells grown *in vitro* and treated with antitubulin antibodies to show the elaborate cytoskeletal structures. Some evidence was presented that transformed cells, examined in a similar fashion, do not exhibit such an organized microtubular system (see text). However, recent data suggest that important factors other than cell transformation may affect the cytoskeletal architecture. × 1150. (Courtesy of Dr. Dan Medina, Baylor College of Medicine, Houston, Texas.)

V. SUMMARY

A variety of morphologic alterations have been shown to be associated with maligancies, including changes in nucleoli, nuclei, chromatin, karyotypes, and cytoplasmic structures. However, no single pathognomonic characteristic has been detected. Rather, a panoply of morphologic changes are noted simultaneously. These reflect the many biochemical processes which occur during malignant transformation and are essential for the histopathological diagnosis of malignancy. As the biochemistry of malignancy is better understood and novel microscopic approaches are developed, pathognomonic differences may be detected allowing more precise diagnosis and contribute to a understanding of the malignant process.

ACKNOWLEDGMENTS

Research supported by Grant CA-10893-P5 from the U.S. Department of Health, Education and Welfare and by Veterans Administration Pathology Research.

REFERENCES

Abercombie, M. (1961). *Proc. Can. Cancer Res. Conf.* **4**, 110.
Abercombie, M., and Ambrose, E. J. (1962). *Cancer Res.* **22**, 525–548.
Asch, B. B., Medina, D., Mace, M. L., and Brinkley, B. R. (1978). *J. Cell Biol.* **79**, Part 2, No. CS271.
Babai, F., and Tremblay, G. (1972). *Cancer Res.* **32**, 2765–2770.
Bernhard, W., and Greenboulan, N. (1963). *Exp. Cell Res., Suppl.* **9**, 19–53.
Bouteille, M., Laval, M., and Dupui-Coin, A. M. (1974). *In* "The Cell Nucleus" (H. Busch, ed.), pp. 5–64. Academic Press, New York.
Brinkley, B. R., Fuller, G. M., and Highfield, D. P. (1975). *Proc. Natl. Acad. Sci. U.S.A.* **72**, 4981–4985.
Brinkley, B. R., Miller, C. L., Fuseler, G. W., Pepper, D. A., and Wible, L. J. (1978). *In* "Cell Differentiation and Neoplasia" (G. Saunders, ed.), p. 419. Raven Press, New York.
Busch, H., and Smetana, K. (1970). "The Nucleolus." Academic Press, New York.
Busch, H., and Smetana, K. (1973). *In* "The Molecular Biology of Cancer" (H. Busch, ed.), pp. 41–80. Academic Press, New York.
Buttner, D. W., and Horstmann, E. (1967). *Z. Zellforsch. Mikrosk. Anat.* **77**, 589–605.
Carter, R. L. (1976). *In* "Scientific Foundations of Oncology" (T. Symington, and R. L. Carter, eds.), p. 172. Yearbook Publ., Chicago, Illinois.
Daskal, Y., and Crooke, S. T. (1979). *In* "Mitomycin C Current Status and New Developments" (S. K. Carter, and S. T. Crooke, eds.), pp. 41–60. Academic Press, New York.
Daskal, Y., Merski, J. A., Hughes, J. B., and Busch, H. (1975). *Exp. Cell Res.* **93**, 395–401.
Daskal, Y., Györkey, F., Györkey, P., and Busch, H. (1976). *Cancer Res.* **36**, 1267–1272.
Daskal, Y., Woodard, C., Crooke S. T., and Busch H. (1978). *Cancer Res.* **38**, 467–473.
De-The, G-Riviere, M., and Bernhard, W. (1960). *Bull. Cancer* **47**, 509.
Edelman, G. M. (1976). *Science* **192**, 218–226.

Edelman, G. M., and Yahara, I. (1976). *Proc. Natl. Acad. Sci. U.S.A.* **73**, 20–47.

Ferreira, A. E. M. (1941). *J. Lab. Clin. Med.* **26**, 1612–1628.

Fonte, W., and Porter, K. R. (1975). *Electron Microsc., Proc. Int. Cong. 8th, 1974* p. 334.

Franke, W. W., and Scheer, U. (1974). *In* "The Cell Nucleus" (H. Busch, ed.), p. 291. Academic Press, New York.

Frenster, J. H. (1974). *In* "The Cell Nucleus" (H. Busch, ed.), pp. 565–580. Academic Press, New York.

Fuller, G. M., and Brinkley, B. R. (1976). *J. Supramol. Struct.* **5**, 497–514.

Gabbiani, G., Csank, B. J., Schneeberger, J. C., Kapanci, Y., Frenchev, P., and Holborow, E. J. (1976). *Am. J. Pathol.* **83**, 457–474.

Ghadially, F. N. (1975). "The Ultrastructural Pathology of the Cell." Buttersworth, London.

Goessens, G. (1976). *Exp. Cell Res.* **100**, 88–94.

Greenstein, J. P. (1954). "Biochemistry of Cancer." Academic Press, New York.

Gyorkey, F., Min, K. W., Krisko, I., and Györkey, P. (1975). *Hum. Pathol.* **6**, 421–444.

Hale, A., Winkelhake, J., and Wever, M. (1975). *J. Cell Biol.* **64**, 398–407.

Heine, U., Sverak, L., Kondratic, J., and Bonar, R. A. (1971). *J. Ultrastruct. Res.* **34**, 375–396.

Luse, S. (1961). *Prog. Exp. Tumor Res.* **2**, 1–35.

McCarthy, W. C., and Haumeder, E. (1934). *Am. J. Cancer* **20**, 403–407.

McNutt, N. S., Cult, L. A., and Black, P. H. (1973). *J. Cell Biol.* **56**, 412–428.

Malech, H. L., and Lentz, T. L. (1974). *J. Cell Biol.* **60**, 473–482.

Miller, C. L., Fuseler, J. W., and Brinkley, B. R. (1977). *Cell Biol.* **12**, 319.

Monneron, A., and Bernhard, W. (1969). *J. Ultrastruct. Res.* **27**, 266–288.

Murad, T. M., and Scarpelli, D. G. (1967). *Am. J. Pathol.* **50**, 335–345.

Norton, W. N., Daskal, Y., Savage, H. E., Seibert, R. A., Busch, H., and Lane, M. (1977). *Virchows. Arch. B.* **23**, 353–361.

Oberling, C. H., and Bernhard, W. (1961). *In* "The Cell" (J. Brachet, and A. E. Mirsk, eds.), Vol. 5, p. 405. Academic Press, New York.

Penman, S. (1966). *J. Mol. Biol.* **17**, 117–130.

Perry, R. P. (1966). *Natl. Cancer Inst., Monogr.* **23**, 527–546.

Petrov, P., and Sekeris, C. E. (1971). *Exp. Cell Res.* **69**, 393–401.

Pianese, G. (1896). *Zieglers Beitr.* **142**, Suppl. 1.

Pollack, R., Ofborn, M., and Weber, K. (1975). *Proc. Natl. Acad. Sci. U.S.A.* **72**, 994–998.

Porter, K. R. (1966). *In* "Principles of Biomolecular Organization" (G. E. Wolstenholme, and M. O'Conner, eds.), p. 308. Little, Brown, Boston, Massachusetts.

Reddy, J., and Svoboda, D. (1968). *Lab. Invest.* **19**, 132–145.

Schenk, P. (1974). *Z. Krebsforsch.* **84**, 241.

Smetana, K., Gyorkey, P., and Busch, H. (1970). *Exp. Cell Res.* **60**, 1600–1603.

Swift, H. (1959). *Symp. Mol. Biol.* pp. 266–303.

Unuma, T., and Busch, H. (1967). *Cancer Res.* 1232–1242.

Warner, J. R., Girard, M., Latham, H., and Darnell, J. E. (1966). *J. Mol. Biol.* **19**, 373–382.

Watson, M. L. (1962). *J. Cell Biol.* **13**, 162–167.

Wetzel, B. (1976). *IITRI Proc. Scanning Electron Microsc.* Part II, p. 136.

Yasuzumi, F., Hyo, Y., Hoshiya, T., and Yasuzumi, F. (1976). *Cancer Res.* **36**, 3574–3577.

Young, J. S. (1959). *J. Pathol. Bacteriol.* **77**, 321–339.

Part II
Carcinogenesis

7

MOLECULAR AND CELLULAR MECHANISMS OF CHEMICAL CARCINOGENESIS

I. Bernard Weinstein

I. INTRODUCTION AND HISTORICAL BACKGROUND

Recent laboratory and epidemiologic studies provide evidence that the majority of human cancers are due to exposure to exogenous or environmental factors rather than inborn or genetic factors. This is an extremely optimistic message in terms of cancer prevention, since it implies that in theory the majority of human cancers could be prevented by appropriate modifications of the human environment including our personal habits and diet. To proceed intelligently in this important area of cancer prevention, however, we must understand certain basic principles about the cellular and molecular mechanisms of chemical carcinogenesis. This understanding has particular importance in terms of designing reliable short-term laboratory tests for predicting which chemicals in our complex environment might be associated with human cancer causation. This chapter will review the current status of our knowledge on basic mechanisms of chemical carcinogenesis. In addition, we will discuss the interaction between multiple

CANCER AND CHEMOTHERAPY, VOL. I

factors in the carcinogenic process and, finally, the current status of short-term tests for monitoring potential environmental carcinogens.

This field recently celebrated, so to speak, its bicentennial. Approximately 200 years ago a British surgeon, Sir Percival Pott, made the first observation linking an environmental factor, in this case occupational hazard, to the causation of human cancer (Pott, 1775). Sir Percival observed that chimney sweepers in England in the eighteenth century were at risk of developing a high incidence of cancer of the skin, specifically, the skin of the scrotum. Sir Percival reasoned that the soot, which lodged in their trousers, must be a carcinogen. This is one of the earliest associations between an environmental or occupational chemical factor and cancer causation. Curiously, the field lay dormant for about 150 years until two Japanese investigators Yamagiwa and Ichikawa (1918), described the first experimental induction of cancer by chemicals. They discovered that if they repeatedly painted coal tar (the type of material Percival Pott had implicated in human cancer causation) on the skin of rabbit ears then, after several months, these animals developed skin cancer. This approach also provided the first bioassay for chemical carcinogens, and it opened the field to experimental studies. As a matter of fact, until recently, our bioassays have not differed appreciably from that used by these early investigators. Even today the most reliable assay for a chemical carcinogen is to determine whether the compound when applied to the skin or fed orally to experimental animals induces cancer.

Yamagiwa and Ichikawa succeeded for several important reasons. First, they found that repeated rather than single applications of the material was required; second, that there was a long lag between the exposure of the skin to the carcinogen and the appearance of skin tumors; and third, it was essential to employ a susceptible host and tissue. We will emphasize these three themes during our subsequent discussion.

Since the skin painting procedure provided a bioassay it became possible to isolate chemical compounds and identify the actual chemical carcinogens. In the 1930s a British group, led by Kennaway, fractionated coal tar and succeeded in isolating a series of highly active pure chemicals which were polycyclic aromatic hydrocarbons (Haddow, 1974). A typical representative of this group is the compound benzo(a)pyrene (Fig. 1). It is now known that this compound is widely distributed in the human environment and that it can induce tumors in several species and tissues (Boyland, 1950; Committee on Biologic Effects of Atmospheric Pollutants, 1972).

II. DIVERSITY OF CHEMICAL CARCINOGENS

Table I lists chemicals or industrial processes which are currently recognized as human carcinogens (Heidelberger, 1975; Tomatis *et al.*, 1978). Obviously,

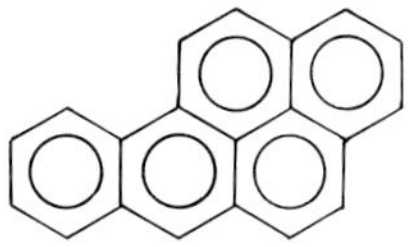

Benzo(*a*)pyrene

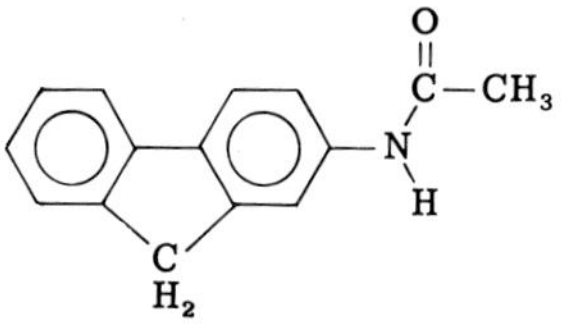

2-Acetylaminofluorene
(*N*-2-fluorenylacetamide)

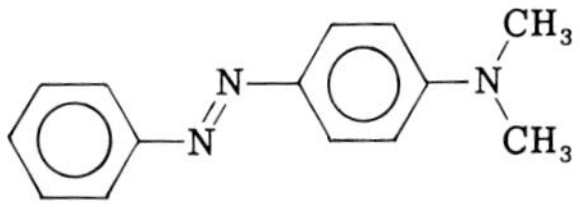

N,*N*-Dimethyl-4-
aminoazobenzene

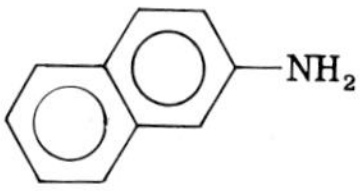

2-Naphthylamine

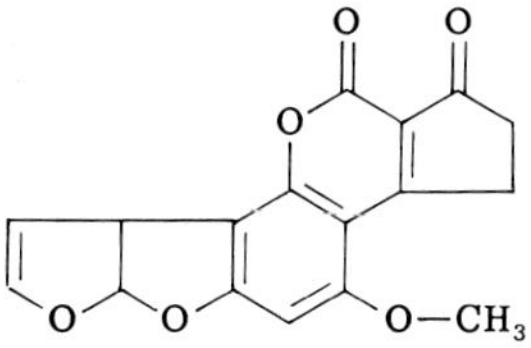

Aflatoxin B$_1$

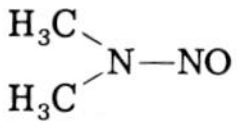

Dimethylnitrosamine

BeO

Beryllium oxide

$H_2C = CHCl$

Vinyl chloride

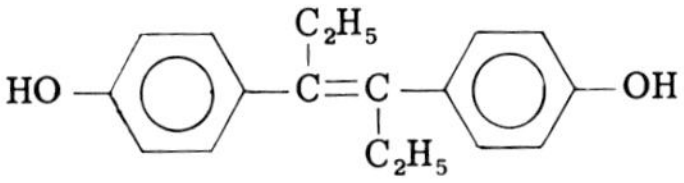

Diethylstilbestrol

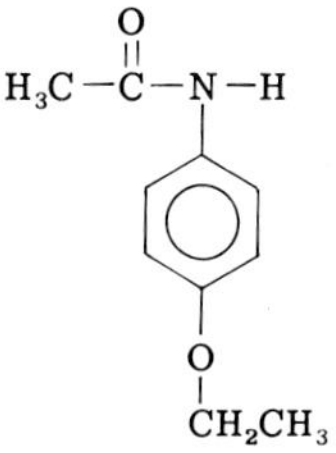

Phenacetin

Fig. 1. Chemical structures of certain types of carcinogens.

TABLE I

Chemicals Recognized as Carcinogens in Humans[a]

Chemical	Site of cancers
Chemical mixtures	
Soots, tars, oils	Skin, lungs
Cigarette smoke	Lungs
Industrial chemicals	
2-Naphthylamine	Urinary bladder
Benzidine	Urinary bladder
4-Aminobiphenyl	Urinary bladder
Chloromethyl methyl ether	Lungs
Nickel compounds	Lungs, nasal sinuses
Chromium compounds	Lungs
Asbestos	Lungs
Arsenic compounds	Skin, lungs
Vinyl chloride	Liver
Drugs	
N,N-bis(2-chloroethyl)-2-naphthylamine	Urinary bladder
Bis(2-chloroethyl)sulfide (mustard gas)	Lungs
Diethylstilbestrol	Vagina
Phenacetin	Renal pelvis
Birth control pill	Benign hepatomas
Naturally occurring compounds	
Betel nuts	Buccal mucosa
Aflatoxins	Liver
Potent carcinogens in animals	
to which human populations are exposed	
Sterigmatocystin	Liver
Cycasin	Liver
Safrole	Liver
Pyrrolizidine alkaloids	Liver
Nitroso compounds	Esophagus, liver, kidney, stomach

[a] Modified from Heidelberger (1975); also see Tomatis *et al.* (1978).

many human carcinogens have not yet been identified. Several aspects of the current list bear emphasis. The first is that these compounds come from highly diverse sources; a second is that in several cases the carcinogenic substance is a chemical mixture. A good example of the latter is cigarette smoke, which contains a number of compounds which when individually tested are carcinogenic in experimental animals, Benzo(*a*)pyrene is one of these, but there are many other types of carcinogens in this complex mixture. Another aspect is that an important source of some of these chemicals are industrial processes, an example of this is 2-naphthylamine. It was recognized several decades ago that workers exposed to this material developed a high incidence of bladder cancer. There are also rather simple carcinogenic substances, such as nickel and chromium compounds. Workers in the smelting industry are at high risk of developing cancer when there is excessive exposure to these materials. There are also asbestos fibers which one would think are relatively inert, yet exposure to them is now known to be associated with certain forms of cancer.

Another very important class of carcinogens is therapeutic drugs (Table II). An example is diethylstilbestrol, a synthetic estrogen which is known to be associated with the induction of human cancer via the transplacental route. It is particularly important that physicians be aware of the fact that several therapeutic drugs are carcinogenic in experimental animals (Hoover and Fraumeni, 1975; Schmähl et al., 1977; Clayson and Shubik, 1976). When prescribing medication for patients, physicians must carefully weigh benefits versus risks, and we must maintain constant surveillance to be certain that the drugs used are not human carcinogens. With the increasing use of long-term therapy in the treatment of chronic diseases, for example, hypertension, this aspect takes on increasing importance.

A final and very important category of carcinogens is naturally occurring

TABLE II

Examples of Diagnostic and Therapeutic Agents with Known or Suspected Carcinogenic Activity in Animals or Humans[a]

Adriamycin
Alkylating agents: chlornaphazin, cyclophosphamide
Androgens
Arsenicals (inorganic)
Dapsone
Diethylstilbestrol
Diphenylhydantoin (Dilantin)
Drugs as precursors of nitrosamines
Estrogens and oral contraceptives
Griseofulvin
Hycanthone
Hydrazines
Isonicotinic acid hydrazide
Metronidazole (Flagyl), and other nitro-heterocycles
Nitrofurans: FANFT {N-[4-(5-nitro-2-furyl)-2-thiazolyl]formamide}
Phenacetin
Phenylbutazone
Radiation: X ray and UV
Reserpine
Tars
Thorotrast

[a] For additional details see Tomatis et al., 1978; Hoover and Fraumeni, 1975; Schmähl et al., 1977; Hiatt et al., 1977; Clayson and Shubik, 1976.

compounds. An example is aflatoxin B_1, the product of a mold which frequently contaminates peanuts, cereals, and grains. It appears to contribute to the high incidence of liver cancer in certain parts of Africa. Thus, there are both man-made or synthetic chemicals as well as naturally occurring carcinogens, such as aflatoxin. As a matter of fact, aflatoxin is the most potent carcinogen known in any experimental animal system. There is increasing awareness of the fact that certain plant and fungal products and certain cooking and food preservation practices may generate carcinogenic substances. Highly potent mutagens have recently been identified in pyrolysis products of certain amino acids (Sugimura *et al.*, 1977).

Not all carcinogens are products of the modern chemical industry. The relative roles of naturally occurring substances, dietary habits, habits related to life-style, and occupational and industrial exposures in the causation of human cancers requires further study.

The broad diversity in chemical structure of the known carcinogens is a major theme in the field of chemical carcinogenesis. It would be relatively easy if it turned out that all carcinogens belonged to a particular class of chemical substances, for example, the polycyclic aromatic hydrocarbons. If this were the case then one could readily identify potential new carcinogens by simply examining their chemical structure and properties. In addition, if one understood the mechanism of action of this class of compounds in biologic systems, one might understand the entire process of chemical carcinogenesis. Unfortunately, the field is much more complex because we are dealing with compounds of diverse structure and because, as will be emphasized later, some compounds may act via different mechanisms or via different stages in the carcinogenic process.

Figure 1 presents chemical structures representative of some of the known types of carcinogens. The polycyclic aromatic hydrocarbon benzo(a)pyrene is carcinogenic in several species and tissues. This compound is representative of a large class of polycyclic aromatic hydrocarbons that are produced during the process of pyrolysis of fossil fuels and other materials. These compounds are present in cigarette smoke, automobile emissions, factory fumes, charcoal broiled meat, etc. N-2-Acetylaminofluorine, an aromatic amine, was originally synthesized as a potential insecticide, but was found to induce liver tumors in animals. It is not marketed, but is a very useful experimental compound in laboratory studies. Dimethylaminoazobenzene is representative of a number of azo compounds, dye stuffs and coloring agents, that may have carcinogenic potential.

The compound dimethylnitrosamine can be formed in the body by the reaction of sodium nitrite with secondary amines. Nitrosamines are potent carcinogens in a variety of experimental animals. Thus, there is considerable concern about the use of sodium nitrate and sodium nitrite as food preservatives.

Diethylstilbestrol is a synthetic estrogen which has produced tumors in a variety of species, including vaginal carcinoma in young women whose mothers were given the compound during pregnancy. The latter example illustrates the phenomenon of transplacental carcinogenesis, which is also well established in experimental animals. In searching out causes of human cancer we must be concerned, therefore, not only with exposure during extrauterine life but also exposure during intrauterine development. In view of the unusual susceptibility of the fetus, and of the young to carcinogens, we must be particularly concerned about protection of pregnant women from carcinogens that might be present in the diet, medication, cosmetics (for example, hair dyes), workplace, etc.

Chlorinated aliphatic compounds, such as vinyl chloride and carbon tetrachloride, as well as chlorinated cyclic compounds, such as polychlorinated biphenyl (PCB), are widely distributed in our environment. Several of these compounds have induced tumors in experimental animals, and workers exposed to vinyl chloride have developed angiosarcomas of the liver. The widespread occurrence of some of these compounds as pollutants in the environment and their limited biodegradeability is a source of increasing concern. The chemical structures shown in Fig. 1 are only a few of the known carcinogens. They further document the theme of chemical diversity of carcinogens.

III. EPIDEMIOLOGIC EVIDENCE

Within the past two decades there has been increasing evidence that a major fraction (perhaps 50–80%) of human cancers are due to exogenous environmental factors rather than endogenous hereditary factors (Hiatt *et al.*, 1977). There are several lines of evidence for this conclusion. The first has to do with worldwide studies on the incidence of specific forms of cancer in different countries. An example is shown in Fig. 2 which compares the mortality for colon cancer in different parts of the world (Levin *et al.*, 1974). The variations are striking. In Japan the incidence is quite low, whereas in the United States it is quite high. As a matter of fact, in the United States cancer of the colon and rectum is the major form of cancer. On the other hand, in Japan there is a high incidence of gastric cancer, whereas in the United States gastric cancer occurs at a much lower incidence. Studies done on migrant populations have indicated that when the Japanese leave Japan and move either to Hawaii or the United States, within one or two generations they acquire a high incidence of cancer of the colon and low incidence of stomach cancer, even though they continue to marry Japanese (Hiatt *et al.*, 1977). These results provide evidence that cancer of the colon and stomach are largely due to exogenous factors and not to genetic or heredity factors.

A second type of evidence relates to time trends. Figure 3 indicates that during the past several decades there has been a dramatic decrease in the incidence of

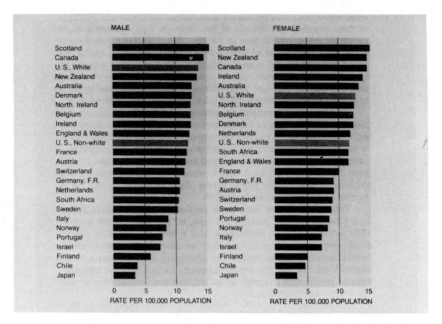

Fig. 2. Age-adjusted mortality rates for malignant neoplasms of the intestine (excluding rectum) in various countries, 1966–1967. (From Levin *et al.*, 1974.)

stomach cancer in United States males (Levin *et al.*, 1974). On the other hand, there has been a shocking increase in lung cancer (Levin *et al.*, 1974). In 1930 lung cancer was a relatively rare disease. Today, it is the most prevalent cancer in the American male, and it is increasing rapidly in the American female. The genetic composition of the human species could not have changed significantly in the past few decades, yet the types of cancer that we suffer have changed dramatically. It is not known what change in environmental factors led to the reduction in stomach cancer in the United States population, although changes in the method of food preservation have been suggested. There is overwhelming evidence that the current epidemic in lung cancer is largely due to cigarette smoking. It is of interest that during the same time period there has been little variation in the overall incidence and mortality rates of colon or breast cancer in the United States. This suggests that these cancers relate to factors that have been present in our environment for at least several decades, such as dietary factors, rather than recently introduced synthetic chemicals or changes in lifestyle.

It would be remiss not to dwell on the problem of cigarette smoking. Figure 4 compares the annual per capita consumption, and the annual mortality from lung cancer per 100,000 population from the period 1930–1970 (Cairns, 1975). Cigarette smoking was not a prevalent habit until the early 1900s. Since then there has been a marked increase in cigarette consumption, and this has been paralleled

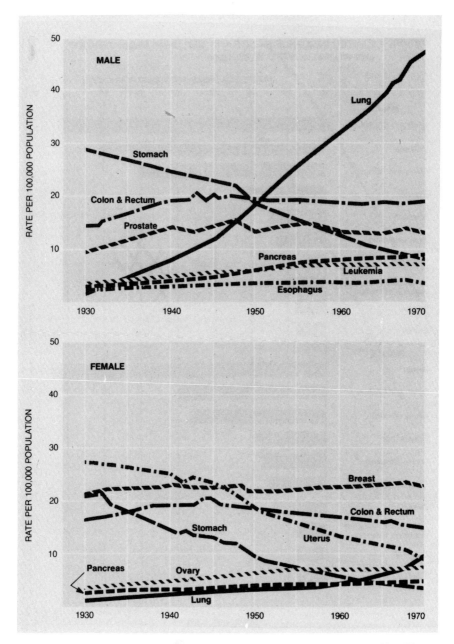

Fig. 3. Time trends in cancer mortality rates by site and sex: United States 1930–1970 (age adjusted to United States 1940 population). (From Levin *et al.*, 1974.)

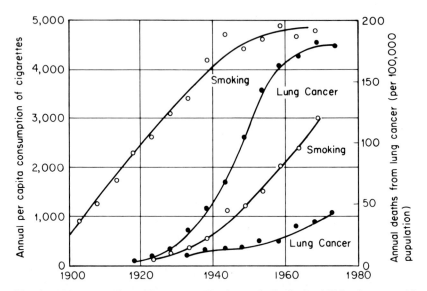

Fig. 4. Cigarette smoking and lung cancer. The data are for England and Wales. In men smoking began to increase at the beginning of the twentieth century, but the corresponding trend in deaths from lung cancer did not begin until after 1920. In women smoking began later, and lung cancers are only now appearing. From "Cancer: Science and Society" by John Cairns. W. H. Freeman and Company. Copyright © 1978.

with a striking increase in lung cancer. There is a distinct lag of approximately two decades between the two curves. This lag between exposure and the occurrence of cancer is characteristic for a number of carcinogens. The first set of curves describes the situation in males; the second set in females. American females took up the cigarette habit later than males, but cigarette consumption is now rapidly increasing in females and (as unfortunately predicted) within a lag of one or two decades, lung cancer is now increasing in the American female population. As a matter of fact, it is increasing at a shocking rate, 8% per year. In the American male it is increasing at a rate of 1% per year. Cigarette smoking is thus a major health problem, accounting for 20 to 30% of all human cancers in the United States. In addition it is associated with an increased risk of cardiovascular and pulmonary diseases. Impaired fetal development can also occur when pregnant women smoke cigarettes.

IV. BASIC BIOLOGIC AND BIOCHEMICAL PRINCIPLES OF CARCINOGENESIS

Table III lists the major biologic principles pertaining to chemical (and radiation) carcinogenesis. In terms of human exposure it is important to emphasize the

TABLE III

Chemical Carcinogens—Basic Biologic Facts[a]

1. Carcinogenesis is *dose dependent*—the larger the dose the greater the incidence of tumors and the shorter the lag. There is no evidence of a *threshold dose* below which a carcinogen is safe.
2. There is a *long lag* between exposure and the appearance of tumors. In humans this is about 5–30 years. In various species the lag is generally proportional to the lifespan of the species. Carcinogens can act transplacentally, with tumors appearing only later in the adult progeny.
3. Conversion of a normal tissue to a malignant neoplasm is a *multistep process*.
4. The action of certain types of carcinogens, so-called *initiating agents,* is markedly enhanced by *promoting agents, hormonal agents,* and various *cofactors*.
5. Cellular *proliferation enhances* carcinogenesis.
6. Neoplasms induced by the same chemical carcinogen often display *antigenic diversity,* as well as a general *diversity of phenotypes* in terms of growth rate, degree of differentiation, cell surface properties, enzyme profiles, etc.

[a] See Weinstein (1976).

apparent lack of a threshold, the increasing incidence with increasing dose, and the long lag between exposure and the appearance of tumors. These principles are well illustrated in the case of cigarette smoking and lung cancer (see Section III and Fig. 4), the lag in the occurrence of leukemias (and even longer lag for carcinomas) in Hiroshima survivors, the occurrence of cancers in patients following radiation for therapeutic or diagnostic purposes, and various occupationally related cancers. The multistep nature of the process appears to be largely the explanation for the lag. This and the role of promoting agents and other cofactors will be discussed later in this chapter. The diversity in phenotypes between individual tumors, even those produced by a pure carcinogen in the same tissue in inbred species, is a puzzling aspect in terms of the biology of cancer. It suggests that there is a certain degree of randomness in the carcinogenic process. A similar diversity of phenotypes is also seen in tissue culture when one compares individual clones of transformed cells. This diversity has thwarted efforts to identify a single biochemical or immunologic characteristic that might provide a universal marker for the detection of cancers or one that might be used as a target or strategy in cancer therapy.

Table IV lists several basic facts related to the biochemistry of carcinogens. The major concepts presented in Table IV are those of metabolic activation and covalent binding to cellular macromolecules. It is now clear that many environmental carcinogens are not active as such, but require metabolic activation, that is, conversion to highly reactive electrophilic species which can then react with nucleophilic residues in cellular macromolecules (proteins and nucleic acids) to form covalent adducts (Miller, 1978).

TABLE IV

Chemical Carcinogens—Basic Biochemical Facts[a]

---

1. They include both man-made and natural products that have extremely diverse chemical structures (see Table I).
2. They are subject to both metabolic activation and detoxification *in vivo*.
3. The metabolically activated forms are highly reactive electrophiles that bind covalently to nucleophilic residues in cellular proteins and nucleic acids.
4. The binding to protein is quantitatively greater than binding to nucleic acids and has a specific activity of about 1 residue of carcinogen per 10^3–10^4 amino acid residues. The amino acid residues are usually the S of methionine or cysteine, N-1 of histidine, or C-3 of tyrosine. Numerous proteins are attacked, both nuclear and cytoplasmic, although a few proteins (example, the "h_2"), whose specific function(s) are not known, are preferential targets.
5. Both RNA and DNA are targets and the specific activity is about 1 residue of carcinogen per 10^4–10^5 nucleoside residues. Most carcinogens bind preferentially to guanine, but adenine, cytosine, and thymine are also targets.
6. The binding to DNA is fairly random in terms of gene specificity. Both main band and satellite DNA are involved, as is mitochondrial DNA. There is some evidence for cross-linking.
7. The binding to RNA appears to involve all species of RNA; tRNA often has a higher specific activity than rRNA.

---

[a] See Weinstein (1976).

Benzo(a)pyrene well illustrates this principle (Fig. 5) (Weinstein *et al.*, 1976, 1978, 1979). The substance itself is not highly reactive chemically, and when simply mixed with nucleic acids or proteins it will not bind to them covalently. However, the endoplasmic reticulum obtained from a variety of tissues and species, including humans, contains a group of enzymes, the so-called P-450 system or aryl hydrocarbon hydroxylase (AHH) system, which converts benzo(a)pyrene to a variety of derivatives, including phenols and dihydrodiols. The intermediates in this oxidative process are epoxides which are subsequently hydrated by an enzyme epoxide hydrase. The normal role of this system is to convert lipid-soluble substances to more water-soluble substances which can be excreted. In other words, it functions as a detoxification pathway. In a sense, carcinogenesis can be thought of as an error in drug detoxification. On the way to being detoxified, highly reactive intermediates such as benzo(a)pyrene dihydrodiol-epoxide can accumulate, and, unless further metabolized, will react with cellular nucleic acids to form covalent adducts, thereby disrupting macromolecular synthesis and function.

The pathway shown in Fig. 5 interacts with a variety of other biochemical pathways and indirectly with many aspects of intermediatary metabolism. Cellular levels of nicotinamide adenine dinucleotide phosphate (NADPH), flavine cofactors, glutathione, and other factors impinge on the function of this system.

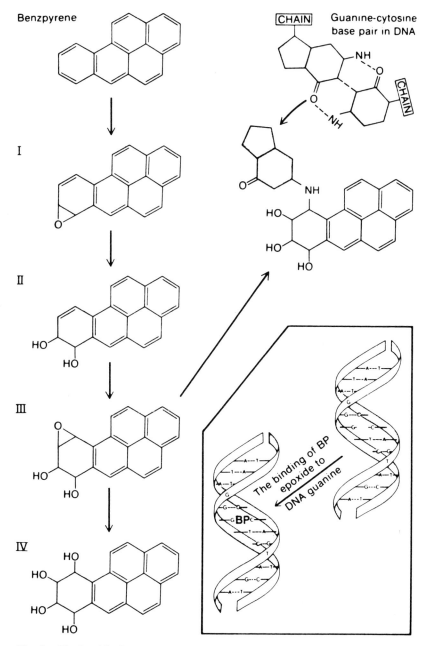

Fig. 5. The detoxification and metabolic activation of benzo(*a*)pyrene. The detoxification of the carcinogen benzo(*a*)pyrene (BP) goes through several steps, as it is made more water-soluble prior to excretion. One of the intermediates in this process (III) is capable of reacting with guanine in DNA (as shown in the diagram). This leads to a distortion in the structure and function of the DNA molecule. (From Cairns, 1978.)

The enzymes in this pathway are also induced by their substrates and by a variety of drugs. Considerable genetic variation as well as tissue–tissue variation exist in the inducibility and absolute levels of these enzymes. Thus, the host's genetic background, previous exposure history, nutritional status, parallel exposure to other agents, and tissue-specific factors will influence the likelihood that benzo(a)pyrene will flow through this pathway and attack cellular macromolecules or alternatively will be detoxified and excreted so that it is not carcinogenic.

V. CARCINOGEN MODIFICATION OF NUCLEIC ACIDS—STRUCTURAL AND FUNCTIONAL CHANGES

Recent studies indicate that the critical metabolite of benzo(a)pyrene is not a simple epoxide but a dihydrodiol epoxide with the structure shown in Fig. 5 (Weinstein *et al.*, 1976, 1978). It results from the oxidation of the 7,8-positions to an epoxide, conversion of this to the corresponding dihydrodiol and then further oxidation to yield the 7,8-dihydrodiol 9,10-oxide. A specific isomer of the latter compound has been demonstrated to be highly mutagenic, to transform cells in culture, to react with nucleic acids *in vitro* and to be carcinogenic in the intact animal.

The complete chemical structure of the adduct formed between benzo(a)pyrene dihydrodiol epoxide and nucleic acids has also been elucidated (Fig. 5) (Weinstein *et al.*, 1976, 1978; Jeffrey *et al.*, 1976). The major derivative consists of a guanine residue linked via its 2-amino group to the 10-position of benzo(a)pyrene. There is evidence that this structure is the major benzo(a)pyrene–nucleoside adduct present in both rodent and human cells after exposure to the parent compound benzo(a)pyrene (Weinstein *et al.*, 1976, 1979; Brown *et al.*, 1979).

The complete structures of nucleic acid adducts formed by several other carcinogens have also been elucidated (Miller, 1978; Weinstein, 1977, 1978). Several carcinogens are methylating or ethylating agents. For example, dimethylnitrosamine results in the methylation of nitrogen and oxygen atoms in nucleic acid nucleosides, and the formation of phosphotriesters. Current evidence suggests that alkylation of the O^6-position of guanine by methylating or ethylating agents is the critical modification with respect to mutagenesis and carcinogenesis. Because the O^6-position is involved in hydrogen bonding in Watson–Crick base pairing, alkylation of O^6 would interfere with hydrogen bonding and produce base-pairing errors during nucleic acid replication.

The situation with the considerably larger polycyclic carcinogens is more complex, as illustrated by the aromatic amine carcinogen N-2-acetylaminofluorene (AAF) which, like benzo(a)pyrene, undergoes metabolic activation (Fig. 1). Activation of AAF occurs on the amino group, and the major nucleic acid adduct involves linkage to the C-8 position of guanine residues. This presents steric, or space-filling, problems in terms of accommodating the bulky AAF residue within the nucleic acid helix. Therefore, conformational distortions in the DNA double-stranded structure occur at sites of AAF modification. For AAF to attack the C-8 position of the guanine residue, the guanine must rotate around its glycoside bond and slip out of the double-stranded helix. The planar carcinogen then binds to guanine and becomes inserted into the helix, occupying the former position of the displaced guanine, so that it now lies coplanar to the next adjacent base. We have termed this altered conformation "base displacement" (Weinstein and Grunberger, 1974; Grunberger and Weinstein, 1976). More recent studies have furnished evidence that the conformation of nucleic acids at sites of modification by benzo(a)pyrene differs from that with AAF. It appears that the benzo(a)pyrene residue covalently bound to guanine is not coplanar to the next adjacent base but lies outside the DNA helix, probably in the minor groove of the helix (Pulkrabek et al., 1977; Weinstein et al., 1979).

How would base displacement affect Watson–Crick base pairing? If the AAF-modified strand of DNA is called upon to serve as a template for DNA or RNA synthesis, when replication reaches the site of AAF modification there will be no guanine residue in the appropriate position for base pairing. Because the AAF residue cannot base-pair, the replication mechanism would stop or skip this position and move on. If the latter occurs, the newly replicated daughter strand will lack a base in the corresponding position. This prediction is fulfilled in that AAF and related compounds are potent frameshift mutagens in the Ames *Salmonella typhimurium* mutagenesis assay. *In vitro* studies also provide evidence that AAF and BP modified nucleic acids are impaired in their template activities (Weinstein et al., 1976, 1978; Weinstein and Grunberger, 1974; Grunberger and Weinstein, 1976; Hsu et al., 1977).

The effects of carcinogen modification of nucleic acids on macromolecular synthesis are summarized in Table V. Fortunately, nature has evolved highly efficient mechanisms so that the damage to DNA produced by radiation and carcinogens is not a *fait accompli* [for review of DNA repair, see Hanawalt et al. (1978)]. Complex enzyme systems can recognize damaged regions of DNA and excise and then repair them. Distortions in the three-dimensional structure of DNA produced by carcinogens are recognized by appropriate nucleases that then excise the modified regions and acjacent bases, after which a DNA polymerase using the intact complementary strand as a template fills in the gap and a ligase enzyme reconnects the polynucleotide DNA chain. This type of repair is termed "excision repair" or "unscheduled DNA synthesis," and it is thought normally to function with high fidelity. The host is thus protected if excision repair occurs before replication of the damaged DNA occurs. Therefore, the extent of cell replication during the period of exposure to a carcinogen, the genetic background of the host in terms of its efficiency of repair, the presence of other agents that

TABLE V

Chemical Carcinogens—Early Effects on Macromolecular Synthesis[a]

---

1. Replication: The binding to DNA induces unscheduled DNA synthesis (excision repair). Most but not all carcinogens are mutagens. They can induce errors in base pairing, frame shift errors, deletions, and chromosomal breakage.
2. Transcription: There is an early inhibition of RNA synthesis which is somewhat preferential for the 45 S ribosomal RNA precursor. Effects on RNA processing have not been studied extensively.
3. Translation: There is often an early inhibition of protein synthesis associated with release of ribosomes bound to the endoplasmic reticulum and disaggregation of polysomes. Function of carcinogen-modified tRNA or mRNA is inhibited.
4. Regulation: Enzyme induction may be blocked. The pattern of transcription is altered, fetal genes depressed, etc. Effects on chromatin structure and function remain to be elucidated. Latent oncornaviruses may be activated.

---

[a] See Weinstein (1976).

might interfere with DNA repair, and other factors will influence the carcinogenic process. In certain forms of the human disease xeroderma pigmentosum, a hereditary defect exists in DNA repair which apparently explains the unusual susceptibility of these patients to skin cancer induced by solar radiation. Ultraviolet light produces thymine dimers and other lesions in DNA which patients with this disease fail to repair.

A second type of DNA repair mechanism, called "postreplication repair," seems prone to a high error frequency, and it has been suggested that it may also play a crucial role in mutagenesis and carcinogenesis. Current research in bacteria indicates that damage to DNA by a variety of agents can result in the induction of an "error-prone" DNA replication mechanism, as well as a highly pleiotropic response which may include activation of latent viral genomes (Hanawalt et al., 1978; Witkin, 1976). Protease(s) seems to play an important role in this process, and this phenomenon warrants intensive investigation in mammalian cell systems. A bacterial assay for potential mutagens and carcinogens called the Inductest is based on this phenomenon and is currently being evaluated as a possible predictor of carcinogens as an alternative to the Ames Salmonella typhimurium mutagenesis assay (Moreau et al., 1976).

If, as discussed above, DNA repair does not occur completely and with high fidelity, then when the carcinogen-damaged DNA replicates, errors are likely to occur in the daughter strand and mutations will occur in the daughter cell. This provides a basis for some of the short-term tests for carcinogens which assay for mutagenicity (see Table XI). Carcinogens are also known to induce aberrations in the chromosomes, and these effects are often cited as evidence for the somatic mutation theory of carcinogenesis. However, we should not close our minds to the possibility that the attack on DNA by carcinogens might produce other types of aberrations in the cell function which may play a critical role in the carcinogenic process. DNA must not only replicate but must also serve as the template for RNA synthesis. A number of laboratories have shown that DNA modification by chemical carcinogens interferes not only with DNA replication but also with RNA transcription. It is possible, therefore, that serious distortions in gene transcription and the pattern of gene expression result from carcinogen modification of cellular DNA (Weinstein, 1976; Weinstein *et al.*, 1979). In addition to binding covalently to cellular DNA, carcinogens also bind to cellular RNA and protein (Table IV). The binding to RNA interferes with its functions during translation and protein synthesis.

An area which we understand very poorly at the present time, but one which may be of key importance in carcinogenesis, is the regulation of gene expression during development and differentiation. The DNA does not exist naked in the cell, but is closely associated with histones and other chromatin-associated proteins. It is apparent that the structure of chromatin plays an important role in the control of gene transcription. Possibly distortions in chromatin structure produced by carcinogens interfere with normal chromatin functions thus impairing patterns of normal gene expression (Weinstein *et al.*, 1979).

In view of the above considerations, we must emphasize that despite the simplicity of the mutation theory of carcinogenesis, at the present time it is not clear whether chemical carcinogens cause the conversion of a normal cell to a tumor cell by (1) inducing mutations and/or chromosomal abnormalities; (2) influencing cell selection, for example, by suppressing immunologic surveillance or other host defense mechanisms; (3) activating or enhancing the activity of viruses or virus-related genes; (4) inducing aberrations in differentiation at the epigenetic level; or (5) some as yet unsuspected mechanism (Weinstein, 1976).

Table VI lists current evidence favoring either the somatic mutation or the aberrant differentiation theories of carcinogenesis (Weinstein, 1976). It is apparent that none of the current evidence is decisive. Personally, I am impressed with the broad disturbances in the control of gene expression manifested by tumors as well as the increasing number of examples demonstrating the capacity of tumor cells to "revert" to a more normal phenotype. Therefore, I favor the theory of aberrant differentiation. Hopefully, recent exciting advances in methodology in cell culture systems should facilitate elucidation of the actual mechanism of chemical carcinogenesis. The results could have profound implications in terms of both cancer prevention and treatment. If, for example, it is found that carcinogenesis is due to an aberration in differentiation and not a mutation, then there will be a sound theoretical basis for approaches to cancer therapy which include the design of agents that "reprogram" tumor cells so that they either (1) revert to a more normal growth pattern, (2) assume a growth pattern which normal host defense or tissue involution mechanisms will respond to, or (3) go into a sequence of terminal differentiation. Just to indicate that these ideas are not

TABLE VI

Evidence Favoring Somatic Mutation or Aberrant Differentiation as Mechanisms of Carcinogenesis[a]

Somatic mutation	Aberrant differentiation
1. The tumor phenotype is stable	1. Differentiation and/or commitment stable
2. Carcinogens attack DNA	2. a. Carcinogens attack RNA and protein
	b. DNA binding and carcinogenicity do not always correlate
3. Many carcinogens are mutagens	3. a. Some mutagens are not carcinogens (base analogues, hydroxylamine, acridines)
	b. Carcinogens are teratogens
	c. The efficiency of transformation in cell culture is higher than random mutation rates
4. Defective DNA repair is associated with increased tumor incidence, e.g., in xeroderma pigmentosum	4. Not all patients with xeroderma pigmentosum have the same defect in DNA repair. Cause and effect relationship is not established
	5. Tumors display broad disturbance in gene expression (hormone synthesis, fetal genes, isozymes)
	6. TS mutants, revertants, and teratomas suggest reversibility of the tumor phenotype and totipotency of the tumor cell genome

[a] See Weinstein *et al.* (1975).

without justification, I have listed in Table VII current examples of such phenomena. These examples indicate that at least certain cancer cells retain most if not all of the information present in normal cells and that under appropriate circumstances the pattern of gene expression and state of differentiation of cancer cells can be reprogrammed (Weinstein, 1976).

VI. MULTISTEP CARCINOGENESIS, TUMOR PROMOTION, AND COFACTORS

In the above discussion, we dealt largely with the early interactions between carcinogens, such as benzo(a)pyrene, and cells. The critical event in the initial encounter between these types of agents and cells appears to be metabolism and covalent binding to cellular macromolecules. Let us now consider the later steps in the carcinogenic process and the role of promoters and certain cofactors.

It is well recognized that carcinogenesis is a multistep process in its development and a multifactor process in terms of causation (Slaga *et al.,* 1978; Foulds,

TABLE VII

Examples of Reversion or Redifferentiation of Tumor Cells[a]

In the animal
1. Crowngall tumor (plant) grafted onto normal plant yields normal seeds
2. Lucké renal carcinoma (frog) nuclei transplanted into enucleated egg yield embryos with well-differentiated tissues
3. Anaplastic embryonal carcinoma (mouse) converts to highly differentiated teratoma
4. Teratocarcinoma cells (mouse) transferred into recipient blastocysts participate in the formation of a normal mouse
5. In endometrial carcinoma (human) progesterone induces formation of decidua and secretory glands in the tumor
6. Neuroblastoma (human) may regress or convert to ganglioneuromas
7. Hormone-induced regression of breast, prostate, and uterine cancer (human)

In cell culture
1. Reversion of virus or chemically transformed cells to "normal" cells
2. Reversible change in transformed cell phenotype in temperature-sensitive (TS) mutants
3. Differentiation of leukemia cells into macrophages and granulocytes
4. Dimethyl sulfoxide induction of hemoglobin synthesis in erythroleukemia cells
5. Induction of phenotypic reversion by cAMP, bromodeoxyuridine (BUdR), and glucocorticoids.

---

[a] See Weinstein (1976).

1969). When a tissue is exposed to a chemical carcinogen, nothing obvious may happen within the first few days, weeks, or months. After a period of time, however, hyperplasia and/or dysplasia ensue, and eventually there may be the appearance of a benign tumor. Benign tumors are tumors that do not invade and metastasize. It is of considerable interest that if one interrupts the administration of the carcinogen or uses a very low dose in certain experimental carcinogenesis systems, many of these benign tumors will regress spontaneously. On the other hand, benign tumors can progress and become fully malignant tumors which cause invasion and metastasis. (It is not always clear, however, that malignant tumors arise from preexistent benign tumors).

From a clinical point of view, malignant tumors are the most serious lesions because they are not readily amenable to surgery or radiotherapy. Thus, an understanding of these later steps, particularly those responsible for the development of a malignant metastasizing tumor, are extremely important. What factors influence the transistion from normal to benign and from benign to malignant, and what is the cellular and biochemical basis for these steps? Our understanding of these aspects is much more limited than our understanding of the initial events in carcinogenesis, although encouraging progress is being made.

The most convenient system for demonstrating these multistep aspects is the

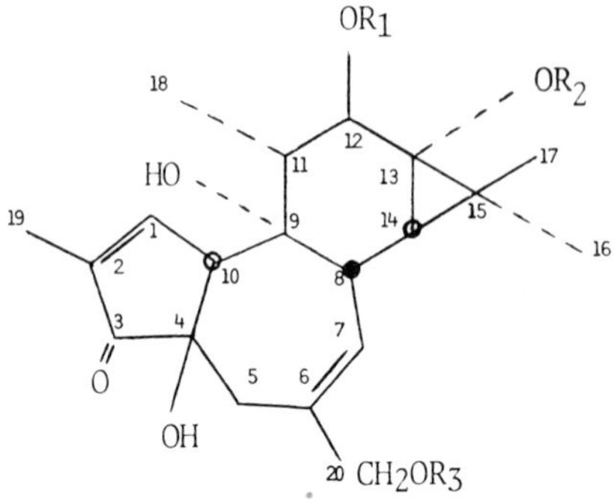

$$PHORBOL: \quad R_1 = R_2 = R_3 = H$$

$$CROTON\ OIL\ FACTOR\ A_1\,(TPA)\ :\quad R_1 = CO(CH_2)_{12}\ CH_3$$

$$R_2 = COCH_3:\ R_3 = H$$

Fig. 6. Structure of phorbol esters. TPA is one of the most active components of croton oil as a promoter of the ''two-stage'' mouse carcinogenesis assay.

two-stage mouse skin carcinogenesis system (Slaga *et al.*, 1978; Berenblum, 1975). It is known that if one applies to mouse skin a small dose of a carcinogen, e.g., benzo(*a*)pyrene, it binds to DNA as described above but no tumors occur. If one follows this with the repeated application of a tumor-promoting agent, such as phorbol ester (Fig. 6), then tumors occur. One can delay the addition of the promoting agent for many months after exposure of the tissue to the initiating carcinogen and still tumors will occur; thus, there is a long-term memory of the initiating event. The promoting agents themselves produce no or only few tumors, and they must be applied after and not before the initiating agent. These and other characteristics of initiating and promoting agents are summarized in Table VIII. For recent reviews on tumor promotion the reader is referred to Weinstein *et al.* (1979), Slaga *et al.* (1978), Berenblum (1975), Van Duuren (1969), and Boutwell (1974).

Recent studies in tissue culture have revealed certain remarkable biologic properties of the phorbol esters (Weinstein *et al.*, 1979). It has been found that when added to normal cell cultures, these agents induce a series of phenotypic changes which mimic those characteristic of tumor cells. This mimicry of transformation is summarized in Table IX. It appears that these compounds have the interesting capacity to turn on some of the very same genes which are in tumor cells.

A second property of the tumor-promoting agents in tissue culture is inhibition of differentiation (Weinstein *et al.*, 1979). Examples of this effect are listed in

TABLE VIII

A Comparison of Biologic Properties of Initiating Agents and Promoting Agents[a]

Initiating agents	Promoting agents
1. Carcinogenic by themselves—"solitary carcinogens"	1. Not carcinogenic alone
2. Must be given before promoting agent	2. Must be given after the initiating agent
3. Single exposure is sufficient	3. Require prolonged exposure
4. Action is "irreversible" and additive	4. Action is reversible (at early age) and not additive
5. No apparent threshold	5. Probable threshold
6. Yield electrophiles—bind covalently to cell macromolecules	6. No evidence of covalent binding
7. Mutagenic	7. Not mutagenic

[a] See Weinstein *et al.* (1979).

TABLE IX

Phenotypic Effects of Phorbol Ester Tumor Promoters in Cell Culture: Mimicry of Transformation[a]

Cell surface and membrane changes
    Altered Na/K ATPase
    Altered morphology
    Increased phospholipid synthesis
    Altered fucose-glycopeptides
    Decreased LETS protein
    Increased uptake ^{32}P, ^{86}Rb, deoxyglucose
    Altered receptors
    Altered fluorescence polarization
Growth properties
    Increased saturation density
    Altered cell–cell orientation
    Decreased serum requirement
Enzymatic
    Increased plasminogen activator synthesis
    Increased ornithine decarboxylase
    Increased prostaglandin synthesis

[a] See Weinstein *et al.* (1979).

Table X. Since it appears that an important aspect of the carcinogenic process has to do with disturbances in differentiation and in the behavior of stem cells, it is likely that these effects of tumor promoters are related to their role in the carcinogenic process.

Current evidence indicates that, in contrast to initiating carcinogens, the initial site of action of the tumor promoters is the cell surface membrane (Weinstein *et al.*, 1979; Slaga *et al.*, 1978; Van Duuren, 1969). Within a few minutes after exposure to phorbol ester, cells in culture display altered cell surface morphology, altered lipid metabolism, increased nutrient uptake, and changes in the function of certain cell surface receptors (Weinstein *et al.*, 1979). Thereafter, there are effects on cytoplasmic and nuclear functions.

The mechanism by which prior exposure of a cell to an initiating carcinogen acts in concert with the promoting agent to produce a stable alteration in cellular growth and differentiation is not clear at the present time. Figure 7 stresses the possibility that an important aspect of the action of promoting agents is to disturb the normal mechanisms of stem cell differentiation. Shown schematically is the normal pattern of division of a basal cell in the adult epidermis. It would appear that each time such a stem cell divides, it gives rise to one daughter cell which remains a stem cell and another daughter cell that undergoes terminal differentiations, becomes keratinized, dies, and is sluffed. Thus, there is balanced growth; the net number of cells in the adult epidermis remains constant, but there is continuous cell division and tissue renewal. We have postulated that an important action of a tumor promoter is to block this mode of division, thus a stem cell undergoes exponential division, so that both daughter cells continue to divide exponentially. If the stem cell affected is one which has been altered by an initiating carcinogen, then this process generates a clone or small population of initiated cells. This clone of cells with its altered phenotype could then give rise to a benign and eventually a malignant tumor. I must emphasize that this is a speculative model.

TABLE X

Examples of Inhibition of Differentiation by Phorbol Ester Tumor Promoters[a]

Cell culture system	Type of differentiation
Murine erythroleukemia	Erythroid
Chicken embryo myoblasts	Myogenesis
Chicken embryo chondroblasts	Chondrogenesis
Murine 3T3	Lipocytes
Murine neuroblastoma	Neurite
Murine melanoma	Melanogenesis

[a] See Weinstein *et al.* (1979).

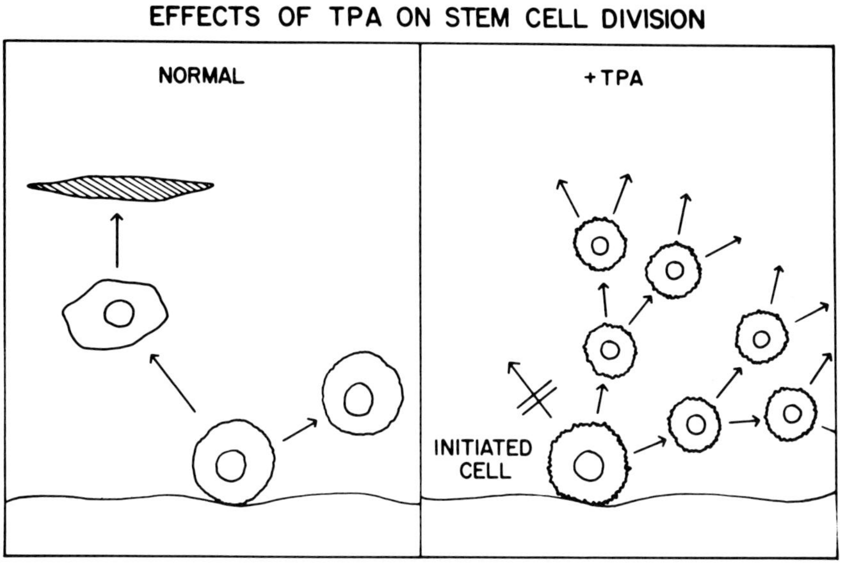

EFFECTS OF TPA ON STEM CELL DIVISION

Fig. 7. Schematic representation of the normal mode of asymmetric stem cell division in epidermis and the hypothesis that the tumor promoter TPA induces exponential growth of an initiated stem cell thus yielding a clone of such cells from which tumors can arise.

In addition to tumor promoters, there are numerous other exogenous cofactors, as well as endogenous host factors, that influence the carcinogenic process, although their mechanisms of action are poorly understood at the present time. Some of these factors may influence carcinogen metabolism or DNA repair as discussed above. Such factors may account in part for species and organ susceptibility.

In considering the roles of diverse factors in the carcinogenic process, it is important to distinguish several types of effects. Two or more agents that can act independently as carcinogens can also act together in the same host synergistically, a phenomenon termed "syncarcinogenesis" (Hecker, 1975). "Cocarcinogens" are defined as agents which do not have carcinogenic activity when assayed alone but enhance the action of carcinogens when given *simultaneously* with a known carcinogen (Van Duuren, 1969). They differ from "promoters" whose administration can be delayed until long after the carcinogen. The specific properties of promoters are best defined on mouse skin and these are listed in Table VIII.

Numerous cofactors are known, i.e., agents which do not have carcinogenic activity alone, but which can enhance the carcinogenic process. Many of these have not been sufficiently studied to know whether their action is similar to that of promoters. Various factors that contribute to the carcinogenic process include nutritional aspects (i.e., the role of dietary fat in colon and breast cancer), alcohol consumption, vitamin deficiency, age, sex, tissue regeneration, cell proliferation, and endogenous metabolic, immunologic, and genetic factors.

Hormones constitute a distinct and important class of agents in carcinogenesis. There is little evidence that they bind covalently to DNA or other cellular macromolecules. It seems more likely, therefore, that they enhance carcinogenesis by modulating gene expression, rather than by inducing damage to the genetic material. In this sense, tumor promotion on mouse skin may be similar to, or a special case of, hormonal carcinogenesis.

Both RNA and DNA viruses can interact synergistically with chemical carcinogens to enhance tumor formation *in vivo* and cell transformation in cell culture (Fisher and Weinstein, 1978; Fisher *et al.*, 1978). The known examples include viruses which on their own have oncogenic activity as well as viruses which appear to lack oncogenic activity except in concert with chemical carcinogens or radiation. There is the possibility that the high incidence of hepatomas in Asia and Africa may be due to an interaction between a chemical carcinogen such as aflatoxin and hepatitis B infection. The latter agent might act by providing a prolonged proliferative stimulus.

VII. CARCINOGEN DETECTION

Finally, let us briefly consider recent developments in the area of carcinogen detection and bioassay (Fisher and Weinstein, 1978; Hollstein *et al.*, 1979; Ames, 1979). This is a subject which one reads about almost daily in the newspapers. The recent animal studies with saccharin have, for example, raised several questions. How reliable are animal bioassay data? If tumors occur in rats given an agent at very high dose, can one simply estimate human risks by simple linear extrapolation to the lower doses to which humans are exposed. How reliable are short term *in vitro* tests, etc.?

Table XI lists the major methods used for detecting potential carcinogens. At the present time animal bioassays are the most reliable laboratory method available for determining whether chemical substances are carcinogenic, but they are expensive, cumbersome, and time consuming. To obtain significant results, large numbers of animals must be used, and they must be studied for their entire lifetime. With the thousands of compounds that must be assayed, animal bioassays are not sufficient to handle the task of surveillance of the human environment for potential carcinogens. Therefore, there is a major effort to develop *in vitro* short term tests. It is important to stress the fact that carcinogens can differ over a millionfold in terms of their potency. Ideally, we would like to predict not only whether a compound is a potential carcinogen but also its potency. It is most

TABLE XI

Methods for Detecting Carcinogens

In vivo
1. Clinical observations—by "astute" physicians and patients
2. Epidemiologic studies
3. Experimental animal bioassays

Short-term tests
1. Mutagenesis assays
   A. Bacteria—Ames test
   B. Mammalian cell culture
   C. Other eukaroytes—yeast, *Drosophila*
2. Assays for cell transformation
3. Assays for DNA binding, damage and repair—and binding to other macromolecules
4. Assays for chromosomal abnormalities and sister chromatid exchange
5. Provision for metabolic activation

---

important, of course, to identify the potent carcinogens and eliminate or reduce their level in the human environment.

There are several unresolved questions in terms of interpreting carcinogen assay data. Is there a linear relationship, over a wide range of doses, between dose and cancer incidence? Which animal species or *in vitro* system is most predictive of the response of humans? How does one extrapolate the results of laboratory assays to the human situation? Does the assay have the same specificity and sensitivity as that of human tissues exposed to the same test compound? These are major issues that require resolution if we are to rationally proceed in this area. At the same time, prudence dictates that positive results obtained in laboratory assays be taken seriously and that, wherever possible, human exposure to such agents be eliminated or reduced. In this regard, it is important to emphasize that animal bioassays have frequently predicted that a compound is carcinogenic and this was later verified in human studies. In addition, most of the known human carcinogens are positive in one or more animal bioassays.

Two types of short-term tests for carcinogens appear to be particularly promising at the present time. The first assays for mutagenesis using bacterial or mammalian cells. The most widely used and validated short-term test is a bacterial mutagenesis assay using specific tester strains of *Salmonella typhimurium,* the so-called Ames assay. This assay employs an extract of rat liver to activate the test substance. A large number of known carcinogens have been tested in this system, and there appears to be a rather good correlation between carcinogenicity and mutagenicity in this assay (Fisher and Weinstein, 1978; Hollstein *et al.,*

1979; Ames, 1979). However, hormones, promoters, and several other types of compounds are negative in this assay because, as discussed above, they are not mutagens. Short-term tests for these agents remain to be developed. Mutagenicity can also be assayed utilizing mammalian cells in culture (Fisher and Weinstein, 1978; Hollstein et al., 1979; Ames, 1979). The second type of assay is to determine whether the exposure of normal mammalian cells in culture to the test substance results in their transformation to tumor cells (Fisher and Weinstein, 1978; Hollstein et al. , 1979; Ames, 1979). This procedure can now be performed with rodent fibroblasts, and efforts are underway to develop similar procedures with epithelial cells and with human cells.

With several compounds it is possible to measure by direct biochemical methods whether or not they damage DNA or chromosomes or whether they induce DNA repair. In all of the *in vitro* assays, it is important that the system provides for metabolic activation of the test substance.

Hopefully, the various short-term assays now being developed and validated will markedly enhance the detection of potential environmental carcinogens. At the present time, as in the time of Percival Pott, the astute physician continues to play a major role in providing clues to human cancer causation. These clues coupled with modern epidemiologic techniques, the rapidly expanding knowledge of carcinogenic mechanisms, and the newer short-term *in vitro* assays will no doubt lead to major advances in cancer prevention.

ACKNOWLEDGMENTS

The author is indebted to numerous research colleagues at Columbia University who made valuable contributions to studies and concepts described in this chapter, particularly Drs. Dezider Grunberger, Alan Jeffrey, Koji Nakanishi, Michael Wigler, Hiroshi Yamasaki, Lih-Syng Lee, Paul Fisher, Alan Mufson, and Jeffrey Laskin. These studies were supported by Grant CA-21111 and Contract No. 1-CP-2-3234 from the National Cancer Institute, Bethesda, Maryland, by Grant RD-50 from the American Cancer Society, and by the Alma Toorock Memorial for Cancer Research.

REFERENCES

Ames, B. N. (1979). *Science* 204, 587–593.
Berenblum, I. (1975). *Cancer* 1, 323–344.
Boutwell, R. K. (1974). *Crit. Rev. Toxicol.* 2, 419.
Boyland, E. (1950). *Biochem. Soc. Symp.* 5, 40.
Brown, H. S., Jeffrey, A. M., and Weinstein, I. B. (1979). *Cancer Res.* 39, 1673–1677.
Cairns, J. (1975). *Sci. Am.* 233, 64–72.
Cairns, J. (1978). "Cancer Science and Society." Freeman, San Francisco, California.
Clayson, D. B., and Shubik, P. (1976). *Cancer Detect. Prev.* 1, 43–77.
Committee on Biologic Effects of Atmospheric Pollutants (1972), p. 30. Natl. Acad. Sci., Washington, D.C.

Fisher, P. B., and Weinstein, I. B. (1978). *In* "Carcinogens in Industry and Environment" (J. M. Sontag, ed.). Dekker, New York (in press).

Fisher, P. B., Weinstein, I. B., Eisenberg, D., and Ginsberg, H. S. (1978). *Proc. Natl. Acad. Sci. U.S.A.* **75**, 2311–2314.

Foulds, L. (1969). "Neoplastic Development," Vol. 1. Academic Press, New York.

Grunberger, D., and Weinstein, I. B. (1976). *In* "Biology of Radiation Carcinogens" (J. M. Yuhas, R. W. Tennant, and J. B. Regan, eds.), pp. 175–187. Raven Press, New York.

Haddow, A. (1974). *Perspect. Biol. Med.* **17**, 543.

Hanawalt, P. C., Friedberg, E. C., and Fox, C. F., eds. (1978). "DNA Repair Mechanisms." Academic Press, New York.

Hecker, E. (1975). *In* "Handbuch der allgemeinen Pathologie" (E. Grundmann, ed.), Vol. 4, pp. 651–676. Springer-Verlag, Berlin and New York.

Heidelberger, C. (1975). *Annu. Rev. Biochem.* **44**, 79–121.

Hiatt, H. H., Watson, J. D., and Winsten, J. A., eds. (1977). "Origins of Human Cancer." Cold Spring Harbor Lab., Cold Spring Harbor, New York.

Hollstein, M., McCann, J., Angelosanto, F. A., and Nichols, W. W. (1979). *Mutat. Res.* **65**, 133–226.

Hoover, R., and Fraumeni, J. F. (1975). *J. Clin. Pharmacol.* **15**, 16–23.

Hsu, W. T., Lin, E. J. S., Harvey, R. G., and Weiss, S. B. (1977). *Proc. Natl. Acad. Sci. U.S.A.* **74**, 3335.

Jeffrey, A. M., Jenette, K. W., Blobstein, S. H., Weinstein, I. B., Beland, F. A., Harvey, R. G., Kasai, H., Miura, I., and Nakanishi, K. (1976). *J. Am. Chem. Soc.* **98**, 714.

Levin, D. L., Devesa, S. S., Godwin, J. D., and Silverman, D. T. eds. (1974). "Cancer Rates and Risks," 2nd ed., DHEW Publ. No. (NIH) 76-691. USDHEW, Washington, D.C.

Miller, E. (1978). *Cancer Res.* **38**, 1479–1496.

Moreau, P., Bailone, A., and Devoret, R. (1976). *Proc. Natl. Acad. Sci. U.S.A.* **73**, 3700.

Pott, P. (1775). "Chirurgical Observations," Section on Cancer Scroti. Hawes, Clarke & Collins, London.

Pulkrabek, P., Leffler, S., Weinstein, I. B., and Grunberger, D. (1977). *Biochemistry* **16**, 3127–3132.

Schmähl, D., Thomas, C., and Auer, R. (1977). "Iatrogenic Carcinogenesis." Springer-Verlag, Berlin and New York.

Slaga, T. J., Sivak, A., and Boutwell, R. K., eds. (1978). "Carcinogenesis," Vol. 2. Raven Press, New York.

Sugimura, T., Nagao, M., Kawachi,T., Honda, M., Yahagi, T., Seino, Y., Sato, S., Matsukura, N., Matsushima, T., Shirai, A., Sawamura, M., and Matsumoto, H. (1977). *In* "Origins of Human Cancer" (H. H. Hiatt, J. D. Watson, and J. A. Winsten, eds.), p. 1561–1577. Cold Spring Harbor Lab., Cold Spring Harbor, New York.

Tomatis, L., Agthe, C., Bartsch, H., Huff, J., Montesano, R., Saracci, R., Walker, E., and Wilbourn, J. (1978). *Cancer Res.* **38**, 877–885.

Van Duuren, B. L. (1969). *Prog. Exp. Tumor Res.* **11**, 31–68.

Weinstein, I. B. (1976). *In* "Advances in Pathobiology," Vol. 4, "Cancer Biology, II. Etiology and Therapy" (C. M. Fenoglio and D. W. King, eds.), pp. 106–117. Stratton Intercontinental Med. Book Corp., New York.

Weinstein, I. B. (1977). *Colloq. Int. C.N.R.S.* **256**, 2–40.

Weinstein, I. B. (1978). *Bull. N.Y. Acad. Med.* [2] **54**, 366–383.

Weinstein, I. B., and Grunberger, D. (1974). *In* "Chemical Carcinogenesis" (P.O.P. Ts'o and J. Di Paolo, eds.), Part A, p. 217. Dekker, New York.

Weinstein, I. B., Yamaguchi, N., Gebert, R., and Kaighn, M. E. (1975). *In Vitro* **2**, No. 3, 130–141.

Weinstein, I. B., Jeffrey, A. M., Jennett, K. W., Blobstein, S. H. Harvey, R., Harris, C., Autrup, H., Kasai, H., and Nakanishi, K. (1976). *Science* **193**, 592–595.

Weinstein, I. B., Jeffrey, A. M., Leffler, S., Pulkrabek, P., Yamasaki, H., and Grunberger, D. (1978). *In* "Polycyclic Hydrocarbons and Cancer (P. O. P. Ts'o and H. Gelboin, eds.), Vol. 2, pp. 4–36. Academic Press, New York.

Weinstein, I. B., Yamasaki, H., Wigler, M., Lee, L. S., Fisher, P. B., Jeffrey, A. M., and Grunberger, D. (1979). *In* "Carcinogens, Identification and Mechanisms of Action" (A. C. Griffin and C. R. Shaw, eds.), pp. 399–418. Raven Press, New York.

Witkin, E. M. (1976). *Bacteriol. Rev.* **40**, 869–907.

Yamagiwa, K., and Ichikawa, K. (1918). *J. Cancer Res.* **3**, 1.

8
VIRAL CARCINOGENESIS
Fred Rapp

I. INTRODUCTION

Ellermann and Bang (1908) demonstrated that visceral lymphomatosis of chickens could be passed between animals by transmission of cell-free extracts. Extensive research in viral oncology was initiated when Rous (1911) demonstrated that a naturally occurring sarcoma from a chicken could be passed to other animals by inoculation with a cell-free tumor filtrate. This was followed by the work of Shope (1932, 1933) and Bittner (1936) on papillomas of rabbits and mouse mammary tumors. Slow progress was due, in part, to the lack of understanding of the general properties of viruses and also to the generally primitive laboratory techniques available. With the discovery of antibiotics and improved cell culture media in the early 1950s, cell culture became a useful and vital laboratory technique and marked the beginning of concentrated research in virology. New technological advances have taken the study of viral carcinogenesis from its early unsophisticated beginning to an established science.

CANCER AND CHEMOTHERAPY, VOL. I

197

Early investigators, modeling their studies after principles established for bacteria, felt the need to demonstrate Koch's postulates in order to demonstrate etiology. The infectious etiology of a disease fulfilling Koch's requirements is depicted in Fig. 1, which shows the necessary steps required to establish the virus etiology of a spontaneous tumor. A tumor filtrate prepared by passage through a membrane filter is followed by replicating a putative virus in cell culture. Upon subsequent inoculation of this virus into an animal of identical species, a tumor is produced. The subsequent isolation of the same virus from the experimentally induced tumor results in the fulfillment of Koch's postulates. This procedure is limited since it is ethically impossible to meet the requirements of Koch's postulates for human cancer. Also, in order to prove a virus etiology, there can be no second virus present in either the cell cultures or tumor tissue. Finally, as will be discussed below, many tumors contain only a fragment of the virus genome, and infectious virus cannot, therefore, be reclaimed.

Within the past 30 years, there has been increasing evidence that viruses produce neoplasia. These include DNA- and RNA-containing viruses and involve several virus groups.

It is probable that many of the cancers studied require multiple factors for establishment of disease. Evidence against the existence of ''cancer viruses'' has accumulated in recent years. Scientists now believe that many viruses produce many types of infections and diseases but produce cancer only as a rare event.

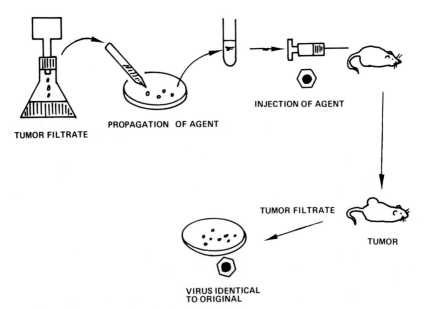

Fig. 1.   Classic steps to demonstrate the virus etiology of a tumor.

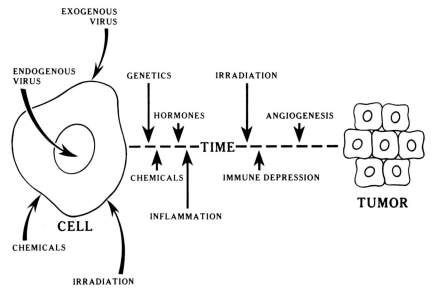

Fig. 2. Multiple influences on transformation and development of a tumor.

Many scientists have regarded cancer in humans as an acute infectious disease, which it is not. Unlike Marek's disease of chickens, cancer in humans has not been shown to be an acute infectious disease with symptoms appearing within a certain (and relatively short) period of time. It is more logical to postulate that cancer in humans is a chronic infectious disease with other factor(s) contributing to the expression of the disease (Fig. 2). The assumption that cancer in humans is a chronic infectious disease implies the existence of an agent that remains latent until it is stimulated, activated, or triggered by some internal or external factor. Following transformation, other factors may be required for tumor progression.

II. ONCOGENIC DNA AND RNA VIRUSES

Tumor viruses contain either double-stranded DNA or single-stranded RNA, with an icosahedral capsid which may or may not be surrounded by a lipid envelope. Oncogenic adenoviruses and papovaviruses (both DNA viruses) replicate in the following way: virus particles adsorb to virus receptors on the cytoplasmic membrane, enter the target cell, replicate their DNA in the nucleus, and transcribe virus messenger RNA for cytoplasmic biosynthesis of virus proteins. New virus particles assemble in the nucleus and are released following cell lysis. Transformation is usually accompanied by repression of late steps in virus replication with no release of infectious virus.

Molecular hybridization techniques have been used to establish that a certain virus is actually responsible for initiating and maintaining the transformed state. Radioactively labeled virus DNA and RNA have been used as probes for virus nucleic acids present in transformed cells. A hybridization experiment to detect virus DNA that has been integrated into a region of the mammalian cell chromosome is depicted in Fig. 3. Using this technique it is possible to detect that every transformed cell contains copies of the virus genome. Thus, the DNA sequences are integrated, and integration seems to be a necessary condition for stable transformation of mammalian cells by certain viruses.

Herpesviruses have double-stranded DNA with a lipid envelope that surrounds an icosahedral capsid. Replication occurs in the following way: the herpesvirus initially adsorbs to cell-specific receptors, and the virus envelope and cell membrane fuse. Replication of the virus begins after early shut-down of host DNA synthesis. Nucleocapsids are assembled in the nucleus, while particles that acquire a lipid envelope from the nuclear membrane exit through the endoplasmic reticulum.

RNA tumor viruses have been subdivided into either B-type or C-type particles based on budding and maturation features. B-type particles have an external spike-covered membrane and a solid spherical nucleoid. C-type morphology, however, is typical of all known leukemia and sarcoma viruses. As the viruses bud they are accompanied by the appearance of crescent-shaped nucleocapsids below the cell surface. These later condense into centrally located spherical nucleoids.

RNA tumor viruses also contain an enzyme, reverse transcriptase, which transcribes DNA from the single-stranded RNA template. The resulting heteroduplex is probably replicated by DNA-dependent DNA polymerase to produce a double-stranded DNA molecule that circularizes and is then inserted into the host chromosome (Fig. 4). These sequences are conserved and replicated with each round of cellular DNA synthesis as provirus DNA. The virus messenger RNA transcribed from the provirus DNA can serve either as messenger

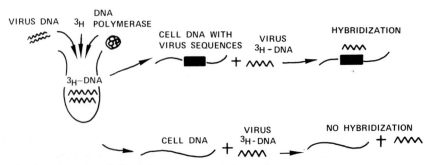

Fig. 3.   Molecular hybridization to reveal virus DNA sequences associated with cellular DNA.

PRODUCTION OF THE INTEGRATED
VIRAL GENOME

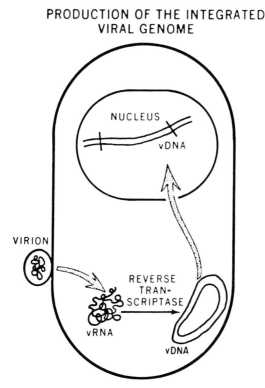

Fig. 4. Transformation of cells by C-type RNA-containing retroviruses. vDNA, viral DNA; vRNA, viral RNA. Modified from D. Baltimore (1978).

RNA for the synthesis of virus proteins or as the genetic material incorporated into progeny particles.

III. RETROVIRUSES

For almost 70 years, RNA tumor viruses, now referred to as retroviruses, have been implicated in several malignancies in a number of animal species. Only recently, however, has sufficient evidence emerged that suggests they may also be involved in the etiology of cancer in man. The most convincing reason to justify the extensive research on these viruses, which produce sarcomas and leukemias in experimental animals, is that these tumors are the most common forms of cancer in children.

This discussion of retroviruses will consider three groups: those that induce leukemia but do not transform cells *in vitro,* those that are endogenous but not pathologic in their natural host, and, lastly, those that produce sarcomas, are usually defective, transform cells *in vitro,* and produce infectious progeny only in the presence of a helper virus.

A. Mouse Mammary Tumor Virus

Bittner (1936) discovered mouse mammary tumor virus (MMTV) in the milk of certain high-incidence cancer mouse strains. Prior to this, it was postulated that the tendency might be transmitted by cytoplasmic inheritance, placentally, or in the milk. It is now known that this tumor virus is transmitted through the milk of mothers carrying the virus. Therefore, if mice born to a high-incidence mouse are isolated and nursed by low-incidence mice, the result will be a low incidence of mammary tumors. Conversely, when offspring from low-incidence mice are nursed by high-incidence mice, a high incidence of mammary tumors is observed. Virus is also passed in seminal fluid and the gametes. It is now apparent that the genome of the virus is incorporated into the chromosome of every mouse cell. There is a great difference in the way the virus is expressed in different strains. It is now known that tumor development is dependent on hormone stimulation and that genetic differences are of prime importance in determining susceptibility or resistance to the virus.

Particles morphologically identical to the mouse B-type particles and containing reverse transcriptase and 60–70 S RNA have been found in samples of human milk (Moore and Charney, 1975). It has been reported that RNA extracted from human breast cancer tissue contains sequences that hybridize with DNA sequences complementary to MMTV RNA (Spiegelman, 1974) (Fig. 5). However, definitive studies await the development of the elusive cell culture system that

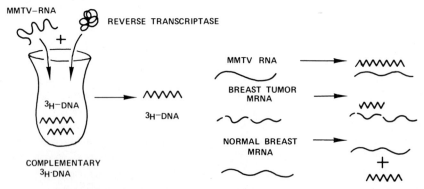

Fig. 5. Demonstration of RNA sequences in human breast tumor tissue hybridizing with DNA prepared from mouse mammary tumor virus (MMTV). Normal human breast tissue does not contain these sequences.

would enable replication of comparable putative human viruses isolated from breast tissue or from milk.

B. Leukemia and Sarcoma Viruses

Avian leukemia viruses (ALV) and sarcoma viruses are endemic in chickens and produce naturally occurring leukemias and sarcomas, respectively. The mode of transmission is horizontal and vertical, although endogenous virus DNA sequences have been detected in all chickens so far. Apparently, these virus genes are inherited having been transmitted via the gametes.

ALV are widespread in chickens and cause leukemias and other diseases of blood-forming tissues. Clinically, they produce conditions of lymphoblastosis, erythroblastosis, and myeloblastosis, sometimes manifesting only one of these conditions, but most frequently in combination. The study of leukemia viruses and cell transformation by ALV is not possible *in vitro* because cell culture systems that will permit the replication of chicken cell blood progenitors do not currently exist. Until this is possible, molecular and biochemical studies on the transformation events will be difficult. Adding to the complexity of this system is that many isolates of ALV may be mixtures of different viruses, each producing their own type of leukemia. Avian myeloblastosis virus is a strain that produces only one type of disease and has become a favorite for biochemical studies because of the high yields of virus.

Rous sarcoma virus (RSV) was the first virus to be classified as an etiologic agent of a solid tumor. This was accomplished by Rous (1911), who successfully induced sarcomas in chickens with a cell-free filtrate. Within the next few years, he isolated new viruses from other spontaneous chicken tumors and firmly established the viral etiology of a number of tumors from chickens.

The first strains of RSV had restricted host range. However, with continued passage of this virus, the host range has been augmented to include ducks, turkeys, guinea fowl, pigeons, rats, and even normal human cells in culture. An important observation was made by Keogh (1938), who grew RSV on the chorioallantoic membrane as a quantitative assay for RSV. After direct inoculation of virus on the membrane, small tumors developed; the number of these tumors was directly proportional to the concentration of the virus suspension. Thus, it was demonstrated that infection with a single RSV particle could transform a normal cell into a cancer cell.

Occasionally, it was observed that chicken embryo fibroblasts were completely resistant to RSV. This was found to be caused by two factors: (1) the cells also contained leukemia viruses that multiplied in the fibroblasts without causing obvious morphological changes, and (2) inherited chromosomal genes control the sensitivity of the cells to infection.

An RSV strain, known as the Bryan strain, has been intensively studied for many years. This strain produces high yields of virus when each cell is infected with large numbers of virus particles. When the cells are infected with only single virus particles, they are transformed and induce tumors that do not yield virus progeny. Several years later, it was demonstrated (Rubin and Vogt, 1962; Temin, 1962) that the simultaneous presence of a related leukemia virus was responsible. Only when cells were simultaneously infected with the Bryan strain and the leukemia virus did progeny particles containing an RSV genome result. The Bryan strain is defective and is dependent upon a helper leukemia virus for infection, can transform cells once it has penetrated them, and is defective only in its ability to replicate.

The evidence for a DNA provirus was first proposed by Temin (1964). He suggested that infecting RNA genomes were used as templates to make DNA templates, which were then integrated as proviruses into one or more chicken chromosomes. Temin and Mizutani (1970) and, independently, Baltimore (1970) made this prediction a reality when they detected an RNA-directed DNA polymerase in mature particles of RNA viruses. Although it is still not clear how the DNA provirus is integrated into cellular DNA, studies with avian tumor virus-infected cells show that these cells acquire provirus DNA that is capable of coding for the synthesis of virus progeny. It now appears that only one gene of these viruses, the *src* (for sarcoma) gene (Brugge *et al.*, 1978) is required for transformation (Fig. 6), and this gene appears to code for a phosphokinase with an approximate molecular weight of 60,000 daltons. How a single gene with this enzyme activity so perturbs the cells to render it malignant is the subject of intensive study.

The viral etiology of mouse leukemia was first demonstrated experimentally by Gross (1951). Leukemia resulted when filtrates from leukemic mouse tissues were inoculated into newborn mice of a nonleukemic strain. Further studies on spontaneous leukemias of low-incidence mice strains demonstrated that mouse leukemia virus (MLV) is transmitted in a latent form from one generation to another directly through the embryos. Gross (1951) postulated that the basic difference between high- and low-incidence strains is the frequency at which the latent virus can be activated to cause leukemia. However, it is possible that the virus may be activated occasionally, skipping several generations.

When mice of a low-incidence strain were exposed to large amounts of X rays,

RETROVIRUS GENE MAP

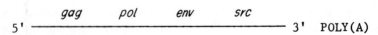

Fig. 6.   The genome of an avian sarcoma tumor virus. The *src* gene is required for transformation and oncogenicity. The other genes are needed for virus replication.

leukemia frequently developed. Infectious MLV particles have been isolated from these X-ray-induced leukemias. However, tissue extracts from nonirradiated mice failed to show any infectious material. X-Ray treatment seems to be responsible for the appearance of the MLV particles.

Many attempts to find viruses that cause other forms of cancer in mice followed the isolation of the Gross leukemia virus. Unfortunately, many of the extracts prepared from sarcomas and carcinomas yielded only leukemias after inoculation into newborn mice and not the types of cancer associated with the original extract. The many different isolates of MLV have often been named after the scientists who first isolated them.

Murine sarcoma viruses (MSV) were discovered in London in 1964 by Harvey, who was able to produce sarcomas and leukemias after obtaining a virus preparation of Moloney strain that had been passaged in rats. Hartley and Rowe (1966) observed that MSV is a defective virus that multiplies only in the presence of a related leukemia virus. Strains of MSV are analogous to the Bryan strain of RSV; they transform cells in the absence of a leukemia helper virus, but cannot produce infectious progeny without the helper virus.

Feline leukemia virus (FeLV) was first isolated by Jarrett et al. (1964) and can be found in about 60% of all cats with leukemia. Feline sarcoma virus (FeSV) has been isolated from several cat fibrosarcomas, and FeLV and FeSV exhibit typical C-type virus morphology (Snyder and Theilen, 1969). They contain 60–70 S RNA and reverse transcriptase which is antigenically related to the respective enzyme in mouse and hamster C-type particles. They have a unique group-specific antigen which is typical of all mammalian C-type particles. The finding that FeSV and FeLV grow in human cells raised the possibility that some human leukemias might be a result of infection with FeLV. Although epidemiologic studies suggest that there is no relation between outbreaks of leukemia and the presence of cats in these homes, reasonable measures should be observed when working with these viruses in the laboratory. Feline leukemia viruses react in a manner similar to the avian and murine leukemia viruses, in that they infect and replicate in, but do not transform, fibroblasts. Feline sarcoma viruses can infect and transform fibroblasts of cats and other species. Laboratory experiments have demonstrated that stocks of FeSV contain FeLV and that these stocks will not only infect newborn cats but will also induce solid tumors upon inoculation into adult cats. The tumors that develop in the adult cats do not persist and usually regress due to cell-mediated immunity. Feline leukemia is an infectious disease among cats, and horizontal transmission has been demonstrated with experimentally and naturally infected cats. Horizontal transmission does not preclude the possibility that vertical transmission also occurs. However, an experimental vaccine capable of preventing neoplasia by these viruses has been developed and suggests that horizontal transmission is the key element in spread of the virus to exposed and susceptible cats.

In 1971, the first isolation of a C-type virus from a subhuman primate occurred when Theilen *et al.* (1971) reported the detection of a C-type virus in a naturally occurring fibrosarcoma of the woolly monkey. The woolly monkey virus, also referred to as simian sarcoma virus, was later shown to produce lymphosarcomas when inoculated into secondary primate hosts. The second isolation was from naturally occurring lymphosarcomas and myelogenous leukemia of the gibbon ape (Kawakami *et al.*, 1972). The gibbon ape leukemia virus has been capable of producing myelogenous leukemia in young gibbon apes after introduction of cell-free extracts from leukemia cells. The importance of these findings in the woolly monkey and gibbon ape will be considered when the human leukemias and sarcomas are discussed.

C. Human Retroviruses

The quest for a human C-type virus has become extremely intense in the last fifteen years. The search for these viruses has also gained notoriety, and new claims for the discovery of such a virus in humans are now regarded with suspicion. The hope for a human RNA tumor virus as a counterpart to animal viruses is based on the accumulation of scientific information that now documents the presence of C-type viruses in many species of animals.

Priori and her colleagues (1971) detected a C-type virus in a stable culture of ESP-1 cells derived from a child with Burkitt lymphoma. Within the same year, Gilden and his colleagues (1971) detected murine group-specific antigenicity in these ESP-1 cells, and Gallo and his group (1971) demonstrated that the reverse transcriptase activity in ESP-1 cells could be inhibited by antiserum to murine reverse transcriptase. These observations reduced this "human C-type virus" to a murine virus that had probably contaminated the cultures of ESP-1 cells.

Another example of a similar occurrence was the RD-114 virus. McAllister and co-workers (1971) inoculated kittens *in utero* with a stable line of human sarcoma cells (RD). Two tumors that developed in these kittens contained C-type viruses; prior to passage in these kittens, the RD cells contained no detectable C-type particles. A stable line of cells, the RD-114 cell line, established from one of these tumors, also contained C-type viruses. As a result of biochemical and molecular experimentation with RD-114 virus, doubts were raised that questioned the validity of this human tumor virus. Since that time, the origin of RD-114 has been debated. The virus could be a latent human virus activated after passage in kittens, or a cat virus that was acquired by the RD cells during their passage in kittens.

Several lines of investigation are producing results that foretell the existence of human C-type viruses. Many of these tests are sophisticated biochemical and molecular assays which have provided the following information: (1) an enzyme similar to RNA reverse transcriptase has been identified by antibody to reverse transcriptase from primate tumor viruses, but not by antibody to reverse transcriptase against cats or avian retroviruses or to DNA polymerase in humans, (2) human leukemia cells have retrovirus nucleic acid sequences in common with mouse and monkey retrovirus nucleic acid, and (3) some antigens present in murine and primate retroviruses have now been detected in several human cancers, although similar antigens are now being detected in normal human tissues. Additional hopes for the discovery of a human C-type virus were raised with the disclosure by Gallo and Gallagher (1975) that they had successfully isolated a C-type human virus from a patient with acute myelogenous leukemia (AML). They have been able to establish the continuous production of C-type virus in a number of cultures of leukocytes from one patient with AML. However, this virus contains group-specific antigens and reverse transcriptase that are related to the oncogenic primate viruses, simian sarcoma virus, and Gibbon ape leukemia virus and cross-hybridizes with these viruses to a very significant degree. This again forces the issue of possible contamination of the human cultures by a virus from another species. However, similar viruses have been isolated by a number of investigators from normal and malignant human cells, but their origin and role in human disease have yet to be clarified.

IV. ONCOGENIC DNA VIRUSES

A. Papovaviruses

Papovaviruses are unenveloped DNA-containing viruses which induce solid tumors in experimental rodents. They comprise two distinct groups on the basis of size: the papilloma viruses have larger capsids and larger genomes than the remaining members of the papovavirus group. The genome of all papovaviruses is circular, and it is estimated that simian virus 40 (SV40) and polyoma virus code for about ten proteins. All have oncogenic potential, except K virus of the mouse. The papovaviruses have four subgroups: papilloma, polyoma, vacuolating, and K viruses.

Ciuffo (1907) demonstrated that human warts could be transmitted with cell-free filtrates, and Shope (1932) initiated his studies on papillomas of wild cottontail rabbits. These naturally occurring and experimentally induced tumors of rabbits rarely became malignant. When the virus was injected into domestic rabbits, two important observations were made: tumors readily progressed to malignant carcinomas, and, infectious virus, which was recoverable from wild cottontail rabbits, was no longer found in the tumors of domestic rabbits. Based on these studies, viral oncologists justified their investigations of cancers in which viruses were not detectable as infectious agents.

Human papilloma viruses, also known as wart viruses, produce painful, disfiguring skin lesions as well as benign tumors in man. The propagation and study of human papilloma viruses have remained elusive due to the rare observation of any cytopathic effect in cultured cells and the lack of a suitable cell culture system. Recent studies using molecular hybridization techniques may prove useful in establishing the pathogenesis of disease due to these viruses (zur Hausen *et al.*, 1974).

Polyoma virus was named for its ability to induce a wide range of tumors when injected into several species of rodents. Although the virus is widespread in mouse populations, it does not appear to be oncogenic in its reservoir host. When injected into newborn animals, it produces adenomas of the parotid gland, large noninvasive sarcomas, and hemangioendotheliomas. The type of tumor that develops depends on the type of cell infected.

The simian vacuolating virus, SV40 was discovered by Sweet and Hilleman (1960) while working with rhesus monkey kidney cells in the testing and production of poliomyelitis vaccines. Girardi and his colleagues (1962) were the first to demonstrate the oncogenic protential of this virus in newborn hamsters. SV40 produced sarcomas in newborn hamsters, but there was no evidence of metastases. This virus has been studied as a model cancer-causing virus and also for its possible long-term effects in humans, since many people were exposed to the virus as a result of contaminated poliovirus and adenovirus vaccines.

A human papovavirus has also been isolated from brain tissue of patients with progressive multifocal leukoencephalopathy (Padgett *et al.*, 1971). This SV40-like virus usually produces disease in individuals with other disorders, particularly in the immunologically compromised host. Whether it is oncogenic in humans remains to be established.

B. Adenoviruses

Adenoviruses can be divided into subgroups on the basis of antigenic cross-reactivity, DNA hybridization characteristics, ability to transform cells of various animal species, and ability to agglutinate rhesus monkey and rat erythrocytes. All adenoviruses except the avian adenoviruses share common group-specific complement-fixing antigenic determinants and also possess type-specific determinants. Human adenoviruses contain a large, linear duplex DNA. They replicate their DNA in the nucleus, synthesize virus proteins in the cytoplasm, and assemble progeny in the nucleus.

Trentin and his colleagues (1962) induced sarcomas in hamsters using human adenovirus type 12. Adenoviruses can also transform cells *in vitro* and induce tumors when inoculated into newborn animals .There are 31 serotypes of human adenoviruses, and many have been isolated from tissue specimens in which the presence of the virus was inapparent or latent. There is no evidence that any of the known adenoviruses are oncogenic in humans.

C. Herpesviruses

The third group of DNA-containing viruses with oncogenic potential are the herpesviruses. Because of their widespread prevalence in the human population and their existence in almost every species, the herpesviruses have become a major focus of interest.

Morphologically, all herpesviruses have basically the same structure: a DNA core within an icosahedrally multilayered capsid. The nucleocapsid is enveloped by one or more membranelike structures that contain lipids and glycoproteins.

An interesting characteristic of herpesviruses is their ability to remain within the body in a latent state. Virus persists in the host after a primary infection and remains undetected. Recurrent attacks after the initial primary infection are probably caused by latent virus and not by reinfection from an exogenous source. It is still not clear where the virus persists in this latent form, although the cells of the central nervous system and peripheral blood leukocytes seem to be favored. It is possible that latent herpesvirus exists as whole virus, a subviral unit, or as virus DNA. It is still not understood how the virus persists and causes disease in the presence of neutralizing antibody titers and the complex immune system of the body.

Productive herpesvirus infection is accompanied by cell death; in contrast to this, malignant transformation occurs only in a nonproductively infected cell that is able to divide and grow. It is, therefore, of great interest that almost all herpesviruses examined can stimulate cell DNA synthesis and mitosis.

The frog herpesvirus was first reported by Lucké (1938) who recognized an association between the herpesvirus of the leopard frog and the subsequent development of renal adenocarcinoma. Recent studies have implicated the Lucké virus as the etiologic agent of these tumors (Naegele *et al.*, 1974). The virus has not been replicated in cell culture, and only circumstantial evidence is available to suggest that this virus acts alone in initiating cell transformation.

There are two types of Lucké tumor cells: summer cells which are taken from tumorous frogs during the summer or are maintained in the laboratory at 20°–25°C and are virus-free, and winter cells which are isolated from tumor-bearing frogs in the winter, or are maintained in the laboratory at 4°–9°C and contain virus particles. This suggests that this virus is temperature sensitive, and recent studies have demonstrated that it is activated by low temperature and is latent in the summer.

Lucké virus particles develop when tumor fragments from summer frogs are transplanted into the anterior eye chamber of leopard frogs and control frogs not carrying the virus and maintained at 7.5°C (Mizell *et al.*, 1968). When summer tumor explants were incubated on agar slants at 7.5°C for 3 months, virus induction occurred (Breidenbach *et al.*, 1971). Activation of the virus at low temperature is independent of the intact host. Virus replication disappears when winter tumor explants are maintained above 11.5°C (Skinner and Mizell, 1972).

Several important questions remain concerning the viral etiology of the Lucké frog tumor: what role does temperature sensitivity play in the interaction between virus replication and cell transformation? Under what conditions do tumors develop? What is the mechanism restricting this virus to tumor induction in only certain types of frogs?

Marek's disease (Marek, 1907), a malignant and highly infectious disease of chickens, was the first neoplasia to be associated with a herpesvirus. This is a lymphoproliferative disease that produces lymphomas and, sometimes, neuropathy in infected fowl. Marek's disease virus (MDV) replicates only in feather follicle epithelial cells and is transmitted by dust and dander, with disease resulting from infection via the respiratory tract.

The economic loss to the poultry industry of chickens developing lymphomas has been significant enough to merit the development of vaccines. A nonpathogenic herpesvirus of turkeys (HVT) is now used extensively to immunize chicks (Fig. 7). The critical factor for the success of this vaccine is the response of host immunity to the immunizing virus. Several theories exist to explain how this might prevent the development of tumors. Some investigators believe that it is a primed immune system capable of humoral and cell-mediated immunity which eliminates the transformants before proliferation occurs. Others suggest that the wild-type MDV contains both defective and infectious particles. The defective particles might be neutralized before infection. If infectious particles escape neutralization, a persistent infection could result. It is possible that both theories are in force. The importance of Marek's disease for the virologist is that Koch's postulates have been fulfilled and a virus etiology has been established for this naturally occurring neoplasm. Future research will reveal whether the development of a vaccine for cancer in chickens has any application and significance for the prevention of cancer in man. Similar investigations have also shown that herpesviruses are oncogenic in rabbits, cattle, and guinea pigs.

There are two known monkey herpesviruses with oncogenic potential: *Herpesvirus saimiri* (HVS) (Meléndez *et al.*, 1968), which occurs naturally in the squirrel monkey and *Herpesvirus ateles* (HVA) (Meléndez *et al.*, 1972a), which occurs in the spider monkey. Both viruses produce mild infections in their natural hosts but cause fatal leukemias and lymphomas in other species. It is presumed that the immunological response is critical in determining susceptibility to the development of the lymphoma and parallels the findings with Marek's disease. Studies by Klein *et al.* (1973) suggest that resistance to the oncogenicity of HVS may be a result of the rapid development of neutralizing antibodies following infection. Squirrel monkeys infected with HVS will develop neutralizing antibodies two to four times faster than similarly treated owl and marmoset monkeys, which develop lymphomas. Meléndez and his colleagues (1972b) found that owl monkeys inoculated with HVS developed fatal lymphomas, while

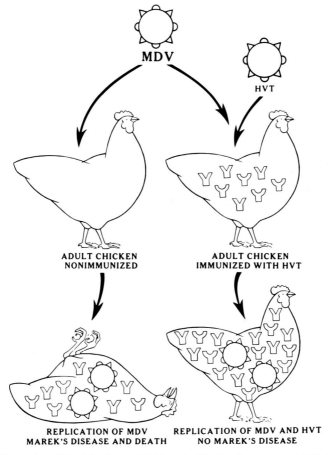

Fig. 7.   Prevention of Marek's disease of chickens by Marek's disease virus (MDV) by inoculation with an attenuated herpesvirus of turkeys (HVT).

those receiving HVA developed a self-limiting lymphoproliferative disorder. It appears that immunological factors are critical in controlling the transition of a cell from a transformed state to malignancy. There is no doubt that Koch's postulates have been fulfilled for HVS and that a virus etiology of malignant lymphomas in marmoset monkeys (Laufs and Fleckenstein, 1972) has been established.

Three human herpesviruses, Epstein-Barr virus (EBV), herpes simplex virus (HSV), and cytomegalovirus (CMV) have been investigated for many years. Since herpesviruses are ubiquitous in the human population, scientists are suspicious of their possible association with cancer. These viruses can produce mild infections in children, but may also recur and cause several types of disease in normal and immunologically compromised adults. The observations that herpesviruses persist in a latent state in the host after a primary infection and are able to recur are perhaps their most important characteristics. Studies have shown that these latent viruses can be activated by emotional or environmental stimuli. Since these viruses are common and exhibit multipotentiality with regard to the type of disease states produced in humans, they are now recognized as likely human tumor virus candidates.

The herpesvirus most closely associated with human cancer so far is EBV. Initially detected (Epstein *et al.,* 1964) in tumor cells from an African patient with Burkitt lymphoma (BL), this virus has more recently been linked to infectious mononucleosis and nasopharyngeal carcinoma (NPC). Burkitt lymphoma is a malignant tumor of the jaw afflicting children in equatorial West Africa. Early epidemiological studies suggested that this disease was probably the result of an infectious agent possibly coupled with the presence of an insect vector. It has been suggested that BL develops in individuals who cannot restrict the proliferation of virus-stimulated lymphocytes, and it is also possible that holoendemic malaria injures the reticuloendothelial system and accounts for the prevalence of this disease.

Although virus has not been detected in tumor biopsy material from BL patients, EBV DNA can be detected by nucleic acid hybridization. This same material also expressed EBV-associated antigens. The membrane antigen and the Epstein-Barr nuclear antigen are detectable, although virus capsid antigens have not been found. Cloning experiments have demonstrated that all cells contain the EBV genome and have the potential to produce virus antigens or intact virus. Studies have revealed the production of serum antibodies to virus antigens in individuals exposed to EBV. It is now known that change in antibody titer to these antigens can be correlated with the diagnosis, prognosis, and changing status of the patient.

Nasopharyngeal carcinoma, an epithelial tumor prevalent among the Southern Chinese, has also been linked to EBV. This association is based on findings that EBV DNA is almost always present in NPC cells (zur Hausen *et al.,* 1972) and that patients with this disease have abnormally high titers of anti-EBV antibody. A genetic factor may be involved in this disease and may represent an example of a cofactor acting in concert with a virus to produce a specific human malignancy.

Herpes simplex viruses are the most common of all the human herpesviruses. These viruses have been divided into two subtypes on the basis of site of infection in the body, base composition of the DNA, growth characteristics in culture, and immunological specificity. Herpes simplex virus type 1 (HSV-1) is usually isolated from oral lesions, while herpes simplex virus type 2 (HSV-2) is isolated from genital lesions. A herpesvirus, when it infects a cell, will cause either a productive or nonproductive infection. If nonproductive infection occurs, the virus and cell will survive, but replication will not take place and infectious progeny will not be made. A productive infection will result in virus progeny, but cell death will occur.

Herpes simplex viruses are now associated with a number of cancers in humans. The most striking relationship is that between HSV-2 and cervical carcinoma. Seroepidemiologic studies have contributed the most to this association, since direct evidence has been almost impossible to obtain. Women with cervical carcinoma more frequently produce antibodies to HSV-2 than matched controls of healthy women (Rawls *et al.*, 1969). Recent studies suggest that HSV-2 genetic information may be present in cervical carcinoma cells (Frenkel *et al.*, 1972; McDougall and Galloway, 1978), and the presence of herpesvirus-specific antigens (Royston and Aurelian, 1970) has also been noted. Furthermore, as venereal spread of HSV-2 increases, there appears to be a concomitant rise in carcinoma *in situ* of the cervix.

Animal studies have demonstrated the oncogenic potential of HSV-1 and HSV-2 (Duff and Rapp, 1971, 1973). *In vitro* transformation of normal cells by these viruses and the subsequent induction of tumors in susceptible hosts by these cells have clearly demonstrated the oncogenicity of these viruses. The transforming potential of HSV cannot normally be expressed in infected cells because these viruses are cytopathic and highly virulent in newborn rodents. To overcome these problems, a procedure using ultraviolet (UV) irradiation or photodynamic inactivation has been employed. Ultraviolet light inactivates virus by damaging virus nucleic acid. As a result, infectious progency are not produced, all particles are defective for replication, and infected cells in culture can be transformed at a low frequency. When cultures of primary hamster embryo fibroblasts are exposed to inactivated virus, foci of transformed cells appear within 2–4 weeks. Transformed cells can then be inoculated into newborn hamsters with the subsequent development of tumors (Fig. 8). Whether these *in vitro* experiments mirror *in vivo* phenomena remains an unresolved problem. However, use of these models has already revealed that herpesviruses require less than 5% of their genome to transform cells, and *in situ* hybridization using labeled HSV-2 DNA (McDougall and Galloway, 1978) has detected (Fig. 9) virus mRNA in human cervical, but not in normal, cells. This finding strengthens the association of HSV with this tumor and will undoubtedly stimulate further work in this area.

Human CMV has been shown to be etiologically associated with prostatic cancer in humans, and it shares many of the properties associated with the other suspected oncogenic herpesviruses. Albrecht and Rapp (1973), exposed hamster embryo fibroblasts to UV-inactivated CMV. Some of the resulting clones formed permanent lines that were oncogenic in newborn hamsters. This virus can also stimulate cell DNA synthesis (St. Jeor *et al.*, 1974), a property of most on-

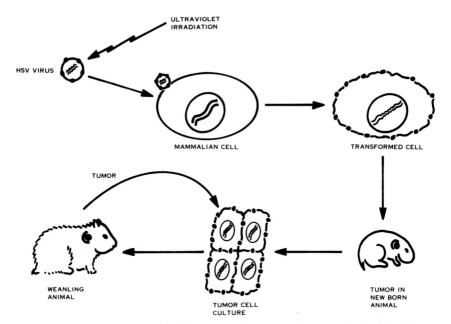

Fig. 8. Schematic representation of events to demonstrate the oncogenic potential of herpes simplex virus (HSV).

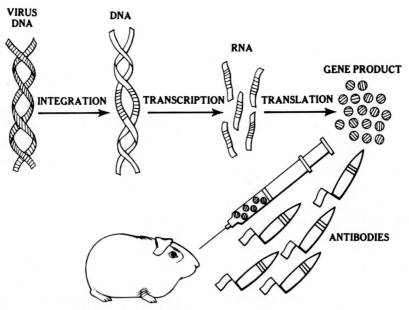

Fig. 9. Amplification of virus DNA integrated with host DNA by transcription to mRNA and translation of the RNA into virus-specific gene products.

cogenic viruses. Recently, it was also observed that human CMV can convert *human* cells into permanent cell lines which are then malignant when transplanted to nude mice. Obviously, this observation is of great relevance to human disease. Several studies within the past few years have shown that CMV, like HSV-2, is venereally transmitted; continuing observations may be instrumental in soon linking CMV to some types of cancer in humans.

D. Hepatitis B Virus

In recent years, the physical and biochemical properties of the virus responsible for hepatitis B (serum hepatitis) have been largely resolved despite failure to establish an *in vitro* system for propagation of this virus. In part, this is due to the "lucky" circumstance that chronic carriers produce large quantities of the virus which can be harvested from the blood and further analyzed. These studies have demonstrated that the infectious unit is the Dane particle with smaller core particles and filamentous forms also produced. The DNA is circular, with one of the two strands nicked and with a relatively small molecular weight of 2×10^6 daltons. It might be expected that such DNA has transforming properties, but this does not yet appear to have been achieved *in vitro*. However, a number of studies have regularly linked this virus, especially in long-term chronic carriers, with hepatocarcinoma. What remains to be established is whether the malignancy is a direct result of virus transformation, a response to liver injury induced by the virus, or a number of other factors acting in concert with the virus to produce the ultimate disease.

V. DISCUSSION

Many viruses are capable of producing tumors in experimental systems, and a number of naturally occurring malignancies of animals (i.e., feline leukemia, bovine leukemia, Marek's disease of chickens, renal adenocarcinoma of the frog) are virus-caused. Human viruses clearly are able to convert cells heritably to malignancy, and neoplasia in humans is becoming more strongly associated with viruses as new evidence solidifies the links. Evidence for the existence of virus information in tumor cells can now be sought by a number of techniques. In the final analysis, it may be most sensible to look for both gene products (i.e., antigens, reverse transcriptase, core proteins) and for virus nucleic acids that are amplified during transcription (Fig. 9). Such technology has already linked a number of viruses with a variety of human malignancies. However, all evidence being assembled will require careful analysis to resolve the complex problem of the etiology of neoplasia.

REFERENCES

Albrecht, T., and Rapp, F. (1973). *Virology* **55**, 53–61.
Baltimore, D. (1970). *Nature (London)* **226**, 1209–1211.
Baltimore, D. (1978). *Hosp. Pract.* **13**, 49.
Bittner, J. J. (1936). *Science* **84**, 162.
Breidenbach, G. P., Skinner, M. S., Wallace, J. H., and Mizell, M. (1971). *J. Virol.* **7**, 679–682.
Brugge, J. S., Steinbaugh, P. J., and Erikson, R. L. (1978). *Virology* **91**, 130–140.
Ciuffo, G. (1907). *G. Ital. Mal. Veneree* **42**, 12.
Duff, R., and Rapp, F. (1971). *J. Virol.* **8**, 469–477.
Duff, R., and Rapp, F. (1973). *J. Virol.* **12**, 209–217.
Ellermann, V., and Bang, O. (1908). *Zentralbl. Backteriol., Parasitenkd., Infektionskr., Hyg., Abt. I Orig.* **46**, 595.
Epstein, M. A., Achong, B. G., and Barr, Y. M. (1964). *Lancet* **1**, 702–703.
Frenkel, N., Roizman, B., Cassai, E., and Nahmias, A. (1972). *Proc. Natl. Acad. Sci. U.S.A.* **69**, 3784–3789.
Gallo, R. C., and Gallagher, R. E. (1975). *Science* **187**, 350–355.
Gallo, R. C., Sarin, P. S., and Allen, P. T., Newton, W. A., Priori, E. S., Bowen, J. M., and Dmochowski, L. (1971). *Nature (London) New Biol.* **232**, 140–142.
Gilden, R. V., Parks, W. P., Huebner, R. J., and Todaro, G. J. (1971). *Nature (London)* **233**, 102–103.
Girardi, A. J., Sweet, B. H., Slotnick, V. B., and Hilleman, M. R. (1962). *Proc. Soc. Exp. Biol. Med.* **109**, 649–660.
Gross, L. (1951). *Proc. Soc. Exp. Biol. Med.* **76**, 27–35.
Hartley, J. W., and Rowe, W. P. (1966). *Proc. Natl. Acad. Sci. U.S.A.* **55**, 780–786.
Harvey, J. J. (1964). *Nature (London)* **204**, 1104–1105.
Jarrett, W. F., Martin, W. B., Crighton, G. W., Dalton, R. G., and Stewart, M. F. (1964). *Nature (London)* **202**, 566–567.
Kawakami, T. G., Huff, S. D., Buckley, P. M., Dungworth, D. L., and Snyder, S. P. (1972). *Nature (London), New Biol.* **235**, 170–171.
Keogh, E. V. (1938). *Br. J. Pathol.* **19**, 1.
Klein, G., Pearson, G., Rabson, A., Ablashi, D. V., Falk, L., Wolfe, L., Deinhardt, F., and Rabin, H. (1973). *Int. J. Cancer* **12**, 270–289.
Laufs, R., and Fleckenstein, B. (1972). *Med. Microbiol. Immunol.* **158**, 135.
Lucké, B. (1938). *J. Exp. Med.* **68**, 457–467.
McAllister, R. M., Nelson-Rees, W. A., Johnson, E. Y., Rongey, R. W., and Gardner, M. B. (1971). *J. Natl. Cancer Inst.* **47**, 603–607.
McDougall, J. K., and Galloway, D. A. (1978). *In* "Persistent Viruses" (J. G. Stevens, G. J. Todaro, and C. F. Fox, eds.), pp. 181–188. Academic Press, New York.
Marek, J. (1907). *Dtsch. Tieraerztl. Wochenschr.* **15**, 417.
Meléndez, L. V., Daniel, M. D., Hunt, R. D., and Garcia, F. G. (1968). *Lab. Anim. Care* **18**, 374–381.
Meléndez, L. V., Hunt, R. D., Daniel, M. D., Fraser, C. E. O., Barahona, H. H., King, N. W., and Garcia, F. G. (1972a). *Fed. Proc., Fed. Am. Soc. Exp. Biol.* **31**, 1643–1650.
Meléndez, L. V., Hunt, R. D., King, N. W., Barahona, H. H., Daniel, M. D., Fraser, C. E. O., and Garcia, F. G. (1972b). *Nature (London), New Biol.* **235**, 182–184.
Mizell, M., Stackpole, C. W., and Halperen, S. (1968). *Proc. Soc. Exp. Biol. Med.* **127**, 808–814.
Moore, D. N. A., and Charney, J. (1975). *Am. Sci.* **63**, 160–168.
Naegele, R. F., Granoff, A., and Darlington, R. W. (1974). *Proc. Natl. Acad. Sci. U.S.A.* **71**, 830–834.

Padgett, B. L., ZuRhein, G. M., Walker, D. L., and Eckroade, R. J. (1971). *Lancet* **1**, 1257–1260.

Priori, E. S., Dmochowski, L., Myers, B., and Wilbur, J. R. (1971). *Nature (London), New Biol.* **232**, 61–62.

Rawls, W. E., Tompkins, W. A. F., and Melnick, J. L. (1969). *Am. J. Epidemiol.* **89**, 547–554.

Rous, P. (1911). *J. Exp. Med.* **13**, 397–411.

Royston, I., and Aurelian, L. (1970). *Proc. Natl. Acad. Sci. U.S.A.* **67**, 204–212.

Rubin, H., and Vogt, P. K. (1962). *Virology* **17**, 184–194.

St. Jeor, S. C., Albrecht, T. B., Funk, F. D., and Rapp, F. (1974). *J. Virol.* **13**, 353–362.

Shope, R. E. (1932). *J. Exp. Med.* **56**, 803–822.

Shope, R. E. (1933). *J. Exp. Med.* **58**, 607–624.

Skinner, M. S., and Mizell, M. (1972). *Lab. Invest.* **26**, 671–681.

Snyder, S. P., and Theilen, G. H. (1969). *Nature (London)* **221**, 1074–1075.

Spiegelman, S. A. (1974). *J. Am. Med. Assoc.* **230**, 1036–1042.

Sweet, B. H., and Hilleman, M. R. (1960). *Proc. Soc. Exp. Biol. Med.* **105**, 420–427.

Temin, H. M. (1962). *Cold Spring Harbor Symp. Quant. Biol.* **27**, 407–414.

Temin, H. (1964). *Natl. Cancer Inst., Monogr.* **17**, 557–570.

Temin, H. M., and Mizutani, S. (1970). *Nature (London)* **226**, 1211–1213.

Theilen, G., Gould, D., Fowler, M., and Dungworth, D. L. (1971). *J. Natl. Cancer Inst.* **47**, 881–890.

Trentin, J. J., Yabe, Y., and Taylor, G. (1962). *Science* **137**, 835–841.

zur Hausen, H., Diehl, V., Wolf, H., Schulte-Holthausen, H., and Schneider, U. (1972). *Nature (London), New Biol.* **237**, 189–190.

zur Hausen, H., Meinhof, W., Scheiber, W., and Bornkamm, G. W. (1974). *Int. J. Cancer* **13**, 650–656.

Part III
Animal Models of
Human Cancer: Their
Use and Limitations

9

TRANSPLANTED ANIMAL TUMORS
William T. Bradner

I. INTRODUCTION

The animal tumor models with greatest similarity to human neoplastic diseases are spontaneous or induced tumors of specific organ sites. However, their extremely slow and variable growth as well as excessive cost have made them totally impractical as primary screening tools. Transplanted animal tumors have the advantage of relatively rapid and uniform growth as well as consistent responses to therapy associated with each type. Thus, they have been widely applied in the search for new antitumor drugs, but lack of direct clinical correlation in therapeutic response has led to a constantly evolving combination of tumor systems used in various laboratories in an attempt to improve this correlation. This chapter will briefly review the history which led to current test systems and outline how they are applied.

II. HISTORY

The first major survey of transplanted animal tumors was sponsored by the American Cancer Society in 1953 in an attempt to identify the most predictive systems for detection of antitumor activity (Gellhorn and Hirschberg, 1955). A large number of cooperating groups contributed test data on the systems shown in

CANCER AND CHEMOTHERAPY, VOL. I

TABLE I

American Cancer Society Study, 1953

15 experimental tumors
21 microbiological systems
17 differentiation and development systems
21 biochemical synthesis systems
Tested against
28 tumor inhibitory and noninhibitory drugs

Table I using the same 28 drugs. When the National Cancer Institute established its first large comprehensive cancer chemotherapy program in 1955, it used this study as a basis for selecting the first systems considered as standard for widespread use as primary screens.

Table II shows briefly the evolution of animal tumor screens in the National Cancer Institute (NCI) supported program (see Zubrod *et al.*, 1966; Johnson and Goldin, 1975). Although other tumors were being used by independent investigators, the NCI program had great impact on the course of cancer drug discovery. Each change in the system was based on review of the rapidly accumulating data from new active drugs in the clinic and on selection of the minimum number of tumors which would, together, respond to nearly all the clinical compounds. At the same time, many attempts were being made to test drugs against human

TABLE II

History of Animal Cancer Screens (National Cancer Institute)

1955
  Adenocarcinoma 755
  L-1210 Leukemia
  Sarcoma — 180
1966
  L-1210 Leukemia
  Walker 256 carcinosarcoma
1968
  P-388 Leukemia
  L-1210 Leukemia
1971
  Add: B16 Melanoma
    Lewis lung carcinoma
1976
  P-388 Leukemia
  Tumor panel (8 Tumors)

TABLE III

Human Tumor Screens

A. *In vitro*—tissue culture
B. Embryonated eggs
C. Immune deprived host
    1. Drug, X-ray depressed
    2. Athymic mice
D. Immune deprived site
    3. Retina
    4. Hamster check pouch

tumor tissue maintained in culture or as xenografts, that is, as tumor transplants in rodents.

All of the systems shown in Table III have been tested in a variety of ways for growing human tumors and testing drugs. The results have been uniformly disappointing. Although some correlation in response has been seen between *in vivo* drug testing against a human tumor and therapy of the original patient, no predictability in response has been discerned relative to the same disease in any other patient. What has clearly emerged from drug testing with both transplanted animal and human tumors is that no single experimental system accurately predicts for any human cancer by organ site. However, a useful finding has been that animal tumors do seem to be able to predict activity for classes of drugs, particularly close analogues. This formed the basis for selecting the tumor screening systems currently utilized. Obviously, the number of tumors kept in passage is limited in any one institution so that the tumors used must be relatively sensitive and broadly responsive. More critical screens can be applied secondarily with the cooperation of outside investigators and the NCI program.

III. PRIMARY SCREENING

The ascitic tumors P-388 and L-1210 leukemia are sensitive to a wide variety of antitumor agents, especially when intraperitoneal treatment is used, permitting close contact between drug and tumor cells in early growth stages (Table IV). P-388 is the more sensitive and is used as the primary screen for all unclassified agents and natural products (see Geran *et al.*, 1972, for methodology). The listing on Table IV shows the classes of agents directed against individual tumors even though all the tumors are responsive to most of the agents. In some respects, compound supply can influence primary screening choice. Mitomycin and tricothecane analogues tend to be supplied in very small amounts. Thus tests on the more sensitive P-388 are run. *cis*-Platinums, nitrosoureas, and antimetabo-

TABLE IV

Ascitic Tumors

Tumor	Host	Materials screened
P-388 Leukemia	Mouse	Natural products
		Mitomycins
		Tricothecanes
L-1210 Leukemia	Mouse	Anthracyclines
		Cisplatinums
		Nitrosoureas
		Antimetabolites
Walker 256	Rat	Alkylating agents
carcinoma		Bleomycins

lites are usually available in adequate quantity initially so that use of the faster growing L-1210 is advantageous. The anthracyclines are about equipotent on both tumors and are thus also tested on L-1210 even if available in very small quantities.

Figure 1 shows a flow sheet for testing in our primary screening system and the basis of our particular testing strategy. Materials which are not defined chemically, such as fermentation broths or novel chemical structures unrelated to known chemotherapeutics, are tested directly on P-388. Testing is continued long enough to establish the maximum tolerated dose and the minimum effective dose (if the compound is active). Analogues of known drugs are tested together with a prototype compound against a responding tumor directly if we receive only small amounts or if the compound is not of great interest. Here we wish to determine whether or not there is any antitumor effects before proceeding further. In the case of high priority analogues in good supply, an LD_{50} is determined first and testing of all similar compounds is conducted using increments of the

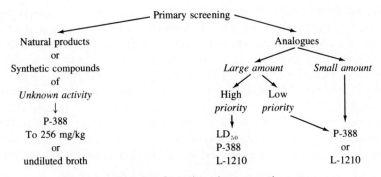

Fig. 1. A flow sheet for testing primary screening system.

TABLE V

Treatment Regimen

A. Schedule dependency
   1. Once daily, 9 days (QD 1→9)
   2. Every third day (L-1210) (Q3D)
   3. Every fourth day (P-388) (Q4D)
   4. Single injection, day 1
B. Route of administration
   1. Intraperitoneal (standard)
   2. Intravenous
   3. Subcutaneous
   4. Oral

LD_{50}. Thus, each compound can be related to another in terms of its effectiveness, regardless of absolute potency. Before further tumor tests are performed, organ-specific side effects are characterized in small animals and must indicate an advantageous toxicity profile. Treatment regimens and routes of administration are shown in Table V.

IV. SECONDARY EVALUATION

Based on the primary screening results with the leukemias (or other compelling biological data for agents not effective on the leukemias) additional more extensive testing is performed to characterize the *in vivo* antitumor properties of each new drug. As a prelude to tests in other tumors, schedule-dependency studies with novel agents are performed so that secondary screening can be performed using the best treatment regimen.

Two solid tumors used frequently are B16 melanoma and Lewis lung carcinoma (Table VI). These are used for secondary evaluation of the products

TABLE VI

Solid Tumors

Tumor	Host	Materials screened
B16 melanoma	Mouse	Anthracyclines
		Bleomycins
		cis-Platinums
		New natural products
Lewis lung	Mouse	Nitrosoureas
		Alkylating agents
		Antimetastatic agents

shown utilizing the best treatment schedule. Often, several analogues will give almost identical responses in tests against the leukemias but will show marked differences on the solid tumors.

Although, as noted earlier, there has been little success with organ-specific tumors in cancer screening, considerable research is continuing and some important examples are shown on Table VII. The NCI has a panel of tumors covering major sites: breast, lung, and colon and includes both mouse and human xenografts of each. Houghton and Houghton (1978) have isolated and characterized individual colon xenografts in an attempt to define chemical–biological parameters of what appears to be a multiple rather than a single disease. Soloway and Sudderth (1978) have developed carcinogen-induced transitional cell carcinomas in mice which appear analogous to the human disease. Both animal and xenografted brain tumors (Shapiro *et al.*, 1978) appear to predict better than average in relation to human therapy.

New agents should be tested on resistant tumors, since identification of secondary and tertiary therapies is of great importance. There are available resistant tumor lines to most every major antitumor drug. Three examples are shown in Table VII.

Various other therapeutic experiments involving animal tumor models are shown in Table VIII. Combination chemotherapy with two or more drugs or combined modality utilizing drugs, radiation, surgery, and/or immunotherapy can be tested in animal systems. Drugs used to ameliorate side effects, such as antiemetics, should be tested in an animal tumor system to be certain that blocking of antitumor activity does not occur. So-called rescue is represented by two different examples. One is the use of high dose methotrexate followed by citrovorum factor (Djerassi *et al.*, 1970). This sequence of administration allows rescue of the bone marrow but not the tumor. The other is simultaneous administration of a specific toxicity-blocking agent which does not interfere with antitumor effects. The example shown is adriamycin plus coenzyme Q10. It has

TABLE VII

Special Tumor Systems

    A. Organ specific tumors
       1. NCI tumor panel
       2. Colon xenografts (Houghton)
       3. Bladder tumors (Soloway)
       4. Brain tumors
    B. Resistant tumors
       1. Bristol L-1210/mitomycin C
       2. NCI P-388/adriamycin
       3. Sloan-Kettering L-1210/*cis*-platinum

TABLE VIII

Experimental Therapeutics

A. Combination chemotherapy
  1. Multidrug
  2. Combined modality
B. Combinations with drugs for side effects
C. Rescue
  1. High doses (methotrexate plus citrovorum factor)
  2. Selective blocking (adriamycin plus coenzyme Q10)

---

been reported that full doses of adriamycin can be given in this manner to animals with no cardiotoxic effects (Bertazzoli and Ghione, 1977).

V. DISCUSSION

It has been more than 70 years since Paul Ehrlich performed initial extensive experiments with transplanted tumors, and over 30 years since the major NCI chemotherapy program began. However, it is in just the last 2 or 3 years that a new, higher level of sophistication has been evident in cancer chemotherapy screening, not only in terms of ranking new analogues but also in the real possibility of organ-specific screens. Hopefully, as these new tools are put into service, better cancer treatments will be identified as a consequence.

REFERENCES

Bertazzoli, C., and Ghione, M. (1977). *Pharmacol. Res. Commun.* **9**, 235–250.

Djerassi, I., Rominger, C. J., Kim, J., Turchi, J., and Meyer, E. (1970). *Proc. Am. Assoc. Cancer Res.* **11**, 21.

Gellhorn, A., and Hirschberg, E. (1955). *Cancer Res., Suppl.* **3**, 1–125.

Geran, R. I., Greenberg, N. N., MacDonald, M. M., Schumacher, A. M., and Abbott, B. J. (1972). *Cancer Chemother. Rep.* **3**, 1–103.

Houghton, P. J., and Houghton, J. A. (1978). *Br. J. Cancer* **37**, 833–840.

Johnson, R. K., and Goldin, A. (1975). *Cancer Treat. Rev.* **2**, 1–31.

Shapiro, W., Basler, G., Horten, B., Norman, C., and Posner, J. (1978). *Proc. Am. Assoc. Cancer Res.* **19**, 153.

Soloway, M. S., and Sudderth, B. (1978). *Proc. Am. Assoc. Cancer Res.* **19**, 167.

Zubrod, C. G., Schepartz, S., Leiter, J., Endicott, K. M., Carrese, L. M., and Baker, C. G. (1966). *Cancer Chemother. Rep.* **50**, 349–540.

10

THE NUDE MOUSE MODEL
Lawrence Helson

I. INTRODUCTION

The First International Workshop on Nude Mice was held in Aarhus, Denmark in 1973. Since then, there has been a Second Workshop in Tokyo, Japan in 1976; a Nude Mouse Symposium in Columbus, Ohio in 1977; and numerous publications in a variety of journals and of scientific conference proceedings. The animal model has been propagated and expanded to all continents for use by investigators in many fields of biomedical research and laboratory animal science in order to study poorly understood human diseases.

This mouse was first mentioned by Isaacson and Lattanach (1962). It was again seen in a colony of albino mice in the Virus Laboratory, Ruchill Hospital, Scotland in 1966. Flanagan (1966) more fully described it and demonstrated that it was due to a recessive gene carried by normally haired mice, and assigned to the mutation the symbol "nu" for nude. It should be mentioned that although the animals appear hairless (Fig. 1), histologic sections of skin do show abortive hair follicles (Fig. 2). The most interesting characteristic of the nude mouse was

CANCER AND CHEMOTHERAPY, VOL. I

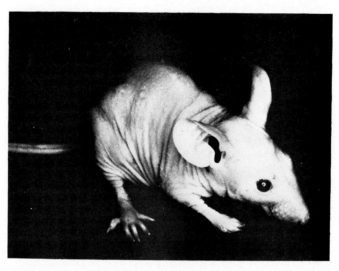

Fig. 1. The nude (nu/nu) mouse.

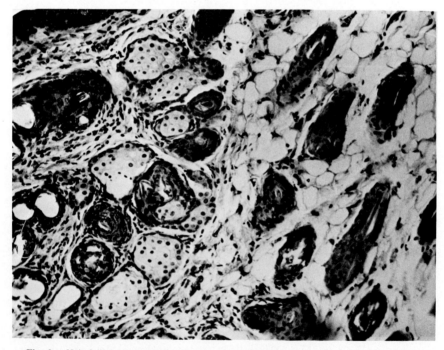

Fig. 2. Hair follicles are present in nude mice. Full development of hair does not take place. Histologic section of skin. Hematoxylin and eosin. × 200.

discovered by Pantelouris (1968). He found that the homozygous mouse nu/nu lacked a thymus and, consequently, was a congenitally immunodeficient animal. This led to its introduction as an animal model which did not require immunosuppressive preparation for heterotransplantation experiments.

The potential of the nude mouse within the context of a model for infectious disease, immunology, and oncology is in continuous and ever expanding exploration and application.

Heterotransplantation of human malignant tissue to nude mice was first reported by Rygaard and Povlsen (1969). They reported a colon cancer which was found to retain its original histological pattern during 32 passages over 4 years. Many other observations of human tumors transplanted to nude mice support the view that fidelity at the histologic level is constant (Nomura *et al.*, 1977). Additional features of primary tumors which can be compared with established heterografts include isoenzyme patterns, secretory products (such as catecholamines, α-1-fetoprotein, and ectopic hormones), and surface markers (such as carcinoembryonic antigen) which are preserved in the majority of

TABLE I

Human Tumors Transplanted to Nude Mice

	Cellular type or organ of origin	
Lymphoma	Undifferentiated small cell	Chronic myelogenous
	Burkitt's type	leukemia
	Diffuse histiocytic	Hodgkin's disease
	Malignant histiocytic	
Carcinoma	Anus	Penis
	Rectum	Testis
	Colon	Prostate
	Stomach	Bladder
	Esophagus	Ovary
	Tongue	Vulva
	Salivary gland	Uterine cervix
	Pharynx	Uterine endometrium
	Nasopharynx	Choriocarcinoma
	Paranasal sinuses	Kidney
	Maxillary sinuses	Adrenal cortex
	Breast	Pancreas
	Liver	
Sarcoma	Osteogenic	Liposarcoma
	Chondrosarcoma	Myogenic
	Ewing's	
Neural crest and central nervous system	Glioblastoma	Meningioma
	Neuroblastoma	Melanoma
	Malignant Schwannoma	Carcinoid
	Primitive neuroectodermal	

heterotransplanted malignant tumors. There are exceptions and variation in specific characteristics. These are preserved in the passage. These may represent the inherent plasticity and adaptation of some tumors (Aubert *et al.*, 1976).

Because of the facile utility of this model and the potential for disorder, a reference center for human tumors transplanted to nude mice was established following the Second International Workshop on Nude Mice. Its goal is to collect and facilitate exchange of information among concerned laboratories. An abbreviated list of tumors successfully transplanted into nude mice at the time of the conference indicates the range of tumors which can be explored (Table I).

The use of the nude mouse in a cancer research laboratory requires methods which are more rigorous than those generally used with standard experimental mice. Essentially, procedures must revolve about the propensity of the mouse to become infected due to its T cell and immunoglobulin A deficiencies. The nude mouse is prone to develop bacterial infections of its Harderian glands and uterine horns and is very susceptible to murine hepatitis virus and protozoan gastrointestinal infections. Commensal organisms may be the most common pathogens for this animal. *Staphylococcus albus* may be found in the Harderian glands and *Giardia muris* in the intestines.

II. CONDITIONS AND PRESERVATION OF TUMOR STOCK

The nude mouse can be bred and studied under three sets of conditions: (1) open shelf or laminar flow shelf with fiberglass bonnets, (2) specific pathogen-free, or (3) germ-free environments. The open shelf or laminar flow shelf is the most practical, since it permits unhindered ease of surgical procedures, bleeding, and other manipulations of the animal. Use of surgical gloves for handling and minimizing length of exposure to environments outside the cage helps reduce infection and prolong the useful life of the animal to 7 to 10 months. Specific pathogen-free or germ-free environments are appropriate for long-term studies, as under these conditions, the animals live their normal lifespan of about 2 years. Plastic isolators are utilized for these conditions. The mice are delivered by Caesarean section and the young introduced into the sterile environment. The major disadvantage of this system is the limitation of manipulation of the mice once in the isolators. Tumors can easily be inoculated, tumor size and mouse weights measured, and mice treated with drugs. However, surgical interventions and serial bleeding procedures are cumbersome. These are the preferred conditions for maintenance of tumors which have not yet been established in cell culture and for preservation of tumor stock.

We found it practical to maintain certain tumors in nude mice in these isolators and upon demand to transfer tumors to animals maintained in open shelf conditions. This technique decreases the possibility of contaminating a unique tumor line with murine hepatitis virus, an event which may frequently occur in mouse stocks used for multiple short-term experiments. An alternative method of preserving human tumors established in nude mice is to place small 1 mm^3 pieces for biopsy in glycerol or cold 10% dimethyl sulfoxide (DMSO) in Eagle's minimal essential medium and store them in liquid nitrogen. Since not all human tumors are susceptible to revival when frozen, multiple aliquots of a freshly growing representative tumor are frozen at the time of the first passage, one of which may be rapidly thawed at 37°C, washed clean of DMSO, and then implanted in a site similar to that in which the first tumor grew. If the frozen tumor is successfully transplanted, the remaining frozen aliquots can be utilized at later dates, and any modification of tumor characteristics occurring over serial transplantation can be compared with the original stored first passage.

Virtually all human tumor lines which are established as monolayers can be cryopreserved. After thawing, these cells may also grow in the nude mice, which would obviate the need for passaging the tumors continuously after freeze-preserving the original tumor tissue. An additional advantage of these techniques is that frozen tumor cells can readily be exchanged among laboratories.

III. SITE OF TUMOR INOCULUM

The easiest and most accessible site of subcutaneous tumor inoculation is the dorsal region of the mouse. Tumors on the ventrum tend to interfere with locomotion, are occasionally bruised, and are prone to infection. There may be variation in tumor growth rates in different subcutaneous locations. Recently, it has been reported that the anterior portion of the body along the midaxillary line was optimal for growth of heterotransplants (Auerbach et al., 1978). This may be true for some tumors, as reported, but does not hold up with systematic investigation. We have not found any consistent optimal growth rates for human neuroblastomas, malignant Schwannomas, and colon cancers in posterior and anterior locations.

Certain sites appear to be particularly useful for initial implantation from patients when the subcutaneous regions do not prove successful. These include the subrenal capsule, the anterior chamber of the eye, and the brain.

Subrenal capsule implantation is a simple operation. The mouse is anesthetized with intraperitoneally injected pentobarbital (100 mg/kg). After painting the skin with Betadyne, a 5-mm right flank incision midway between the fore- and hindlegs is made. The incision is spread to about 8 mm with the blunt sides of a scissors, and the kidney, which is mobile in the mouse, is expressed on to the skin surface using two soft cotton applicators. The renal capsule is gently lifted and a 1 mm^3 piece of tumor is placed under it using sharp forceps. The kidney is replaced and the peritoneum and skin closed with clips. At the time of operation, pieces of tumor can also be placed within the peritoneal cavity and in subcutaneous sites. In 100 animals with 20 different tumors obtained directly from patients, we were unable to establish intraperitoneally growing tumors, but subrenal capsular growth was not infrequent.

For intracerebral inoculation, a small 10-μl volume of tumor cells is inoculated directly into the brain using a 26-gauge short needle. It is injected at a point midway between the eye and the ear, and 2 mm lateral to the saggital line.

Inoculation of tumor into the anterior chamber of the eye can be done with a dissecting microscope in an anesthetized animal using a 30-gauge needle. These latter two sites appear to be very effective for tumors with otherwise low takes in subcutaneous or subrenal capsular sites.

In some studies, tumor tissue derived from patients was systematically implanted subcutaneously, intraperitoneally, and under the renal capsule. In three tumors, two malignant Schwannoma and one adenocarcinoma of the testis, tumor growth occurred only in the subrenal capsular site. These tumors, when large enough, were transferred to other nude mice in these same three sites through five serial transfers. By the fifth serial transfer, the tumor could be grown subcutaneously. This suggested that some kind of adaption by the tumor to the hosts was taking place. The histology and secretory characteristics of these three tumors and their growth rates have not changed over 25 subsequent transfers. This adaption of the tumor to an anatomic site different from its original successful implantation may be analogous to the human condition where primary tumors may remain indolent and then suddenly "adapt" and develop metastases or begin to grow more rapidly.

Tumors, such as brain gliomas, may be primarily grown in the nude mouse brain and then transferred to subcutaneous sites in other mice. Even under these conditions, brain tumor transplants, after a few weeks of growth, may be reabsorbed.

Some tumors do not take, while others regress after starting to grow. Tumor regression may, in part, be due to effective lymphocyte B cell, macrophage, and natural killer cell activity in these nude mice. Splenectomy, pretreatment of the mouse with antisera directed against the mouse lymphocyte, total body radiation, cyclophosphamide, cytosine arabinoside, or corticosteroids have been used to improve tumor takes. Apart from anti-lymphocytic globulin, these other methods do not appear to be of consistant help in facilitating tumor growth and may interfere with later studies and the animal's longevity.

There are other congenital mutations affecting the immune system, such as the asplenic mouse. An asplenic–athymic nude mouse has been recently established. A human malignant melanoma was transplanted to these mice and to nu/nu mice. Compared to the tumor in the nu/nu mouse, the tumor in the asplenic–athymic mouse had an elevated rate of growth and lower inoculation cell number for successful transplantation (Gershwin et al., 1978). It is possible that the "take" rate in these mice for similar sites, compared to that in the nu/nu, may be superior, but this has not been systematically studied.

A heterotransplanted tumor growing in a nude mouse does produce affects within the mouse which may vary according to the tumor's characteristics and its metabolic requirements. All tumor vascularization is presumed to be due to tumor-instigated angiogenesis of the host mouse. Hence, the final tumor architecture is essentially dependent upon a murine vasculature and ground substance material (Fig. 3). In the human, angiogenesis induced by the presence of a tumor is presumed to act similarly. It is possible that heterotransplanted solid tumors and leukemias which do not initiate a tumor angiogenesis factor do not grow larger than the limits of diffusion in the subcutaneous regions of the nude mouse. This, then, might be a critical factor in the "take" of a tumor.

Some human tumors which have been transplanted continue to secrete carcinoembryonic antigen or α-1-fetoprotein, substances which may be measured in the serum of mice (Helson *et al.*, 1979) (Fig. 4). Heterotransplanted neuroblastoma tumors in mice may give rise to immune complexes and changes in com-

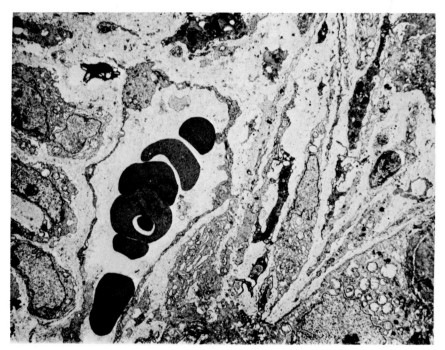

Fig. 3. Electron microscopic section of a murine blood versus coursing through a human colon cancer. The murine endothelium shares a common ground substance with the human cells. Evidence of inflammatory reaction is lacking.

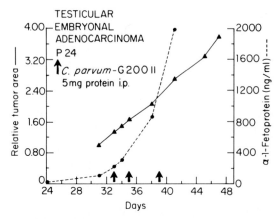

Fig. 4. There is a good correlation between secretion of α-1-fetoprotein into the serum and tumor growth in a nude mouse bearing a human testicular adenocarcinoma. This experiment demonstrates the lack of antitumor effect of a partially purified mouse serum preparation from *C. parvum*-treated CD-1 mice on tumor growth and α-1-fetoprotein secretion in a nude mouse. (From Helson *et al.*, 1979.)

plement as the tumors grow (Brandeis *et al.*, 1978). Although the homozygous nude mouse has no response to sheep red blood cells and has relatively low IgG$_1$, IgG$_2$, and IgA compared to the heterozygote, it does have elevated IgM and IgG surface markers in lymph nodes and spleen. Hence, it is capable of producing a response to foreign antigens or tumor via the B lymphocyte system, natural killer cells, and possibly macrophage activity.

The significance of the immune complexes in the growth of heterotransplanted tumors in nude mice is not understood. Ostensibly, they are considered to be "blocking antibodies" when found in partially suppressed or normal patients bearing spontaneous tumors as reported by Sjögren *et al.* (1971). It has been observed in our laboratory that immune complexes increase with increasing tumor load and may deposit in the kidney glomerular basement membranes. The effects of chemotherapy or tumor ablation on immune complex formation remain to be established.

IV. CHEMOTHERAPY

The development of experimental chemotherapy has relied mainly on syngeneic transplantable spontaneous or induced murine tumors to screen new potential anticancer agents. Because extrapolation to human tumors is limited, these animal screening methods still require extensive human chemotherapeutic trials to establish effectiveness as well as safety. Human cancers have a range of sensitivities, and although heterografts of human tumors in thymectomized and irradiated mice and hamsters have been used, the method has certain objectionable qualities. The major one is that the required pretreatment could effect the host and the metabolism of the new drug. The use of the nude mouse circumvents these objections. However, there are a number of assumptions which must be made and considered in interpreting data from this model. For example, the constancy of the growth of each tumor in each serial transplant may vary. Most tumors fit a Gompertzian growth function, but there may be a drift toward shorter incubation periods following serial inoculation. This may be a manifestation of tumor cell selection, a result of serial passage and transfer between animals without accompanying discernable morphological differences between early and late transfers. This instability may be a characteristic of certain but not all tumors and requires further study. In our laboratory we have passaged two lines (a malignant Schwannoma and an adenocarcinoma of the testis) for 25 passages and find that by using similar tumor inoculums at each transfer the delay (in days) to onset of growth (latency period) varies by not more than 10%.

The actual tumor growth rates in nude mice may be shorter than in the original human host; however, the process of heterotransplantation may, when successful, select for the most potent, rapidly growing, and least fastidious of the tumor cells. Of particular importance is the possibility that the tumor cell population which does grow in the nude mouse represents the generating fraction of the original tumor, and it is these cells which must ultimately be eliminated in order to cure the host. Consequently, screening antitumor agents against these tumor cells may be of signal importance.

The nude mouse has some additional differences from man. For example, it is not dependent upon vitamin C in its food supply; hence studies concerning the antitumor activities of vitamin C are inappropriate in this model. It may metabolize drugs differently than heterozygous mice. For example, it has been reported by Houchens et al. (1977) that the LD_{50} of most anticancer drugs in nude mice are higher than in heterozygotes. This has been attributed to increased hepatic microsomal enzyme activity. The nude mouse as a drug testing model for man should reflect or predict the tumor's behavior vis à vis these same drugs in the clinical setting. Retrospective analysis of four lines of neuroblastoma tumors with varying sensitivities to cyclophosphamide in the clinic and corresponding sensitivities in tumors growing in nude mice were found (Helson et al., 1977). We infer from this that it is reasonable to have a spectrum of the same tumor type from different patients to be tested against any single agent or drug combination. Just how many tumors should compose the battery is unknown. At present, we estimate three to five different tumors with different degrees of sensitivity are adequate.

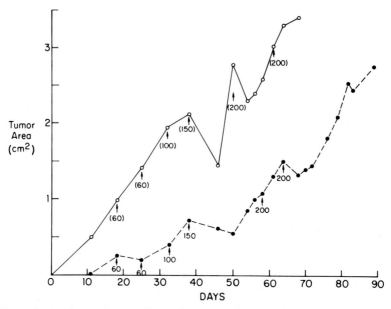

Fig. 5. Repetitive small intraperitoneal doses of cyclophosphamide in an otherwise drug-sensitive neuroblastoma tumor in nude mice lead to resistance. Tumor growth in two nude mice are depicted. Numbers at data points indicate dose of cyclophosphamide (mg/kg).

V. RESISTANCE

One of the major problems in anticancer chemotherapy is the development of drug resistance by the malignant cells. The human tumor-bearing nude mouse lends itself admirably to this problem. A mouse bearing a drug-sensitive tumor can be given drugs at repetitive intervals at less than effective dosages. Ultimately, resistance develops (Fig. 5). The tumors can then be passed back into cell culture or to other mice to test for the persistance of drug resistance. The resistant cells can be cloned and studied for novel proteins and metabolic characteristics which may be related to the mechanism of resistance.

VI. RADIATION THERAPY

The subcutaneous tumor is particularly amenable to radiation therapy since the mouse can be fit simply into a lead shield (Fig. 6). The results of some experiments with radiation combined with chemotherapy are displayed (Fig. 7). Numerous factors affecting radiation effects, such as degree of tissue oxygenation and tumor size, are amenable to study using this model. By implanting two

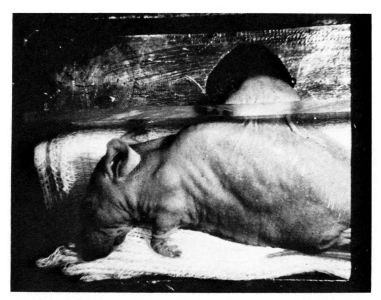

Fig. 6. The lead shield is designed to permit radiation treatment of subcutaneous tumors. Animals are anesthetized during the administration of radiation.

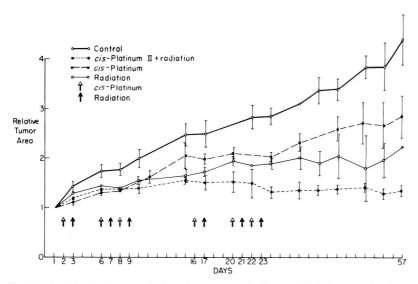

Fig. 7. Combined radiation and chemotherapy with cis-platinum II. Animals bearing human malignant Schwannomas were treated with 500 rad delivered from a cesium-137 source every 4 days every other week for 4 weeks. Groups of eight animals each were treated with radiation, cis-platinum II, or both. The day prior to irradiation, each animal received cis-platinum II (3 mg/kg ip). Control groups are depicted. The combination of radiation and drug appeared to be the optimum treatment.

tumors in animals, abscopal effects can be studied if only one is irradiated. The animal with two tumors facilitates the comparison of chemotherapy plus radiation versus chemotherapy alone in the same animal.

VII. UTILIZATION OF THE NUDE MOUSE

We conclude from a variety of observations in our laboratory and from reports in the literature that the response to chemotherapy and radiation therapy can be adequately evaluated. The practical utilization of the tumor-bearing nude mouse in cancer chemotherapy testing has many pitfalls. It is important to be aware that the variability in tumor growth curves of control animals create difficulties in evaluating minor changes which nevertheless may be of clinical significance. The heterotransplanted tumors in the nude mice appear to have a limited vasculature. Consequently, they tend to undergo spontaneous central necrosis when greater than 1.5 to 2 cm in diameter. Growth rate changes in larger solid tumors are difficult to evaluate because of variabilities in clearance of dead cells. The kinetics of proliferation in the tumors in mice are probably different from the human situation, and consequently extrapolation of data to human tumors in patients should be done with caution as long as correlations between results in these mice and clinical data are not available for review.

Additional factors which may confuse the evaluation of the response are the stromal responses induced by the heterotransplant. Under such circumstances, the tumor may be comprised of cells of mixed origins. The lack of tumor size decrease following treatment may be due to the persistant viability of the host cells. Certainly, after treatment and in the presence of growth stasis, viability testing should be undertaken. One method of testing induced growth rate inhibition is to measure the specific incorporation of radiolabeled thymidine into tumor DNA. Effective chemotherapy inhibits overall growth and may specifically alter thymidine incorporation. This has been shown to be a sensitive method of determining drug effect in nude mice bearing rapidly growing tumors (Helson *et al.*, 1978).

VIII. SCREENING OF NEW ISOTOPES FOR TUMOR
LOCALIZATION

Where a good vascular supply develops, the heterotransplanted tumor is an excellent model to test new tumor localizing agents. The animals can be injected intravenously via the retro-orbital venous plexus or in the tail veins. Depending upon metabolic clearance of isotopes and their half-lives, animals can be scanned

TABLE II

Gallium-67 Uptake 48 Hr after Intravenous Injection of 20 μCi in the Nude Mouse

Tumor	Tumor-to-blood ration	Tumor-to-muscle ratio
Malignant schwannoma	8.8	13.7
Undifferentiated lymphoma	19.7	31.0

using routine thyroid scanning equipment while under pentobarbital sedation. Specific activity of tumors and other organs can be compared. Differential uptake of gallium-67 by malignant Schwannoma and non-Hodgkin's lymphoma in the same mouse has recently been investigated by Yeh and Helson (1978). Constant ratios of tumor–blood or tumor–muscle are found (Table II). This technique permits the screening of new agents at a greatly reduced cost; for example, animals growing four different tumors can be prepared and distribution of isotopes determined at different times following injection (Fig. 8).

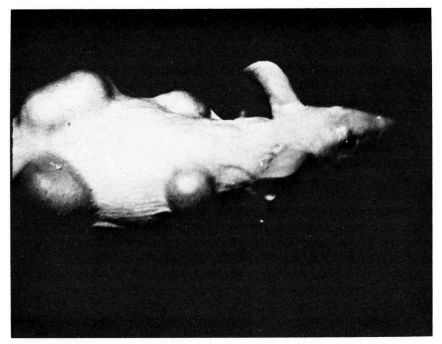

Fig. 8. Nude mouse with four neuroblastomas, the sizes of the tumors are controlled by the primary inoculum size.

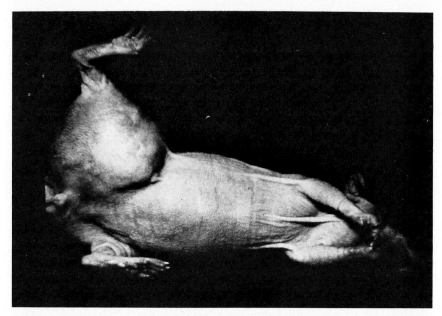

Fig. 9. Nude mouse with neuroblastoma inoculated in the right femur. One month later, it developed a metastasis to the left neck region.

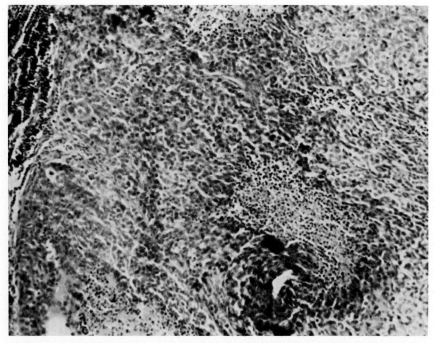

Fig. 10. Histologic section of a neuroblastoma metastasis involving a lymph node of the neck of a nude mouse. Hematoxylin and eosin. × 140.

IX. METASTASES

Metastases from heterotransplanted tumors in nude mice are rare, but they do occur. In neuroblastoma, they may occur when the primary implant is allowed to grow to a very large size (3–4 cm in diameter). In two instances, tumors implanted in and about the lower extremity metastasized to the neck (Fig. 9), salivary glands on the opposite side of the body (Fig. 10), and, in one instance, to the liver. Bone metastases have not been seen. We have been able to implant tumor into the femur of mice (Figs. 11 and 12) where it fills the marrow space and appears to cause bone destruction.

One reason for the general lack of metastases may be derived from the requirements for establishing a heterograft. In a tumorigenic human neuroblastoma, inocula below 10^6 cells rarely form tumors, while larger inocula usually do. If metastases are to be formed from the parent tumor, they require a good outflow vascular channel, one large enough to carry clumps of 10^6 or more cells. Where this occurs tumor emboli must first traverse the lung, where macrophages may inhibit its growth, and the lung for some tumors, such as neuroblastoma in the clinical setting, is a poor site for growth. The malignant Schwannoma,

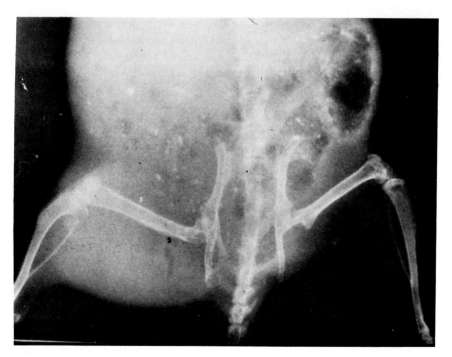

Fig. 11. Radiograph of femur with implanted neuroblastoma and surrounding soft tissue swelling due to tumor mass (see Fig. 10).

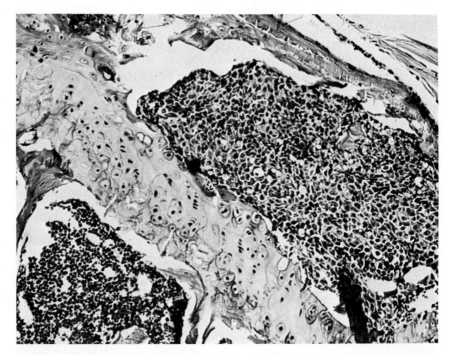

Fig. 12.   Histologic section of femur of nude mouse with implanted neuroblastoma. Hematoxylin and eosin. × 140.

established from a lung metastasis of a patient, can be permitted to grow large enough with contiguous extention to fill the abdomen of the mouse, yet does not metastasize to the lung.

X. CONCLUSIONS

The congenitally, partially immunodeficient nude mouse is a protean research tool. Its potentials in cancer research are just beginning to be appreciated. It is probable that future research will extend current simplistic drug–tumor response models to sophisticated models of tumor pharmacology and biology.

REFERENCES

Aubert, C., Chirieceanu, E., Foa, C., Rorsman, H., Rosengren, E., and Rouge, F. (1976). *Cancer Res.* **36**, 3106–3112.

Auerbach, R., Morrissey, L., and Sidky, Y. A. (1978). *Cancer Res.* **38,** 1739–1744.

Brandeis, W., Helson, L., Khan, A., Liu, Y. P., and Day, N. K. (1978). *Proc. Am. Assoc. Cancer Res.* **19,** 80.

Flanagan, S. P. (1966). *Genet. Res.* **8,** 295–309.

Gershwin, M. E., Ahmed, A., Ikeda, R. M., Shifrine, M., and Wilson, F. (1978). *Immunology* **34,** 631–642.

Helson, L., Helson, C., Rubenstein, R., and Hajdu, S. I. (1977). *Proc. Int. Workshop Nude Mice, 2nd, 1977,* pp. 291–303.

Helson, L., Helson, C., Das, S. K., and Rubenstein, R. (1978). *In* "The Use of Athymic (Nude) Mice in Cancer Research" (D. Houchens and A. Ovejera, eds.), pp. 257–266. Fischer, Jena.

Helson, L., Helson, C., and Green, S. (1979). *Exp. Cell Biol.* **47,** 53–60.

Houchens, D. P., Johnson, R. K., Gaston, M. R., Goldin, A., and Marks, T. (1977). *Cancer Treat. Rep.* **61,** 103–104.

Isaacson, J. H., and Lattanach, B. M. (1962). *Rep. Mouse Newsl.* **27,** 31.

Nomura, T., Ohsawa, N., Tamaoki, N., and Fujiwara, N. eds. (1977). "Proceedings of the Second International Workshop on Nude Mice." Univ. of Tokyo Press, Tokyo.

Pantelouris, E. M. (1968). *Nature (London)* **217,** 370–371.

Rygaard, J., and Povlsen, C. O. (1969). *Acta Pathol. Microbiol. Scand.* **77,** 758–760.

Sjögren, H. O., Hellström, I., Bansal, S. C., and Hellström, K. E. (1971). *Proc. Natl. Acad. Sci. U.S.A.* **68,** 1372–1375.

Yeh, S., and Helson, L. (1978). *J. Nucl. Med.* **19,** 716.

Part IV
Immunotherapy of Cancer

11

IMMUNOTHERAPY: AN INTRODUCTION
Paul Siminoff

I. INTRODUCTION

The idea that immune mechanisms in the host prevent the successful proliferation of malignant cells into frank neoplastic disease was first advanced in 1909 by Paul Ehrlich, one of the founders of modern immunology. Over the ensuing 70 years, a good deal of evidence has been amassed, largely derived from studies in laboratory animals and to some extent in man, to support Ehrlich's concept. Based upon newer information, Thomas and Burnet have reformulated Ehrlich's concept into a theory of immune surveillance which proposes that constantly arising malignant cells in the body are eliminated by immunocompetent cells of the host which recognize the malignant cells as foreign intruders. As a logical outcome of this view, the theory also states that development of cancer results from a breakdown in immune surveillance (Burnet, 1970).

CANCER AND CHEMOTHERAPY, VOL. I

The rationale for cancer immunotherapy then emerges from the theory of immune surveillance and the laboratory and clinical evidence that supports it. Many animal and some human tumors do have certain identities which are not found or expressed in their hosts. Quite frequently, the host is capable of mounting an immune response to the tumor, the intensity of which varies according to the tumor and according to the host. Significantly, immune capability and intensity of the immune response are often related to prognosis of the disease. Finally, it is a cardinal principle of clinical immunotherapy that immune responsiveness of the human cancer patient to his tumor can be manipulated to improve his body's surveillance mechanisms.

This discussion will briefly examine how the immune mechanism functions, how the host responds immunologically to the appearance of malignant cells, what we know about failure of host defense mechanisms, and, finally, some treatment modalities presently employed by clinical immunotherapists in the treatment of human cancers.

II. THE IMMUNE APPARATUS

A. Challenge and Response

Basic to the immune response is the ability of the host to discriminate between self and nonself. The unique identities which determine self reside in special chemical groupings on the surface of cells in the body; some of these are species specific while other identities are strain or individual specific. The introduction into the host of substances or bodies, such as viruses and bacteria, which bear identities foreign to those of the host can give rise to an immune response. Such substances or bodies act as antigens and are potentially capable of stimulating certain host cells to produce antibodies and of stimulating other cells which are involved in cellular immunity.

Two main classes of cells derived from progenitor cells (stem cells) in the bone marrow participate in the immune response; lymphocytes and macrophages (Good, 1972). The lymphocytes mature and acquire functionality via two major arms of the immune apparatus; the thymus and "bursal equivalent" systems (shown in Fig. 1). The "bursal equivalent" refers to the bursa of Fabricius, a primary lymphoidal organ in chickens; under the influence of this organ stem cells proliferate and differentiate into B lymphocytes. The mammalian equivalent of the bursa of Fabricius has not been identified.

After having acquired functionality, B lymphocytes (or B cells) migrate to peripheral lymphoidal tissue, such as spleen and lymph nodes. Under a specific antigenic stimulus, those B cells with selective capacity to respond further differentiate into plasma cells which secrete a population of plasma proteins termed

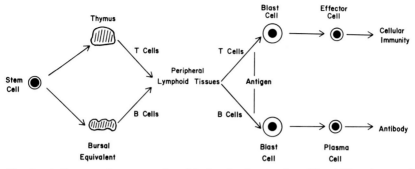

Fig. 1. A diagrammatic representation of the functional maturation of B and T lymphocytes via the "bursal equivalent" and thymus systems, respectively.

antibodies or immunoglobulins capable of combining with the antigen which elicited their formation (see Fig. 2). These antibodies are Y-shaped structures which contain two major fragments: Fab and Fc. The Fab fragment contains the variable (V) regions. The terminal sites of the V region bind antibody (Wang, 1976). Distributed at the membrane surface of B cells are immunoglobulins linked to receptors on the cells via the terminal sites of their Fc moieties. These surface immunoglobulins serve as recognition sites for complementary antigens (Douglas, 1976).

   Those lymphocytes which develop under the influence of the thymus are called T cells (see Fig. 1). During their residence in the thymus, these cells acquire the

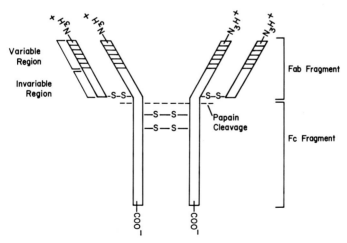

Fig. 2. A simplified representation of the antibody molecule showing the regions contained within the two major fragments, Fab and Fc.

ability to respond to foreign antigens via recognition immunoglobulins present on the T cell surfaces, although not in as great abundance as on B cells. Upon response to antigenic stimulus, T cells transform into lymphoblasts which are the effector cells of such expressions of cellular immunity as rejection of tissue and organ grafts, delayed hypersensitivity reactions, and the direct killing of cancer cells.

The other major class of cells involved in host defense reactions, the macrophage, develops independently of the lymphocyte. Precursor cells in the bone marrow differentiate into mononuclear cells (or monocytes) which circulate in the blood and seed various organs and tissues, as well as serous cavities, e.g., the peritoneal and pleural spaces. The end stage of development, the macrophage, is a phagocytic cell (i.e., capable of ingesting particulate matter) which participates in immunological and nonimmunological killing of bacteria, fungi, and tumor cells (Douglas, 1976; Levy and Wheelock, 1974).

B. Regulation of the Immune Response

A large number of immunological reactions, particularly those involving the so-called thymus-dependent antigens, involve the collaboration of specialized subpopulations of T and B cells (see Fig. 3). Upon presentation of a specific T-dependent antigen, responding T cells differentiate into helper cells and either present the antigen to the B cell or release factors which stimulate the B cell to differentiate into antibody-producing plasma cells. There is evidence that the macrophage can also participate in the T-dependent process, possibly by accept-

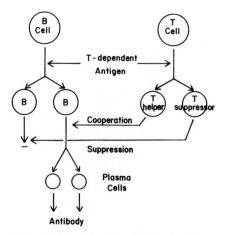

Fig. 3. Cooperative and suppressive interactions between lymphocytes of the two arms of the immune response.

ing the antigen from the T helper cell, processing the antigen, and presenting it to the B cell.

As well as positive collaboration between the two lymphocytic arms of the immune apparatus, there are also negative interactions which result in shutdown of specific immune reactions. The same antigen-responding T cells which form the helper population can also differentiate into suppressor cells which turn off the antigen-responsive B cells. It has also been shown that under certain conditions, B cells and/or antibody can suppress T cell-mediated immune responses to the same eliciting antigen. Phagocytic macrophages can also suppress immune responses by some mechanism requiring cell-to-cell contact between the macrophage and sensitized lymphocytes (Marchalones, 1976).

Thus, the immunological system is a highly tuned self-regulating mechanism in which collaborative interactions between cellular elements of the system help to initiate and amplify the response, while other elements act to shut the system down.

III. HOST RESPONSE TO TUMORS

A. Defense Mechanisms

The ability of the host to make a response to emergent cancer cells appropriate to its survival is highly dependent upon the expression of those antigenic identities on the tumor cells which are not expressed by normal host tissue (Klein, 1974). There are two broad categories of tumor antigens, tumor-associated and tumor-specific (Möller, 1975). Tumor-associated antigens are not directly related to malignant transformation but may be associated with a transforming virus or the tissue from which the tumor cells arose (see Fig. 4). In general as will be seen later in the discussion, immune responses to these associated antigens, for example, the fetal antigens on the human cell, may be useless at best and actually

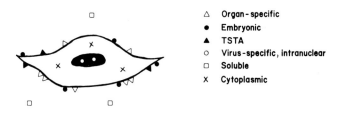

Tumor Cell

Fig. 4. A schematic representation of the distribution of antigens, including tumor-specific transplantation antigen (TSTA) on a tumor cell.

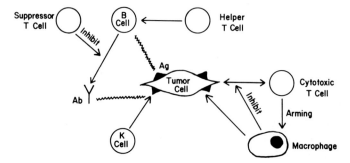

Fig. 5. Schematic representation of the collaborative and suppressive interactions between B cells, T cells, and macrophages in the host's response to tumor cells.

deleterious at worst. On the other hand, the immunologic response directed against tumor-specific antigens, for example, the tumor-specific transplantation antigen on rodent tumor cells, is crucial to host survival and is the operational mechanism in immune surveillance (Byers and Levin, 1976; Klein, 1975).

The immune response to tumor antigens appears to be similar to responses made to other antigens. Interactions between T cells, B cells, and macrophages result in the development of effector cells which are capable of attacking and killing target cancer cells (see Fig. 5). Collaboration between helper T cells and B cells can result in the production of cytotoxic antibody or antibody capable of coating the target cell rendering it susceptible to attack by killer (K) cells. Sensitized T cells can activate macrophages to kill target cells by some immunologically specific mechanism. By the same token, suppressor cell activity can also occur during the immune response to tumors. Suppressor T cells have been identified both in experimental animals and in human cancer patients and may be a significant factor in the progression of neoplastic disease.

1. T Cell Cytotoxicity

T cells are small lymphocytes which contain receptor sites on their surfaces which bind to antigens on the tumor cells (see Fig. 6). This adherence of T cell to target cell results in disturbance of the target cell membrane, its eventual rupture, and lytic death of the cell.

2. Antibody-Dependent Cytolysis (ADC)

Antibody-dependent cytolysis involves nonimmune lymphocytes (or possibly other cells including monocytes, neutrophils, and null cells) with receptors for the Fc fragment of antibody molecules (Möller, 1975). By this mechanism, these so-called K cells bind to specific antibody-coated tumor cells resulting in lysis of the targets.

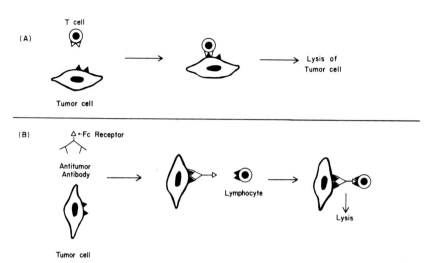

Fig. 6. Mechanisms of tumor-specific cytolysis by sensitized lymphocytes. (A) Direct killing of target cells by T cells. (B) K cell killing of antibody-sensitized target cells.

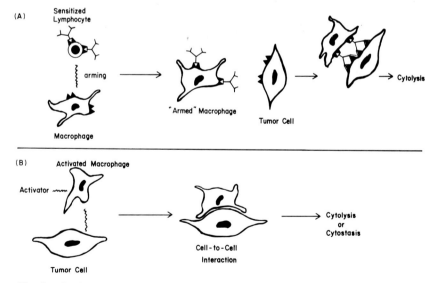

Fig. 7. Cytolytic or cytostatic effect of macrophages on target tumor cells. (A) Immune specific killing of tumor cells by "armed" macrophages which acquire immunoglobulin receptors for tumor-specific antigens upon interaction with sensitized lymphocytes. (B) Activated macrophages kill or inhibit tumor cell growth nonspecifically by a mechanism requiring cell-to-cell contact.

3. Killing by Macrophages

Macrophages may be "armed" by interaction with immune lymphocytes to recognize and kill target tumor cells, possibly by acquisition of recognition immunoglobulins (see Fig. 7). Besides the immunologically specific activation, macrophages can also be stimulated by a number of different agents, e.g., endotoxins, Bacillus Calmette-Guérin (BCG), and interferon, to kill tumor cells. This activation is nonspecific, that is, the macrophage will by some yet mysterious recognition mechanism kill tumor cells selectively without the need for prior encounter and regardless of the source of the tumor cells (Levy and Wheelock, 1974).

4. NK Cells

There has recently been described a group of yet unclassified cells which apparently can kill a broad range of tumors without the need for prior exposure or sensitization. These so-called "natural killer" or NK cells have been demonstrated in both lower animals and man. It is thought that NK cells are important effectors in immunosurveillance.

B. Failure of Defense Mechanisms

Although the host can marshall a formidable array of defensive weapons to prevent establishment in the body of a growing tumor, clearly these defenses break down with an all too alarming frequency in man. A number of working hypotheses have been proposed for the ability of tumors to escape immune rejection (see Table I), and these will be briefly discussed (Byers and Levin, 1976; Klein, 1975).

TABLE I

Escape by Tumors from Immune Rejection

I. Properties of tumor antigen
Nonimmunogenic
Sneaking through
II. Immunosuppression
Genetic, age, stress
Environmental factors
Tumor factors
III. Immunologic enhancement
Blocking factors
Suppressor cells
IV. Genetic defects

1. Properties of the Tumor Antigen

Tumors in animals and man vary in immunogenicity. Some tumors, particularly those induced by oncogenic viruses or carcinogenic chemicals, tend to be strongly immunogenic. On the other hand, many tumors spontaneously arising in man may be weak immunogens (Weiss, 1977) and so escape detection by immunosurveillance mechanisms or stimulate a feeble immune response which may, in fact, promote tumor growth. As a result, emergent malignant cells which proliferate either unnoticed or unrestrained by the immune system may well reach a population size which the host is no longer capable of rejecting.

2. Immunosuppression

The successful growth of tumors may be due to suppressive influences on the host's immune capabilities. These influences may be related to the genetic disposition of the individual, and to effects of aging, stress, and environmental factors, including exposure to carcinogens and oncogenic viruses. The tumor itself may be immunosuppressive. Investigators have shown in a number of experimental models in animals that tumors are capable of producing substances which enter the circulation and severely suppress immune responsiveness to the tumor.

3. Immunologic Enhancement

There is strong evidence derived from studies in animals and humans that certain types of immune responses may actually enhance tumor growth. One well-described phenomenon is the development of blocking factors (see Fig. 8). In this model, soluble tumor antigens (probably tumor-associated) are shed into the surrounding environment. Some of these antigens bind to and thereby block the recognition sites of immune lymphocytes. Some induce tumor-specific antibodies which coat the tumor cell in noncytotoxic fashion and prevent lysis of the coated tumor cell by cytotoxic lymphocytes (Coggin et al., 1974).

Although the existence of blocking factors has inclined many immunotherapists to seek treatments which emphasize cellular immunity to the tumor, recent evidence of suppressor T cell involvement in tumor development indicates that such an approach may be a mixed blessing.

4. Genetic Defects

Inborn defectiveness in the immune system, especially if immune surveillance is compromised, may contribute to the development of at least some human cancers. Genetically determined immunodeficiency diseases in man have a very low frequency; it may be supposed that they contribute proportionately to the incidence of neoplastic disease in man.

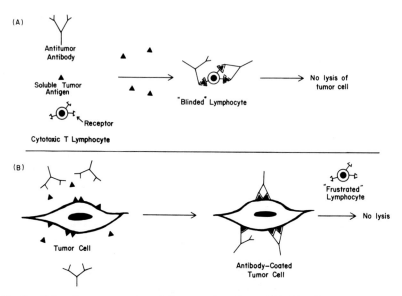

Fig. 8. Schematic representation of the protective effect of blocking factors on target cells against the action of cytotoxic lymphocytes. (A) Antibody to soluble tumor antigens blocks receptor sites on cytotoxic T cells preventing their lytic interaction with target tumor cells. (B) Noncytotoxic antibody binds to surface antigens of the tumor cell shielding it from the cytotoxic lymphocyte.

5. *Tumor Growth*

From the immunologist's point of view, the stages in the growth of a tumor can be related to a sequence of immunologic events. In the early phase, tumors grow slowly under a virtual balance between immunological factors which either limit or promote growth. When the tumor reaches a point where it can produce enough antigen to block effector lymphocytes, there is an acceleration of growth and some metastases. When the host becomes immunologically unresponsive (that is, anergic), metastatic spread becomes severe with likely terminal consequence (Coggin *et al.*, 1974). The challenge, then, to immunotherapy is to prevent anergy or to restore immune responsiveness in the cancer patient.

IV. IMMUNOTHERAPY OF CANCER

Immunotherapy has several objectives: (1) to prevent or reverse immunosuppression caused by other modes of cancer therapy; (2) to restore immune responsiveness compromised by the disease; (3) to enhance immunity to the tumor (Haskell, 1977; Hersh *et al.*, 1977; Mathé, 1976). To achieve these objectives, the immunotherapist has available several different types of immunotherapeutic

TABLE II

Modalities of Immunotherapy of Cancer

1. Passive Serum, cells, transfer factor
2. Active, specific Immunization with tumor cells, purified tumor antigens, oncogenic viruses, bacterial products
3. Active, nonspecific Systemic or local

TABLE II

Modalities of Immunotherapy of Cancer

procedures: (1) passive immunization; (2) active, specific immunization; (3) active, nonspecific immunotherapy (see Table II).

A. Passive Immunotherapy

This strategy seeks to introduce into cancer patients agents, such as serum, cells, or cell products, capable of destroying the tumor (Rosenberg and Terry, 1977). Sera from normal subjects, from "cured" patients with the same type tumor, and from animals hyperimmunized to the tumor type have been used with varying results. Disadvantages of this approach may be the transfer of blocking factors and development of serum sickness.

Both nonimmune and immune lymphoid cells have been transferred to cancer patients with claimed benefits. Bone marrow transplantations have been used to "rescue" patients from lethal doses of drugs or radiotherapy as well as for tumor therapy. One serious complication is attack by the transplanted cells upon the recipient's tissue causing graft versus host disease.

A potential treatment which has not yet been sufficiently explored to allow judgment is the use of "transfer factor." Lysates of leukocytes from immune donors when injected into nonimmune recipients render them immune. The substance mediating this conversion is called "transfer factor." This treatment may avoid some of the problems encountered with other modes of passive immunotherapy.

B. Active, Specific Immunotherapy

Active, specific immunotherapy is designed to elicit immunity to the host's own tumor (Prager, 1978). Irradiated or chemically modified tumor cells, solubilized tumor-associated antigens, oncogenic viruses, or bacterial products cross-reactive with tumor antigens have been used in laboratory studies with varying success. Application of the technique to man has been limited because success requires an immunocompetent patient, there is fear about increasing the tumor load in the patient, and there is uncertainty as to whether such manipulation may enhance or inhibit tumor growth.

C. Active, Nonspecific Immunotherapy

By far, the most widely employed modality is the use of agents, such as Bacillus Calmette-Guérin (BCG), *Corynebacterium parvum,* and levamisole, which actively and nonspecifically restore or enhance immune responsiveness (Hersh *et al.,* 1977; Mathé, 1976). In general, these agents are more likely to be beneficial to immune-compromised patients than to those still competent. It also seems to be the general clinical experience that active, nonspecific immunotherapy, at least at its present stage, is most effective when the primary tumor mass is maximally reduced by other procedures—chemotherapy, radiotherapy, or surgery.

A number of agents in clinical use are listed in Table III. The table also summarizes their modulating effects on the three major cellular components of the immune response—T cells, B cells, and macrophages. Those agents which enhance both T cell and B cell responses and activate macrophages to inhibit tumor cells include BCG, MER, and Krestin. BCG is a live bacterial vaccine generally administered either regionally or directly into accessible lesions. There are a number of reports that BCG when used adjunctively with other therapeutic procedures has reduced or eliminated metastatic disease, at least temporarily, and increased survival of cancer patients. MER is a methanol extraction residue of BCG which may be more immunopotentiating in man than BCG (Mikulski and Muggia, 1977). Krestin, a polysaccharide extracted from a fungus, is presently used in Japan as adjunctive therapy with claimed increase in life span of patients with stomach cancer or acute leukemias.

TABLE III

Effect of Immunomodulators on Cellular Components of the Immune Response[a]

Agent	T cell modulation	B cell modulation	Macrophage activation
BCG ⎱ MER ⎰	↑	↑	+
C. parvum	↓	↑	+
Levamisole	↑	0	−
Thymosin	↑	0	−
Interferon	↓	↑	+
Krestin	↑	↑	+

[a] T and B cells: ↑, enhanced; ↓, depressed; 0, no effect. Macrophages: +, activation; −, no effect.

The killed bacterial vaccine, *C. parvum,* and the antiviral substance, interferon, enhance B cell activity, stimulate macrophages, but depress T cell-associated immune response. *C. parvum* has been used both systemically and by intralesional or regional administration. In man, effectiveness of *C. parvum* is related to immunocompetence (Milas and Scott, 1978). Interferon, which is produced by various cells of the body when confronted by viral invasion or when stimulated by certain substances, has been used in cancer patients with some degree of benefit. The major impediment to more extensive clinical trials is the limited supply of purified human interferon and its relatively high cost of production.

The synthetic antihelminthic compound, levamisole, and thymosin, a family of peptides secreted by the thymus, appear to selectively enhance T cell function. In man, levamisole has given encouraging results when used as a prophylactic against recurrent lung or breast cancers. Limited clinical studies with thymosin indicate it may be used advantageously in situations where other therapy has severely compromised T cell function.

V. DISCUSSION

The concept of immune surveillance, although not universally accepted, provides the underlying rationale for the use of immunotherapy in the treatment of human neoplastic disease. The rationale is reinforced by a wide range of studies in tumor immunology which demonstrate the immunogenicity of many animal and human tumors, however weak, and the ability of hosts to respond immunologically. There is also evidence, although not applicable to all tumors and all individuals, that progressive disease is associated with immunologic anergy. Clinically, the absence of, or reduced, immune responsiveness often signals a poor outcome in the cancer patient.

At its present stage of development, cancer immunotherapy has shown only limited utility (Muggia, 1977). Nevertheless, its potential for specific killing and elimination of cancer cells justifies continued interest in this treatment strategy. As clinical experience and basic knowledge increase, existing deficiencies in immunotherapy may be overcome. First, it is necessary to devise dosing regimens for each agent to assure immune potentiation rather than unresponsiveness. Second, the role of suppressor cell activities must be clearly understood and the dangers of their stimulation during immunotherapeutic intervention circumvented. Finally, the time relationships between immunotherapy and other therapies must be clearly understood so that maximum benefits of both modalities may be obtained (Weiss, 1978).

Our understanding of the immunologic aspects of host–tumor relationships is rapidly enlarging. As the basic science of tumor immunology deepens our understanding of host defense to cancer invasion, there will hopefully be a concomitant increase in the effectiveness of immunotherapy in the treatment of human cancer.

REFERENCES

Burnet, F. M. (1970). *Prog. Exp. Tumor Res.* **13,** 1–27.
Byers, V. A., and Levin, A. S. (1976). *In* "Basic and Clinical Immunology" (H. H. Fundenberg, D. P. Stites, J. L. Caldwell, and J. V. Wells, eds.), pp. 242–259. Lange Med. Publ., Los Altos, California.
Coggin, J. H., Jr., Ambrose, K. R., Dierlam, P. J., and Anderson, N. G. (1974). *Cancer Res.* **34,** 2092–2101.
Douglas, S. D. (1976). *In* "Basic and Clinical Immunology" (H. H. Fundenberg, D. P. Stites, J. L. Caldwell, and J. V. Wells, eds.), pp. 70–87. Lange Med. Publ., Los Altos, California.
Good, R. A. (1972). *Clin. Immunobiol.* **1,** 1–28.
Haskell, C. M. (1977). *Annu. Rev. Pharmacol. Toxicol.* **17,** 179–195.
Hersh, E. M., Gutterman, J. V., and Mavligit, G. M. (1977). *Adv. Intern. Med.* **22,** 145–185.
Klein, G. (1974). *Clin. Immunobiol.* **2,** 219–241.
Klein, G. (1975). *Collect. Pap. Annu. Symp. Fundam. Cancer Res.* **26,** 21–54.
Levy, M. H., and Wheelock, E. F. (1974). *Adv. Cancer Res.* **20,** 131–163.
Marchalones, J. J. (1976). *In* "Basic and Clinical Immunology" (H. H. Fundenberg, D. P. Stites, J. L. Caldwell, and J. V. Wells, eds.), pp. 88–96. Lange Med. Publ., Los Altos, California.
Mathé, G. (1976). "Cancer Active Immunotherapy." Springer-Verlag, Berlin and New York.
Mikulski, S. M., and Muggia, F. M. (1977). *Cancer Treat. Rev.* **4,** 103–117.
Milas, L., and Scott, M. T. (1978). *Adv. Cancer Res.* **26,** 257–306.
Möller, G. (1975). *Collect. Pap. Annu. Symp. Fundam. Cancer Res.* **26,** 8–14.
Muggia, F. M. (1977). *Cancer Immunol. Immunother.* **3,** 5–9.
Prager, M. D. (1978). *Cancer Immunol. Immunother.* **3,** 157–161.
Rosenberg, S. A., and Terry, W. D. (1977). *Adv. Cancer Res.* **25,** 323–388.
Wang, A. C. (1976). *In* "Basic and Clinical Immunology" (H. H. Fudenberg, D. P. Stites, J. L. Caldwell, and J. V. Wells, eds.), pp. 15–31. Lange Med. Publ., Los Altos, California.
Weiss, D. W. (1977). *Cancer Immunol. Immunother.* **2,** 11–19.
Weiss, D. W. (1978). *Isr. J. Med. Sci.* **14,** 1–13.

12
ANIMAL MODELS
Michael A. Chirigos

I. INTRODUCTION

The term immunotherapy has several definitions and is often used to imply the application of immunologic methods to the treatment of a specific disease. For the purpose of this chapter the term will be applied to the treatment of cancer. The numerous attempts to apply one or another immunologic method to the treatment of cancer in animal experimental systems, as well as in human beings, have been reviewed and only a few are referenced (Currie, 1972, 1976; Chirigos, 1978; Feingold et al., 1976; Gutterman, 1977; Mackaness, 1969; Mackaness et al., 1973). The aim of all modalities of cancer treatment is to remove or to destroy the tumor without undue damage to the host. Currently three treatment modalities are extensively employed to remove or arrest tumor growth: surgery, irradiation, and chemotherapy. A fourth approach is the application of immunological methods to treat the cancer, referred to as immunotherapy (Mathé, 1969; Proctor *et al.*, 1976; Sinkovics, 1976; Smith, 1972).

II. POTENTIAL METHODS OF CANCER IMMUNOTHERAPY

A. Active Immunotherapy

Immunization is accomplished by injecting live autochthonous tumor cells which have been altered by one of several methods: killed by irradiation or cytoxic agents, heterogenized by infecting the tumor cells *in vitro* with a nonpathogenic virus, cell-free extracts of tumor cells, tumor cells reacted with neuraminidase.

B. Passive Immunotherapy

This approach involves the transfer of antitumor sera.

C. Adoptive Immunotherapy

Cells which have been sensitized to the tumor are transferred to the tumor-bearing host. The two particular cell types demonstrating antitumor lytic activity are T lymphocytes and macrophages.

Much has been published on the above three approaches demonstrating some degree of either preventive or tumor reductive effect. All three have a common characteristic, that of dealing with tumor antigen either on the tumor cell surface or in a soluble form.

Passive immunotherapy has been abandoned almost completely because success is doubtful, and many investigators fear enhanced tumor growth may occur (Currie, 1972).

D. Nonspecific Immunotherapy

The most promising development in recent years is that of nonspecific stimulation of host resistance by biological and chemical agents. This review will be confined primarily to such biological and chemical agents reported to modulate the host's cellular immune response.

TABLE I

Chemical and Biological Agents Demonstrating Immune Modulating Activity

Chemical	Biological
Levamisole	Thymosin
Pyran copolymer	Bacille Calmette-Guerin (BCG)
Poly(I:C)	Muramyl dipeptides
Poly(A:U)	*Corynebacterium parvum*
BM 12.531	*C. granulosum*
Bestatin	*Staphylococcus aureous*
Isoprinosine	*Streptococcus pyrogenes* (OK 432)
Glucan	*Brucella abortus*
Krestin	*Pseudomonas aerogenosa*
Lentinan	Interferon
Levan	MER (methanol extractable residue)
Dextran sulfate	

III. CHEMICAL AND BIOLOGICAL AGENTS DEMONSTRATING IMMUNE MODULATING ACTIVITY

Table I contains a list of chemical and biological agents which have been reported to exert an immunological response when tested either in an *in vitro* or *in vivo* system. A few of these agents will be discussed in this chapter. The reader is referred to published reviews of many of these agents (Terry and Windhorst, 1978; Chirigos, 1978). Of the biological agents, extensive experimental and clinical work have been conducted with Bacille Calmette-Guérin (BCG), *Corynebacterium parvum* and thymosin. Of the chemicals possessing immunomodulating activity, levamisole has been the most extensively investigated. Figure 1 shows the molecular structure of levamisole, and Fig. 2 shows the structure of pyran copolymer, polyinosinic:polycytidylic acid, and dextran sulfate.

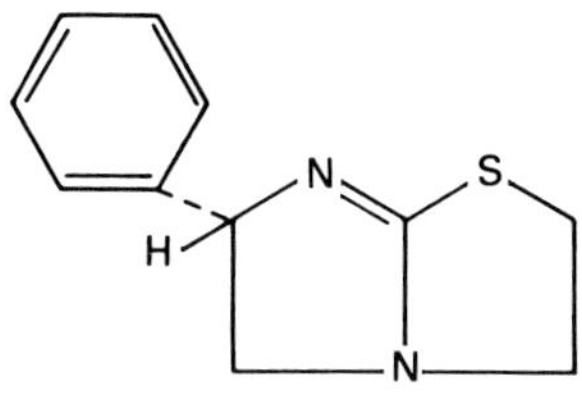

LEVAMISOLE

2,3,5,6-Tetrahydro-6-phenylimidazo[2, 1-*b*] thiazole

Fig. 1. Chemical structure of levamisole. (From Chirigos, 1978.)

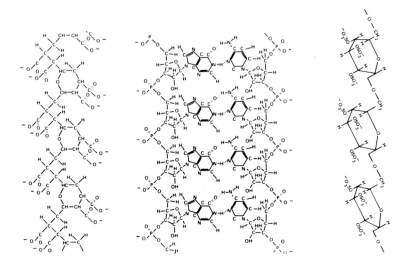

PYRAN COPOLYMER   POLYINOSINIC:POLYCYTIDYLIC ACID   DEXTRAN SULFATE

Fig. 2.   Chemical structures of immunostimulating agents.

IV. ANIMAL MODEL SYSTEMS FOR EVALUATING IMMUNOADJUVANTS

Several *in vivo* and *in vitro* test systems have been developed which have been found useful in assessing the ability of selected agents to modulate the cellular immune response.

A. Delayed Type Hypersensitivity Assay

There are many variations of this test system which is a measure of T lymphocyte (lymphocytes of thymic origin) response. The most often used technique is that of injecting sheep red blood cells (SRBC) into the footpad of mice. Hypersensitivity is measured as the increase in footpad thickness 24 hr after injecting an eliciting dose of SRBCs. Modifications of this technique have been reported for measuring the lymphoproliferative response in a regional lymph node (Mackaness *et al.*, 1973) and the number of plaque-forming cells (PFC) that appear in the popliteal lymph node following footpad inoculation with SRBC (Miller *et al.*, 1973). The procedure for adoptive sensitization by spleen cell transfer has also been described (Mackaness, 1969).

An example of delayed type hypersensitivity is shown in Table II. Mice were

TABLE II

Delayed Type Hypersensitivity Assay

Immunoadjuvant	Dose (mg/kg)	Foodpad thickness (mm)	P value
Brucella abortus	16	0.35	<0.02
	8	0.31	>0.10
	4	0.32	>0.10
B-M 12-531	250	0.32	>0.10
	25	0.33	>0.10
	2.5	0.55	<0.001
Bestatin	40	0.43	>0.01
	10	0.36	>0.10
	1	0.40	>0.10
Pyran copolymer	5	0.48	>0.001
SRBC control	Placebo	0.22	—

injected in the left footpad with 1×10^9 SRBC, and within 1–2 hr the immunoadjuvant was injected intraperitoneally. Four days later the mice were challenged in the right footpad with 1×10^9 SRBC, and the right footpad measured 24 hr later for increased thickness. The results in Table II show that all four immunoadjuvants were effective in enhancing the delayed type hypersensitivity above that obtained in the SRBC control.

The guinea pig has also been used in studying delayed type hypersensitivity. Table III shows the results of reconstituting the immune response in guinea pigs

TABLE III

Effect of Levamisole on BCG Delayed Hypersensitivity in Immunosuppressed Guinea Pigs

Group no.	No. guinea pigs	BCNU[a] Dose (mg/kg)	Day	LMS[b] Dose (mg/kg)	Day	PPD challenge on day zero (µg/dose) read in cm 0.062	0.25	1.0
1	8					0.90	1.18	1.47
2	4	40	−5			0.48	0.87	1.20
3	4	40	−5	20	−2	0.68	1.15	1.50
4	4	60	−5			0.42	0.77	1.10
5	4	60	−5	20	−2	0.58	1.03	1.35

[a] BCNU, 1,3-bis(2-chloroethyl)-1-nitrosourea.
[b] LMS, levamisole.

which have been immunized with BCG and subsequently immunosuppressed with 1,3-bis(z-chloroethyl)-1-nitrosourea (BCNU) treatment. Control animals immunized with BCG and challenged with purified protein derivative (PPD) (group 1) responded with a typical delayed type hypersensitivity response. The intensity of response was markedly diminished in the immunized animals as the result of immunosuppression resulting from BCNU treatment (groups 2 and 4). Suppression was markedly reversed as the result of treatment with levamisole (LMS) in groups 3 and 5. These results are indicative of the ability of LMS to reconstitute the depressed immune response provoked by BCNU treatment.

B. Combined Modality Treatment

Several different types of tumor model systems have been used to assess the effectiveness of immunoadjuvants when used alone or in combination with chemotherapy.

The first example of combined therapy with cytoreductive agents and levamisole is shown in Fig. 3. Mice with systemic Moloneyleukemia virus-induced lymphosarcoma (LSTRA) leukemia treated with BCNU had a twofold

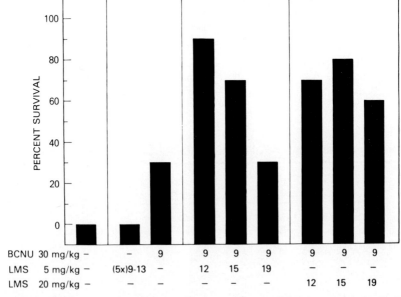

Fig. 3. Effect of monotherapy or combined treatment on the LSTRA murine leukemia. Ten-week-old CDF$_1$ male mice were inoculated with 1×10^5 LSTRA leukemia cells on day 0. BCNU or levamisole (LMS) was administered on indicated days. (From Chirigos, 1978.)

TABLE IV

Tumor Load Response to Chemotherapy and Immunoadjuvant in Leukemic Mice[a]

Cytoxan (mg/kg, day 8)	Levamisole (mg/kg, day 11)	Median survival time (days)	Percent survival
—	—	17.5	0
—	2.5	17.0	0
—	5.0	22.0	0
—	10.0	18.0	1
50	—	24.5	0
50	2.5	20.5	0
50	5.0	21.0	0
50	10.0	22.0	0
100	—	25.5	0
100	2.5	25.5	0
100	5.0	24.0	0
100	10.0	25.0	0
200	—	27.5	10
200	2.5	>100	60
200	5.0	44.0	40
200	10.0	40.0	50

[a] Mice inoculated with 1×10^4 Graffi leukemic cells sc on day 0.

increase in survival time and a 30% survival rate. Levamisole alone was ineffective, but when administered 3 to 10 days after BCNU treatment, a significant number of animals survived. Delaying treatment with levamisole at the 5 mg/kg dose was ineffective and could be attributable to the fact that animals treated with BCNU had begun to relapse. This response seemed to be reversible by a higher dose of levamisole.

Results in Table IV show the response attained when cytoxan or levamisole alone, or combined, effected growth of the Graffi leukemia in mice. Levamisole exerted only minimal effect when used alone. Cytoxan treatment resulted in an increase in survival time with increasing doses. A combined effect was not apparent till cytoxan at 200 mg/kg was combined with Levamisole treatment. Both survival time and the percent survival increased. The synergistic effect with the cytoreductive agent, cytoxan, and the immunostimulator, levamisole, indicates that levamisole was capable of exerting an immunostimulatory effect only when the tumor burden was more effectively reduced by the higher dose of cytoxan.

TABLE V

Timing of Pyran Therapy as an Adjuvant to Chemotherapy against the LSTRA Murine Leukemia[a]

Days of pyran therapy (20 mg/kg/day)	Survival time (days)	Percent survival[b]
Untreated controls	14.0 ± 0.7[c]	0
BCNU alone	23.4 ± 0.5	30
BCNU + pyran, days 6, 7, 8	24.0 ± 1.0	30
BCNU + pyran, days 6, 8, 10	27.4 ± 3.1	30
BCNU + pyran, days 13, 14, 15	>90	70
BCNU + pyran, days 13, 15, 17	>90	80
BCNU + pyran, days 20, 21, 22	>90	80
BCNU + pyran, days 20, 22, 24	>90	90

[a] LSTRA cells (1×10^4) injected sc on day 0. Chemotherapy consisted of BCNU, 30 mg/kg sc, on day 7.
[b] Surviving more than 90 days after tumor inoculation free of disease.
[c] Mean $\pm$ S.E.

Pyran copolymer has been reported to induce interferon when injected into mice, possess antitumor activity, and stimulate macrophage tumoricidal activity. In addition this chemical also acts as an immunoadjuvant.

Table V demonstrates that adjuvant therapy after BCNU with pyran copolymer was effective if treatment was started on day 13 or day 20. Daily or every other day therapy for a total of three doses produced 70 to 90% long-term survivors (cures) compared to chemotherapy alone which produced only 30%. Pyran started on day 6 was no more effective than chemotherapy alone. The time period of 13 to 20 days corresponded to the chemotherapeutic-induced remission period at a time when the early suppressive effects of BCNU had diminished and the tumor load was still at a low level. Treatment prior to remission induction (where tumor load was minimum) was ineffective, thus pyran treatment started on day 6 was ineffective.

Having established the most effective time interval for pyran therapy following BCNU induction of remission, Table VI summarizes the results of tests in which the dose of pyran was varied. Compared to BCNU therapy alone, pyran appeared to be effective as an immunoadjuvant at doses ranging from 0.1 to 100 mg/kg.

To determine whether this approach could be used in a different tumor system, pyran was tested against the Lewis lung carcinoma to determine its activity when used as an adjuvant to chemotherapy against a solid tumor. In Table VII, chemotherapy with 1-(2-chloroethyl)-3-(trans-4-methylcyclohexyl)-1-nitrosourea significantly increased the mean survival time of tumor-bearing animals by 15 days. A single dose of pyran 5 days after chemotherapy further increased

TABLE VI

Dose–Response using Pyran as an Adjuvant to Chemotherapy against LSTRA Murine Leukemia[a]

Treatment		
BCNU	Pyran (mg/kg, day 13)	Percent survival[b]
−	−	0
−	+ (25)	0
+	−	0
+	+ (0.1)	80
+	+ (0.25)	80
+	+ (0.50)	80
+	+ (1.0)	70
+	+ (2.5)	60
+	+ (5.0)	80
+	+ (10.0)	90
+	+ (25.0)	80
+	+ (50.0)	90
+	+ (100.0)	80

[a] LSTRA cells (1×10^4) injected sc on day 0. Chemotherapy consisted of BCNU, 30 mg/kg sc on day 7.

[b] Surviving more than 90 days after tumor inoculation free of disease.

TABLE VII

Pyran Copolymer as an Adjuvant to Chemotherapy against the Lewis Lung Carcinoma

Experimental groups	Survival (%)	Survival time (days)
1. Lewis lung control[a]	0	37.0 ± 1.2[b]
2. MeCCNU[c], 20 mg/kg, Day 9 MeCCNU, 10 mg/kg, Day 16	0	52.0 ± 3.1[d]
3. MeCCNU, 20 mg/kg, Day 9 MeCCNU, 10 mg/kg, Day 16 Pyran copolymer 20 mg/kg, D_{21}	0	62.3 ± 2.9[e]
4. MeCCNU, 20 mg/kg, Day 9 MeCCNU, 20 mg/kg, Day 16 Pyran copolymer, 20 mg/kg, every day, days 21–23	0	60.4 ± 4.6

[a] Tumor inoculated sc in BDF_1 mice as a 10% (w/v) homogenate. Cell count approximately 1×10^6 cells/ml.

[b] Mean ± S.E.

[c] MeCCNU, 1-(2-chloroethyl)-3-(*trans*-4-methylcyclohexyl)-1-nitrosourea.

[d] $p < 0.01$ when compared to group 1 by t test.

[e] $p < 0.05$ when compared to group 2 by t test.

the mean survival time by another 10 days over controls, but multiple treatments did not improve the response over a single dose. Therefore, the beneficial effects of adjuvant therapy with pyran copolymer are not limited to the treatment of leukemias alone.

The Lewis lung carcinoma tumor model was again used in determining the effectiveness of levamisole as an immunoadjuvant to chemotherapy. Three parameters were measured: median survival time, weight of the primary tumor (i.e., the tumor arising at the subcutaneously inoculated site), and the number of lung lesions developing as the result of metastasis from the primary tumor site. Figure 4 shows that levamisole alone was effective only in decreasing lung lesions and tumor weight. The combined treatment of 1-(2-chloroethyl)-3-

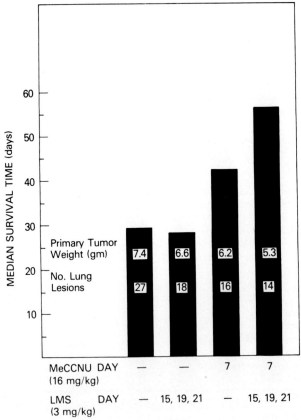

Fig. 4. Effect of levamisole as an adjuvant to chemotherapy against the Lewis lung carcinoma. Tumor inoculated sc in BDF_1 male mice as a 10% (w/v) homogenate. Cell count approximately 1 × 10^6 cells/ml. 1-(2-Chloroethyl)-3-(*trans*-4-methylcyclohexyl)-1-nitrosourea (MeCCNU) and levamisole (LMS) administered intraperitoneally on indicated days. (From Chirigos, 1978.)

(*trans*-4-methylcyclohexyl)-1-nitrosourea (MeCCNU) and levamisole proved more effective than MeCCNU alone, resulting in a significant increase in life span and decreases in primary tumor weight and number of lung lesions.

C. Tumor Response to Levamisole Monotherapy versus Combined Drug and Levamisole

An attempt was made to evaluate if a trend could be demonstrated concerning the ability ot levamisole monotherapy to retard or inhibit tumor growth. Of ten tumor systems tested, levamosole monotherapy did not appear to exert an antitumor effect (Table VIII).

However, when levamisole was combined with chemotherapy, a more beneficial effect was achieved (Table IX). The tumor types listed in Table IX were

TABLE VIII

Negative Cytoreductive Effect of Levamisole on Primary Growth of Several Tumors

Tumor	Host	Results
P 388 leukemia	Mouse	Negative
Moloney LSTRA leukemia	Mouse	Negative
Moloney MCAs-10 leukemia	Mouse	Negative
B16 melanoma	Mouse	Negative
M109 adenocarcinoma	Mouse	Negative
Meth-A fibrosarcoma	Mouse	Negative
MC-7 sarcoma	Rat	Negative
Walker 256 tumor	Rat	Negative
RD-3 tumor	Rat	Negative
CELO-virus induced tumor	Hamster	Negative

TABLE IX

Positive Effect of Levamisole after Cytoreductive Therapy

Tumor	Host	Cytoreductive therapy[a]	Effect
L1210 leukemia	Mouse	MeCCNU	+
Moloney LSTRA leukemia	Mouse	BCNU, Cy	+
Moloney MCAs-10 leukemia	Mouse	BCNU, Cy	+
Graffi leukemia	Mouse	BCNU, Cy	+
3-MC induced fibrosarcoma	Mouse	BCNU, Cy	+
Meth-A fibrosarcoma	Mouse	Cy	+
Lewis lung carcinoma	Mouse	MeCCNU	+
DMBA-induced breast carcinoma	Mouse	None	+

[a] Cy, cytoxan.

selected for representation, of the effects of combined chemotherapy and levamisole treatment because they are often used in drug testing. However, results of cytoreductive therapy combined with levamisole for other tumor types also have been reported. The most important point made through these studies was the importance of initial tumor cytoreductive therapy to be applied prior to administering levamisole.

D. Alveolar Carcinoma M109 Tumor Model

The Madison lung carcinoma (M109), a transplantable line derived from a spontaneous neoplasm in a BALB/c mouse, has been adapted for *in vivo* and *in vitro* studies and makes an excellent model for evaluating the effectiveness of different treatment modalities and lung tumor lesions.

M109 cells grown *in vitro* were harvested during their exponential growth phase by gentle trypsinization, washed twice, and resuspended in serum-free RPMI-1640. The number of single viable cells was determined and adjusted to 5 $\times$ 10^5 cells/ml medium. Tumor cells were injected intravenously into the tail vein of normal BALB/c mice. Inoculum volume per mouse was 0.2 ml (10^5 cells). After 24 hr, the mice were randomly divided into two cages and injected intraperitoneally with either 0.9% NaCl solution or pyran copolymer at 25 mg/kg. The mice were sacrificed on day 15, and the number of pulmonary metastases was determined by inflation with India ink according to the method of Wexler (1966).

Results in Fig. 5 show the results of pyran treatment on M109 lung lesion development. Pyran strikingly reduced the number of pulmonary lesions in at least two separate experiments. These lesions were identified histologically as the M109 carcinoma. In contrast to multiple tumors in the lungs of placebo-treated mice, many lungs from pyran-treated mice remained tumor-free at day 15.

The same tumor lung model was employed to assess the activity of a *Brucella abortus* ether–alcohol extracted material (Bru Pel) which has been reported to be a potent interferon inducer (Feingold *et al.,* 1976).

For determination of whether Bru Pel was similarly effective in potentiating surveillance against M109 pulmonary metastases, Bru Pel was administered as a single intraperitoneal injection either 5 days prior to, on the same day as, or 1 day after intravenous tumor inoculation. Mice were sacrificed on days 14 and 20, and lungs were inflated with India ink to visualize tumor nodules. The results in Fig. 6 show that Bru Pel almost completely suppressed the development of metastatic lung lesions. In contrast to multiple tumors in the lungs of placebo-treated animals, many lungs from Bru Pel-treated mice remained tumor free at day 20. The results also show the *Brucella* lipopolysaccharide (LPS) did not exert any demonstrable effect on retarding tumor lung lesion development. The LPS control

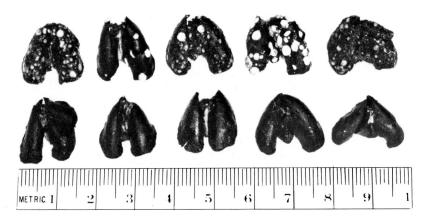

Fig. 5. Influence of pyran copolymer treatment on artificially induced M109 metastases. Mice were given 1×10^5 M109 cells intravenously on day 0 and inoculated with pyran or placebo intraperitoneally on day 1. The lower figure shows India ink-inflated lungs from pyran-treated animals. The lungs are free of identifiable tumor nodules at day 15. In contrast, the upper figure shows lungs from 0.9% NaCl solution-treated mice. Numerous tumor lesions are visualized by India ink treatment.

was an important control to include since several endotoxins (lipopolysaccharides) of bacterial origin have been reported to enhance cellular immune responsiveness.

The potent inhibition of lung metastasis formation by Bru Pel and pyran copolymer indicate a strong cellular immune response. Our preliminary histopathological observations show macrophage accumulation in the interstitium of the lungs from Bru Pel-treated animals encircling the metastatic foci and completely arresting their development. The current data suggest that activated macrophages have a surveillance function in inhibiting or controlling metastatic cell growth. This subject will be covered in more detail in Section IV.F.

E. Vaccine Model and Adjuvants

In order for an immune adjuvant to be effective it must be capable of augmenting cellular and/or humoral immunity whem combined with a vaccine. We have developed a tumor cell vaccine model which is useful in testing adjuvants capable of augmenting the immunity to tumor challenge induced by a suboptimal application of tumor vaccine.

A brief description of preparing the leukemia L1210 tumor cell vaccine for use with adjuvants is as follows. L1210 ascites cells were adjusted to a concentration

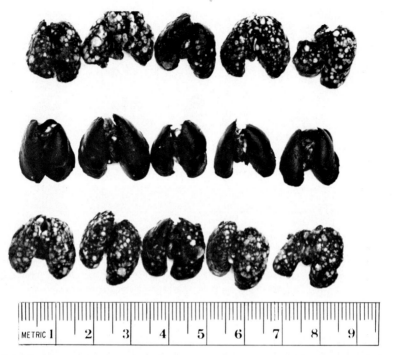

Fig. 6. Effect of Bru Pel and *Brucella abortus* lipopolysaccharide (LPS) treatment on artificially induced M109 pulmonary metastases. Mice were treated intraperitoneally with Bru Pel (100 mg/kg) or *Brucella* LPS (2 mg/kg) 5 days prior to receiving 2×10^4 M109 cells intravenously. Some mice received 0.2 ml Dulbecco's phosphate-buffered saline as placebo. Top row: India ink-inflated lungs from placebo-treated animals on Day 20. Numerous tumor lesions are visualized by India ink treatment. In contrast the middle row shows lungs that are essentially free of identifiable tumor nodules from Bru Pel-treated animals. Lungs from *Brucella* LPS-treated mice (bottom row) appeared like placebo-treated controls.

of 5.0×10^7 cells/ml in Eagles minimal essential media and inactivated by exposure to 5000 R X radiation. Vaccination was done by the intraperitoneal injection of 10^7 cells 7 days before live tumor challenge. At no time did the vaccine produce systemic leukemia. Animals receiving both vaccine and drug treatment received the vaccine 1 to 2 hr after the drug in a separate injection.

Results of several experiments are summarized in Table X. Vaccination with L1210 or pyran treatment alone did not significantly alter the response of the animals to subsequent challenge. However, if pyran and vaccine were both given 7 days before challenge, a markedly enhanced resistance was seen, with about 45% of the animals resistant to 10^4 L1210 cells and the remainder having a marked increase in their average survival time.

Having demonstrated that concomitant administration of pyran and vaccine

TABLE X

Potentiation of Leukemia L1210 Vaccine by Pyran Copolymer

L1210 vaccine (10^7 cells, ipr, on day 7)	Pyran (25 mg/kg, ip, day 7)	L1210 challenge (10^4 cells, ip, day 0)	Survivors[a]/ total	Average survival time (days ± S.E.)[b]
+	−	−	112/112	>70
−	−	+	0/119	10.8 ± 0.1
+	−	+	0/122	11.1 ± 0.2
−	+	+	0/121	12.4 ± 0.1
+	+	+	57/126	27.9 ± 1.3

[a] Animals scored for survival 70 days after viable L1210 challenge.
[b] Calculated from individual days of death of animals dying from systemic leukemia.

resulted in a synergistic response in which the inadequate immunization with L1210 vaccine was strongly improved by pyran, we looked to see if the experimental variables initially chosen were really optimal. To determine the effective dose range of pyran, all other conditions were held constant and the dose of pyran given with vaccine was varied over a wide range. That pyran has a widely effective dosage range in this system is evident in Table XI. Doses less than 1.0

TABLE XI

Potentiation of Leukemia L1210 Vaccine by Different Doses of Pyran Copolymer

L1210 vaccine (10^7 cells, ipr, day 7)	Pyran (mg/kg, day 7)	L1210 challenge (10^4 cells, ip, day 0)	Percent survival[a]	Average survival time (days ± S.E.)[b]
+	−	−	100	>70
−	−	+	0	10.8 ± 0.1
+	−	+	0	11.7 ± 0.4
−	25	+	0	12.4 ± 0.1
+	0.5	+	0	12.9 ± 0.4
+	1.0	+	10	20.7 ± 2.7
+	2.5	+	70	25.0 ± 2.5
+	5.0	+	80	42.0 ± 10.0
+	10.0	+	80	28.5 ± 9.5
+	25.0	+	90	29.0 ± 0
+	50.0	+	60	39.8 ± 7.5
+	75.0	+	50	28.2 ± 5.8
+	100.0	+	30	30.0 ± 3.6
+	200.0	+	25	22.8 ± 5.1

[a] Animals scored for survival 70 days after viable L1210 challenge.
[b] Calculated from individual days of death of animals that died from systemic leukemia.

mg/kg were ineffective, and doses over 100 mg/kg were somewhat toxic. The dose of 25 mg/kg appeared to be an optimal dose.

Subsequent tests have shown other agents capable of acting as adjuvants in the L1210 tumor cell vaccine, e.g., Bru Pel, BCG and lipopolysaccharide. Thus, the L1210 tumor vaccine model could serve as a model for evaluating vaccine adjuvants.

F. Macrophage Assay

The vital role of mononuclear phagocytes in host defense against neoplasia, as well as infectious organisms, has been amply demonstrated. There appears to be a close relationship between the ability of biologic and synthetic agents to enhance host antitumor resistance and their capacity to activate macrophages. Although normal resting macrophages are not cytotoxic to tumor cells, they can be rendered nonspecifically cytotoxic (activated) by soluble mediators (lymphokines) released by thymus-derived lymphocytes upon interaction with either sensitizing antigen or mitogen. Once activated, macrophages display a variety of increased activities, including enzymatic secretion, phagocytosis, bacteriostasis, and the ability to selectively kill transformed cells. There appear to be four separate pathways whereby macrophage are stimulated to kill tumor target cells *in vitro* (Fig. 7). Interferon appears to be intimately involved in each of these schemes that affect macrophage tumoricidal activity.

Normal peritoneal macrophages exposed to interferon *in vitro* showed accelerated spreading on plastic as compared to control culture (Fig. 8).

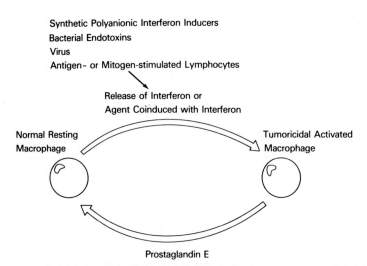

Fig. 7.   Pathways for the induction of nonspecifically tumoricidal (activated) macrophages.

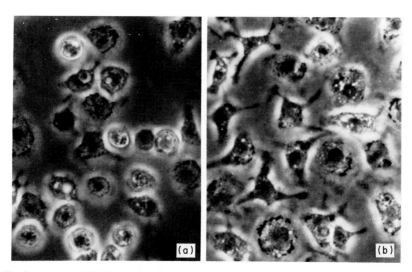

Fig. 8. Normal C57B1/6 peritoneal macrophages after 48 hr cultures in control medium (a) or medium containing 1000 units of interferon (b). Note increased cell spreading and prominent vacuolization following interferon treatment.

Figure 9 shows the assay developed for testing biological or chemical agents for their capability of activating macrophages to exert a tumoricidal effect. The details of this assay have been reported elsewhere (Schultz *et al.*, 1977). Briefly, noninduced peritoneal macrophages are harvested from treated (i.e., with activator) or normal mice. The adherent purified macrophages are washed with Roswell Park Memorial Institute (RPMI)-1640 medium, and approximately 4 × 10^5 macrophages are seeded into 16 mm wells on tissue culture cluster plates in 1.0 ml RPMI-FCS. The cultures are incubated for 90 min, and macrophage monolayers were thoroughly washed with jets of medium before use in experiments.

The MBL-2 lymphoblastic leukemia target cells are maintained as a suspension culture in RPMI-1640 medium supplemented with 20% heat inactivated (56°C for 30 min) fetal calf serum, 100 μg/ml gentamycin solution, 0.075% NaHCO$_3$, and 10 mM HEPES buffer. Viability of the cells is determined by trypan blue exclusion. The ratio of macrophages to target cells is adjusted to 10 : 1 at the beginning of the experiment. All cultures are incubated at 37°C in an atmosphere of 5% CO$_2$ in air, and viable leukemic cells are counted after 48 hr with a hemacytometer. The percent of growth inhibition of MBL-2 tumor target cells is calculated by comparison to MBL-2 cells grown in the presence of normal resting macrophages alone.

Other tumor target cells can also be employed in place of the MBL-2 tumor cell line. We have employed both the MBL-2 and M109 tumor cells in this assay.

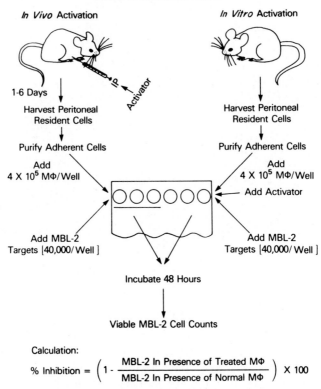

Fig. 9. Scheme of testing agents for macrophage activating capability *in vivo* and *in vitro*. Mφ, macrophage.

Several agents have been tested in this assay employing the M109 tumor cell, and the results obtained compared to their activity when tested *in vivo* against the M109 tumor (Fig. 10). The details of these tests have been reported (Schultz *et al.*, 1976, 1978). The ability of four of the five agents (Fig. 10b) capable of stimulating macrophages to exert a tumoricidal effect on M109 target cells were confirmed to possess tumor retarding activity in M109 tumor-bearing mice (Fig. 10a). Dextrane sulfate although capable of activating macrophages to tumoricidal activity did not demonstrate a tumor retarding effect *in vivo*.

V. DISCUSSION

Based on the results of studies with several experimental tumor and nontumor model systems, the ability of agents exerting a stimulatory effect on the cellular

(a)

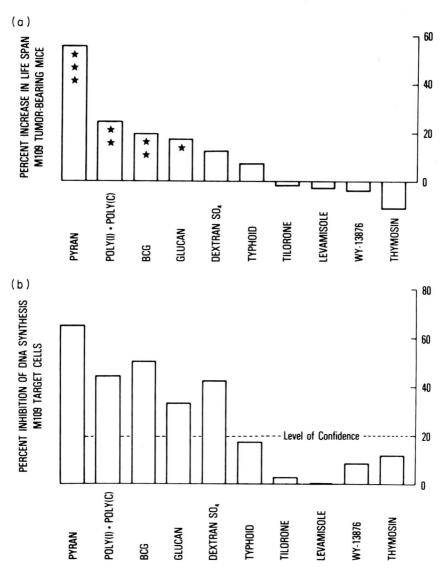

Fig. 10. Comparison of *in vivo* antitumor activity to macrophage tumoricidal activity against the M109 alveolar carcinoma by several agents. The values represent the means obtained from three or more separate determinations. The probabilities are indicated as: * = $P < 0.05$; ** = $P < 0.01$; *** = $P < 0.001$.

elements of the immune system can be quantitatively measured. Of particular importance is the role of immunoadjuvants in immunotherapy. Results from several experimental tumor model systems show that the more effective use of immunoadjuvants appears to be following cytoreductive therapy. Figure 11 represents a general plan for the implementation of immunotherapy, in form of immunoadjuvants, following cytoreductive therapy. Depending upon the tumor type, one of three cytoreductive treatment modalities may be initially used to reduce the tumor burden of the host. Without this intervention the tumor burden will increase in time leading to the death of the host. During the remission period, induced by cytoreductive treatment, immunotherapy can be initiated in a single, multiple, or intermittent regimen. In the event of tumor recurrence, the same or another cytoreductive treatment regimen can be reinstituted, which again can be followed by immunotherapy. The ultimate aim is to reduce the number of tumor cells in the host without irreversible damage to host physiological functions (e.g., extensive bone marrow suppression, liver or kidney toxicity, or cardiac dysfunction by extensive chemotherapy). Immunoadjuvants are beneficial in that they mobilize the cellular components of the immune system by earlier reconstitution of thymus-derived lymphocytes (T cells) and activating

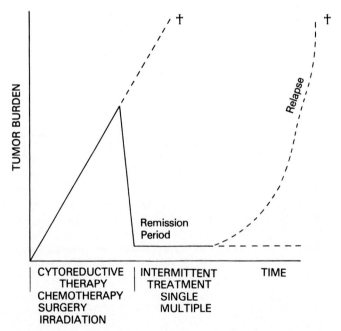

Fig. 11. Scheme for immunoadjuvant treatment when combined with cytoreductive therapy. †, death.

macrophages. Indeed, immunoadjuvants when used judiciously may well prove to be an effective therapy complementing other established treatment modalities.

REFERENCES

Chirigos, M. A., ed. (1978). "Immune Modulation and Control of Neoplasia by Adjuvant Therapy," Vol. VII. Raven, New York.

Currie, G. A. (1972). *Br. J. Cancer* **26**, 141–153.

Currie, G. A. (1976). *Biochim. Biophys. Acta* **458**, 135–165.

Feingold, D. S., Keleti, G., and Youngner, J. S. (1976). *Infect. Immun.* **13**, 763–767.

Gutterman, J. H. (1977). *Cancer Immunol. Immunother* **2**, 1–9.

Mackaness, G. B. (1969). *J. Exp. Med.* **129**, 973–992.

Mackaness, G. B., Auclair, D. J., and Lagrange, P. H. (1973). *J. Natl. Cancer Inst.* **51**, 1655–1667.

Mathé, G. (1969). *Br. Med J.* **4**, 7–10.

Miller, T. E., Mackaness, G. B., and Lagrange, P. H. (1973). *J. Natl. Cancer Inst.* **51**, 1669–1676.

Proctor, J. W., Lewis, M. G., and Mansell, P. W. (1976). *Can. J. Surg.* **19**, 12–22.

Schultz, R. M., Papamatheakis, J. D., Stylos, W. A., and Chirigos, M. A. (1976). *Cell. Immunol.* **25**, 309–316.

Schultz, R. M., Papamatheakis, J. D., and Chirigos, M. A. (1977). *Cell. Immunol.* **29**, 403–409.

Schultz, R. M., Papamatheakis, J. D., and Chirigos, M. A. (1978). *In* "Immune Modulation and Control of Neoplasia by Adjuvant Therapy" (M. A. Chirigos, ed.), Vol. VII, pp. 459–467. Raven, New York.

Sinkovics, J. G. (1976). *Postgrad. Med.* **59**, 110–116.

Smith, R. T. (1972). *N. Engl. J. Med.* **287**, 439–450.

Terry, W. D., and Windhorst, D., eds. (1978). "Immunotherapy of Cancer: Present Status of Trials in Man." Raven, New York.

Wexler, H. (1966). *J. Natl. Cancer Inst.* **36**, 641–645.

13
CLINICAL TRIALS
Michael A. Chirigos

I. INTRODUCTION

Several agents possessing immunostimulatory activity on the macrophage, T cell, or B cell components of the immune system as demonstrated by experimental *in vitro* and *in vivo* tumor or nontumor animal models have been incorporated into phase I and phase II clinical trials. The agents were used in combination with one of the three established cancer treatment modalities. Many of these studies are still in an early stage and evaluation is premature. A few of the more advanced studies have been selected for discussion based on the type of tumor treated and the adjuvant employed.

II. LUNG CARCINOMA

Results of several years of study in experimental tumor systems pointed to Bacille Calmette-Guérin (BCG) as an effective bacterial potentiator of the immune response (Bast *et al.*, 1974). As the result of such studies, BCG was considered a good candidate as an immune adjuvant to augment cytoreductive therapy, whether this therapy was surgery, chemotherapy, or irradiation. Extensive studies have been conducted by Mathé *et al.* (1976, 1977) in which BCG is incorporated as an adjuvant to chemotherapy in the treatment of childhood leukemia.

CANCER AND CHEMOTHERAPY, VOL. I

McKneally *et al.* (1978) recently updated their results of a trial randomizing lung cancer patients following surgical resection to either intrapleural BCG plus oral isoniazid or isoniazid alone. Initially were 47 patients in the treated group and 48 patients in the control group. The two groups were essentially comparable. Sixty-five of the 95 patients in the study have been followed for more than 1 year. Of 26 stage I BCG-treated patients, only two had recurrence, and one of these died. Nine recurrences were found among the 32 stage 1 control patients, and all of them subsequently died. A more recent evaluation of the study is shown in Table I, where the results of a 3 year follow-up are shown. The percent survival in the BCG-treated groups is highly significant. However, no benefit was seen with BCG treatment for patients with stage II and III disease. Of particular interest was that all the BCG-treated patients developed transient elevation of the plasma alkaline phosphatase, indicative of a controlled form of granulomatous hepatitis induced by BCG.

Dimitrov *et al.* (1978) conducted a pilot study in which patients with stage 1 adenocarcinoma or squamous cell lung cancer were randomized after surgery. One group received *Corynebacterium parvum* + adriamycin + cyclophosphamide, and one group did not receive further treatment. At 18 months, no recurrences were evident in the chemoimmunotherapy treated group, while the control group had five recurrences. This study design, however, did not allow an evaluation of what effect *C. parvum* exerted compared to chemotherapy alone. Kerman and Stefani (1977) randomized patients having inoperable, locally advanced lung cancer to receive either radiotherapy (6000 rads) or radiotherapy plus intradermal BCG. Sixteen patients received radiotherapy alone (concurrent control), and 15 patients received both radiotherapy and immunotherapy. The two groups were comparable concerning age, lung cancer histology, and dose of radiotherapy received. The median survival of 52 weeks in the combined treated group was significantly longer than the 33 weeks survival average of those treated with radiotherapy alone. Of interest was that the development of metastases was delayed in the BCG-treated group as well as an improvement in a

TABLE I

Effect of Intrapleural BCG Treatment Postsurgery on Survival of Patients with Stage I Lung Cancer

	Random control $N = 36^a$	Historical control $N = 100$	With BCG $N = 30$
Survival (%)[b]	50	42	95

[a] N = number of patients.
[b] Evaluated at 3 years.

variety of immune parameters. These results suggest that BCG immunostimulation had a beneficial effect on survival and delay of recurrence.

Although several successful responses have been reported for BCG or *C. parvum* immunoadjuvant therapy, many other studies have reported failure of these adjuvants to augment the therapeutic response attained by either chemotherapy, surgery, or irradiation of lung tumors. For more detailed descriptions of clinical studies incorporating BCG or *C. parvum* as immunoadjuvants in treating lung cancer, the reader is referred to two recent reviews (Chirigos, 1978; Terry and Windhorst, 1978).

Another large study was reported in which levamisole was employed as an adjuvant to surgery (Amery, 1978). Two hundred and eleven patients were selected for this study. In most part, the two treatment groups were comparable. Apart from surgery, all patients were treated with tablets containing either 50 mg levamisole or placebo. The dosage was one tablet for 3 consecutive days, every second week, and started 3 days before the operation. This treatment was continued for 2 years, unless relapse was evident, in which case the appropriate chemotherapy was administered. However, until recurrence of tumor, any use of cytostatics, corticosteroids, or irradiation treatment was prohibited. Table II shows the results of the 2-year follow-up of this study. It is evident that, at 2 years, the difference in survival of 88% in the levamisole group to 58% in the placebo group is significant. Of particular interest in this study was the importance of adequate dosing with levamisole. More effective response was noted in patients receiving adequate doses of 50 mg/day at a body weight of 50 kg. The recommended dose is 2.5 mg/kg or 100 mg/m^2 per day. Another interesting aspect of this study was that patients with larger tumors at time of surgery responded better than those that had smaller tumors (Table III). It was not clear from this study whether this is due to a more marked reversal by levamisole of the immune suppression usually associated with the more advanced cancers.

TABLE II

Effect of Oral Levamisole Treatment Pre- and Postsurgery on Survival of Patients with Lung Cancer

Time after surgery (months)	Remission duration NED[a] (%)		Percent survival	
	Levamisole	Placebo[b]	Levamisole	Placebo[b]
12	86	70*	95	83*
18	83	55**	90	63***
24	70	51*	88	58***

[a] NED = No evidence of disease.
[b] *, $p < 0.05$; **, $p < 0.01$; ***, $p < 0.001$.

TABLE III

Effect of Surgery and Oral Levamisole on Duration of Remission According to Lung Tumor Size at Surgery

Time after surgery (months)	Remission duration (%)[a]			
	Tumor size <3 cm		Tumor size >3 cm	
	Levamisole	Placebo	Levamisole	Placebo
12	100	88	79	58
18	90	75	79	44
24	90	75	64	37

[a] No evidence of disease (%).

In a more recent study, Chrétien et al. (1978) reported the beneficial effect of thymosin (Table IV). In patients with small cell carcinoma of the lung receiving intensive chemotherapy (also randomized to receive thymosin 60 mg/m^2, thymosin 20 mg/m^2, or placebo twice weekly), increased survival occurred in patients receiving thymosin at 60 mg/m^2. The increase in survival was greatest in patients with low pretreatment T cell levels (low <775/mm^3). These observations suggest that a more beneficial effect could occur with thymosin, and possibly other immunoadjuvants, in patients with relatively low initial T cell levels. The authors relate the improved response noted in the low T cell level patients treated with thymosin 60 mg/m^2, to results of in vitro studies. In general, among populations with low T cell levels, T cell levels increased in vitro after incubation with thymosin, but among those patients with high T cell levels, the levels decreased after incubation with thymosin.

A parallel finding concerning T cell levels in Hodgkins disease patients for levamisole was reported by Ramot et al. (1978). Incubation of lymphocytes from

TABLE IV

Response of Small Cell Carcinoma of the Lung to Chemotherapy and Thymosin and Relationship to T Cell Levels

Pretreatment T cell levels	Median survival (days)			Probability value
	Chemotherapy alone	Chemotherapy + thymosin (60 mg/m^2)		
High >775/mm^3	285 (11)[a]	350 (9)		$p = 0.28$
Low <775/mm^3	180 (8)	405 (12)		$p = 0.006$

[a] Numbers in parentheses are numbers of patients.

patients with Hodgkin's disease with levamisole resulted in an increase in the number of E-rosette-forming cells (a technique for identifying T cells).

III. BREAST CARCINOMA

Combination chemotherapy has been shown to produce consistently high objective remission rates and overall survival times superior to those achieved by hormonal therapy or single agent chemotherapy. Over the past several years, reports have appeared suggesting that nonspecific immunotherapy with BCG, and *Corynebacterium parvum* is able to prolong the duration of remission and survival of chemotherapy treated patients.

Two separate studies have been reported indicating that the addition of an immunoadjuvant has increased responsiveness to either chemotherapy or irradiation. Table V contains the results reported by Hortobagyi *et al.* (1978). Two hundred and thirty-one evaluable patients with measurable metastatic breast cancer were treated with a combination regimen of 5-fluorouracil, adriamycin, cyclophosphamide, combined with levamisole or levamisole plus BCG. The results were compared to the results attained in 44 patients which received chemotherapy alone. The addition of levamisole, or levamisole plus BCG, resulted in significant differences both in remission duration and median survival time.

In another large study, Rojas *et al.* (1976) reported the effect of radiation combined with levamisole on advanced human breast cancer. Forty-three women with stage III primary breast cancer, considered inoperable, were entered into the study. After being rendered clinically disease free by radiotherapy to the breast, supraclavicular area, and axilla, patients were allocated alternately to a control group (no further treatment), and a levamisole-treated group (150 mg orally three times a week on alternate weeks). Of the 43 patients (23 control and 20 levamisole treated), there was a significant prolongation of the median disease-

TABLE V

Results of Studies of Chemotherapy and Chemoimmunotherapy for Advanced Breast Cancer

Treatment regimen[a]	No. of patients	Response rate (%)	Remission duration (months)	Median survival (months)
FAC	44	72	9.0	17
+ BCG + levamisole	105	73	14.0	>28
+ Levamisole	111	72	13.0	28

[a] F, 5-fluorouracil; A, adriamycin; C, cyclophosphamide; BCG, Bacille Calmette-Guérin.

free interval (9 months versus 30 months), and in survival at 30 months (35% versus 90%) in the control versus Levamisole-treated groups, respectively. Levamisole treatment was found also to increase the percentage and intensity of delayed hypersensitivity skin reactions and in the absolute lymphocyte counts. This last observation is again reminiscent of the increased lymphocyte responses reported by Ramot *et al.* (1978) for levamisole and by Chrétien *et al.* (1978) for thymosin.

IV. MALIGNANT MELANOMA

Bacille Calmette-Guérin (BCG) and *Corynebacterium parvum* have also been reported to augment chemotherapy in the management of malignant melanoma (Morton *et al.*, 1977; Gutterman *et al.*, 1974, 1977). Response rates of patients with disseminated malignant melanoma receiving chemotherapy alone or combined with BCG or *C. parvum* were compared. Twelve years ago, a 15% remission was achieved with dimethyl triazenocarboxamide (DTIC) chemotherapy alone. In subsequent studies the remission rate was increased from 15 to 27% when BCG was combined with DTIC chemotherapy. In more recent studies (Table VI) when DTIC chemotherapy was combined with actinomycin D and *C. parvum*, a 32% increase in survival was observed at 18 months (Gutterman *et al.*, 1978).

V. DISCUSSION

Immunotherapy is developing into the fourth major modality of human cancer treatment. Although it is in its formulative years, immunotherapy already has demonstrated activity in terms of increasing the remission rate or increasing the

TABLE VI

Survival Rates of Patients with Disseminated Malignant Melanoma Responding to Regimens of Chemoimmunotherapy

	DTIC[a]	DTIC + BCG	DTIC + C. parvum	DTIC + actinomycin D + C. parvum
Survival total at 18 months	1/16	4/24	5/10	13/16
Percent increase	—	10	44	75

[a] DTIC, dimethyl triazenocarboxamide.

TABLE VII

Current Clinical Use of Immune Adjuvants in Various Tumor Types

Tumor type	Cytoreductive therapy	Immunoadjuvant	Current results[a]	Reference
Breast carcinoma	Radiation	Levamisole	+	Rojas *et al.* (1976)
Breast carcinoma	Chemotherapy	Levamisole	+	Hortobagyi *et al.* (1978)
Breast carcinoma	Chemotherapy	BCG	+	Hortobagyi *et al.* (1978)
Lung carcinoma	Surgery	Levamisole	+	Amery (1978)
Lung carcinoma	Surgery	BCG	+	McKneally *et al.* (1978)
Lung carcinoma	Chemotherapy	Thymosin	+	Chrétien *et al.* (1978)
Melanoma	Chemotherapy	*C. parvum*	+	Gutterman *et al.* (1974)
Melanoma (cutaneous)	None	Glucan	±	Israel and Edelstein (1978)
Melanoma (cutaneous)	None	Glucan	±	Mansell *et al.* (1978)

[a] Based on number of patients, extended remission duration, and/or extended survival time.

remission and survival durations in a variety of human malignancies. Table VII contains, in summary form, the current clinical use of immune adjuvants in various tumor types. Although, there have been several successes, there have also been many failures. Our understanding of the mechanism(s) through which immunoadjuvants function are now being better understood. As the other conventional modalities of cancer treatment (surgery, radiotherapy, and chemotherapy) are improved and better defined, and the immunological effects of these modalities of treatment are better established, a less empirical and more rational basis for the integration of the use of selected immunoadjuvants in immunotherapy in the overall strategy of cancer treatment will be developed.

REFERENCES

Amery, W. K. (1978). *Cancer Treat. Rep.* **62,** 1677–1683.
Bast, R. C., Zbar, B., Borsos, T., and Rapp, H. J. (1974). *N. Engl. J. Med.* **190,** 1413–1420.
Chirigos, M. A., ed. (1978). "Progress in Cancer Research and Therapy," Vol. VII. Raven, New York.
Chrétien, P. B., Lipson, S. D., Makuch, R., Kenady, D. E., Snyder, J. J., Cohen, M. H., and Minna, J. D. (1978). *Cancer Treat. Rep.* **62,** 1787–1790.
Dimitrov, N. V., Aabo, K., Rao, M., and Hug, H. (1978). *Proc. Am. Assoc. Cancer Res.* **19,** 371.
Gutterman, J. V., Mavligit, G., Gottliev, J. A., Burgess, M. A., McBride, C. M., Einhorn, L., Freireich, E. J., and Hersh, E. M. (1974). *N. Engl. J. Med.* **291,** 592–597.
Gutterman, J. V., Mavligit, G., Benjamin, R., Burgess, M. A., and Hersh, E. M. (1977). *Proc. Am. Soc. Clin. Oncol.* **18,** 300.
Gutterman, J. V., Mavligit, G. M., Richman, S. P., Benjamin, R. S., Kennedy, A., McBride, C.

M., Burgess, M. A., Bartold, S. L., Gehan, E. A., and Hersh, E. M. (1978). *In* "Immunotherapy of Human Cancer" (W. D. Terry and D. Windhorst, eds.), p. 257. Raven, New York.

Hortobagyi, G. N., Yapp, H. D., Blumenschein, G. R., Gutterman, J. V., Buzdar, A. V., Tashima, C. K., and Hersh, E. M. (1978). *Cancer Treat. Rep.* **62**, 1685–1692.

Israel, L., and Edelstein, R. (1978). *In* "Progress in Cancer Research and Therapy" (M. A. Chirigos, ed.), Vol. VII, p. 249. Raven, New York.

Kerman, R., and Stefani, S. (1977). *In* "Neoplasm Immunity: Solid Tumor Therapy" (R. G. Crispin, ed.), pp. 24–35.

McKneally, M. F., Kaver, C. M., and Kausel, H. W. (1978). *In* "Immunotherapy of Cancer: Present Status of Trials in Man" (W. D. Terry and D. Windhorst, eds.), pp. 161–171. Raven, New York.

Mansell, P. W. A., Rowden, G., and Hammer, C. (1978). *In* "Progress in Cancer Research and Therapy" (M. A. Chirigos, ed.), Vol. VII, pp. 255–280. Raven, New York.

Mathé, G., DeVassal, F., Delgardo, M., Ponillart, P., Belpomme, D., Joseph, R., Schwarzenberg, L., Amiel, J. L., Schneider, M., Catton, A., Musset, M., Misset, J. L., and Jasmin, C. (1976). *Cancer Immunol. Immunother.* **1**, 77–86.

Mathé, G., Amiel, J. L., Schwarzenberg, L., Schneider, M., Catton, A., Schlumberger, J. R., Hazot, M., and DeVassal, F. (1977). *Biomedicine* **26**, 29–35.

Morton, D. L., Eilber, F. R., Homes, E. C., Townsend, C. M., Mirra, J., and Weisenburger, T. H. (1977). *In* "Adjuvant Therapy of Cancer" (S. E. Solman and S. E. Jones, eds.), pp. 191–198. Elsevier, Amsterdam.

Ramot, B., Biniaminov, M., and Rosenthal, C. (1978). *In* "Progress in Cancer Research and Therapy" (M. A. Chirigos, ed.), Vol. VII, pp. 141–145. Raven, New York.

Rojas, A. F., Feierstein, J. N., Mickiewiez, E., Glaut, H., and Olivari, A. J. (1976). *Lancet* **1**, 211–215.

Terry, W. D., and Windhorst, D., eds. (1978). "Immunotherapy of Cancer: Present Status of Trials in Man." Raven, New York.

Part V
Antineoplastic Drug Development: Approaches, Design, and Evaluation

14

CHEMICAL APPROACHES TO NEW DRUGS

Terrence W. Doyle

I. INTRODUCTION

Before dealing with the approaches to new drugs which are presently being used, it would be useful to define the goals of such research. The ideal cancer chemotherapeutic agent should be either highly toxic to cancer cells or cause such cells to revert to normal cell types. It should show little or no host toxicity and should have a broad spectrum of activity. In sharp contrast to these goals is the present state of affairs in which most antitumor drugs have a good deal of host toxicity and a narrow spectrum. While chemotherapy has been quite successful for a small number of cancers (e.g., Hodgkin's lymphomas, childhood leukemias), the majority of cancers are resistant to treatment, and even in those tumors which can be treated, the cure rate is low.

The present state of the art is reminiscent of the early stages in the battle against infectious disease. The concept of selective toxicity in which the harmful organism is destroyed while the host is spared may be attributed to Paul Ehrlich. His search for a cure for syphilis culminated in the arsenical, salvarsan. While salvarsan represented a very real breakthrough in 1910, it had numerous

CANCER AND CHEMOTHERAPY, VOL. I

drawbacks, such as high host toxicity. The discovery of the penicillins and other selective antibacterial agents has superceded the use of salvarsan and other toxic agents. Much of the methodology which led to the discovery of the antibiotics is presently being applied to the discovery of antitumor agents and forms the subject of this section. There is no question that we are in the "arsenical" age of cancer chemotherapeutic agents. In many respects the breakthrough, comparable to Fleming's discovery of penicillin, will be more difficult in view of the nature of the target organism.

II. THE ROLE OF CHEMISTRY

Historically the chemist's role in cancer drug discovery may be divided into three main areas.

The first area is natural products research. Here, the chemist is responsible for the isolation and structure determination of novel chemotypes active in one or more tumor models.

The second area is synthesis. The modification of new leads to optimize activity-toxicity ratios forms an important part of the medicinal chemists' job. This also encompasses the total synthesis of new agents based on lead structures or biochemical rationales.

The third area is biochemistry. The determination of a novel chemotype's mechanism of action is an important part of new drug development. Such knowledge aids in the design of new analogues and can be of use in helping to unravel the mysteries of the cell, especially when a drug having a new mechanism of action is discovered. Such biochemical tools may conceivably be of greater use, as such, than as therapeutic agents. In addition to defining the mode of action of new drugs, biochemistry has revealed much about the basic pathways governing cell regulation, which in turn has led to drugs specifically designed to interfere with cellular metabolism. The use of such tools as prescreens is also important (see Chapter 15).

III. SOURCES OF NEW LEADS

For the most part, the new leads have come from random screening programs of natural products (Bradner, this volume, Chapter 15) and synthetics.

The natural products area may be further divided into those from fermentation, plants, and animal sources. Once antitumor activity has been detected in a crude extract (or broth), the process of isolation begins. This is a collaborative effort between chemist and biologist, the latter providing bioassays which are used to guide the fractionation. Once a bioactive substance has been isolated free of contaminants, the job of structure determination commences. With the array of modern spectroscopic tools available to the chemist (especially X-ray spectroscopy when applicable), this is no longer the tedious chore it once was.

That natural product research has been a fruitful area for the anticancer field is readily attested to by a listing of some of the clinically useful antitumor agents originally discovered in nature. From fermentation broths have come the anthracyclines (Fig. 1), adriamycin (Arcamone *et al.*, 1969), daunomycin (Arcamone *et al.*, 1968), and carminomycin (Brazhnikova *et al.*, 1974); the bleomycins (Fig. 2) (Takita *et al.*, 1978), the tallysomycins (Konishi *et al.*, 1977) (Fig. 3); and the mitomycins (Hata *et al.*, 1956) (Fig. 4). The higher plants have provided a number of antitumor agents in current use, the *vinca* alkaloids, vinblastine and vincristine (Nobel *et al.*, 1958; Johnson *et al.*, 1960) (Fig. 5); the podophyllotoxins, VP-16 and VM-26 (Keller-Juslen *et al.*, 1971) (Fig. 6);

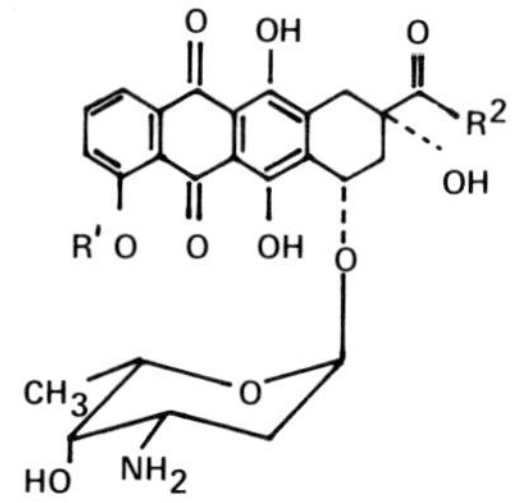

R' = H R^2 = CH_3 Carminomycin (Carubicin)
R' = R^2 = CH_3 Daunorubicin
R' = CH_3 R^2 = CH_2OH Doxorubicin (Adriamycin®)

Fig. 1

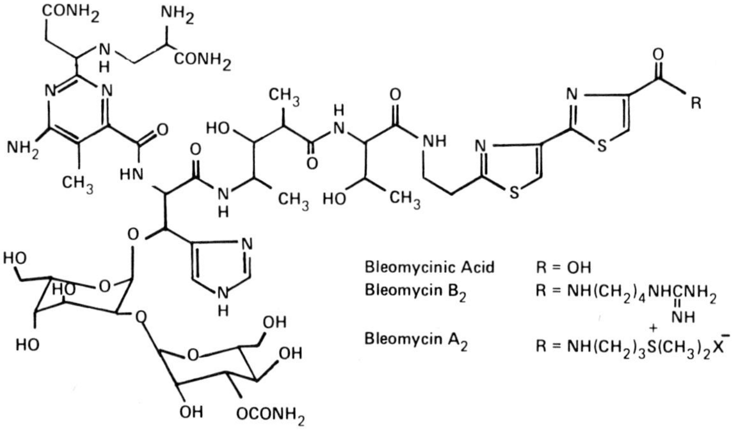

Bleomycinic Acid   R = OH
Bleomycin B_2 R = $NH(CH_2)_4NHCNH_2$
                                          NH
Bleomycin A_2 R = $NH(CH_2)_3S(CH_3)_2X^-$

Fig. 2

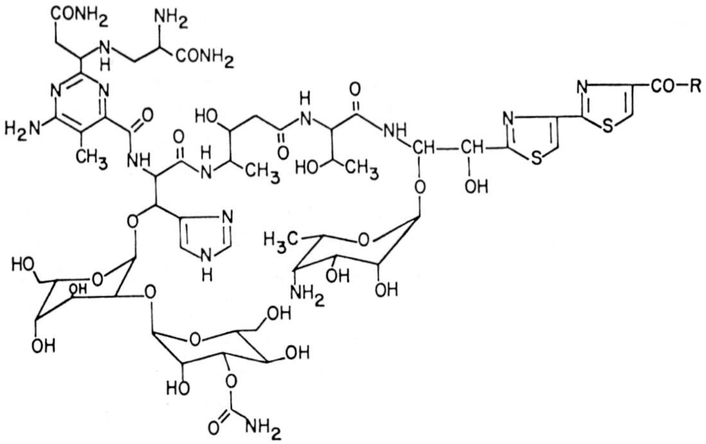

$$R = NHCH_2CH_2CH_2CHCH_2CONH(CH_2)_3NH(CH_2)_4NH_2$$
$$\quad\quad\quad\quad\quad\quad NH_2$$

Fig. 3

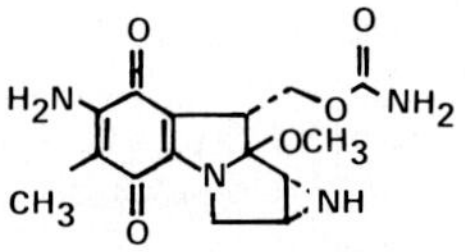

Mitomycin C (Mutamycin®)

Fig. 4

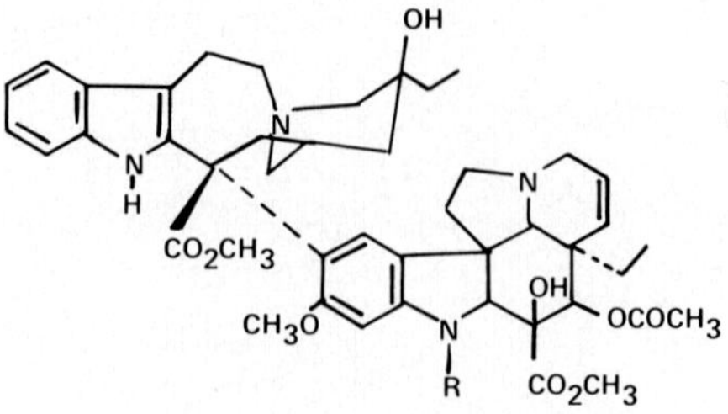

R = CH₃   Vinblastine (Velban®)

R = CHO   Vincristine (Oncovin®)

Fig. 5

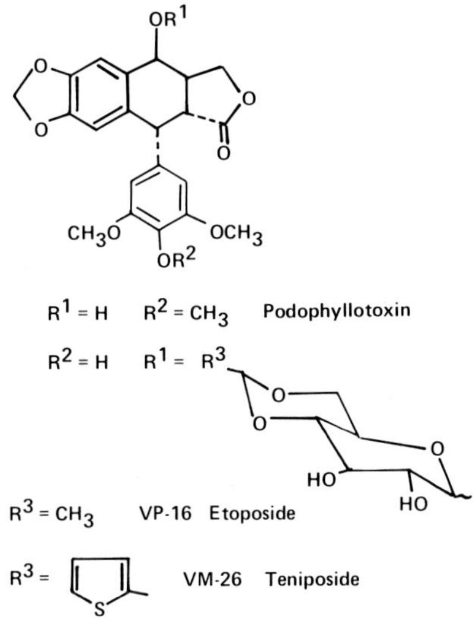
OR1
CH3O
OCH3
OR2
R1 = H R2 = CH3 Podophyllotoxin
R2 = H R1 = R3
HO
HO
R3 = CH3 VP-16 Etoposide
R3 =
VM-26 Teniposide

Fig. 6

and maytansine (Kupchan *et al.*, 1972a, b, 1974, 1975, 1977) (Fig. 7). The animal kingdom has yet to provide a clinically useful antineoplastic agent; however, the area is relatively unexplored. In one case, the discovery of the pyrimidine arabinosides (Fig. 8) spongouridine and spongothymidine from sponges (Bergman and Feeney, 1950; Bergman and Burke, 1955) may have inspired the synthesis of ARA-C.

The synthesis screening programs have also produced their share of antitumor agents including nitrogen mustards (Fig. 9), nitrosoureas (Fig. 10), and cisplatin (Fig. 11) (Rosenberg, 1971) as well as a number of other compounds which have found limited use, such as DTIC, mitotane, procarbazine, and Hydrea (Fig. 12).

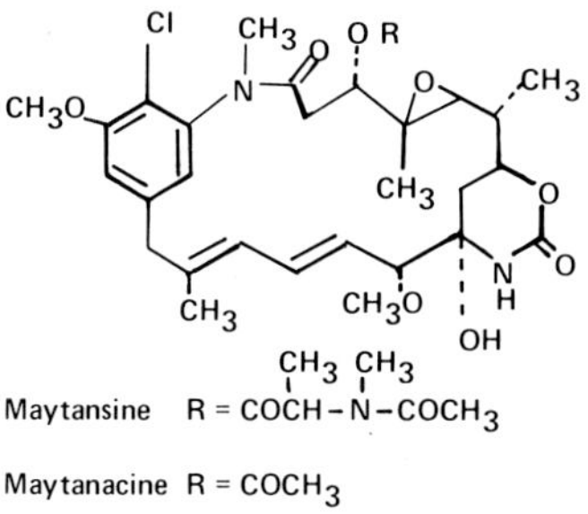
Cl
CH3
OR
CH3O
CH3
CH3
CH3O
OH
Maytansine R = COCH(CH3)–N(CH3)–COCH3
Maytanacine R = COCH3

Fig. 7

Nucleosides

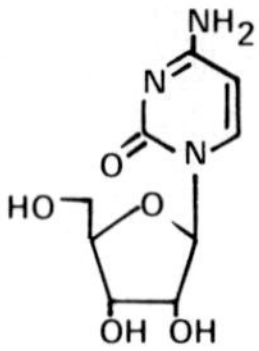

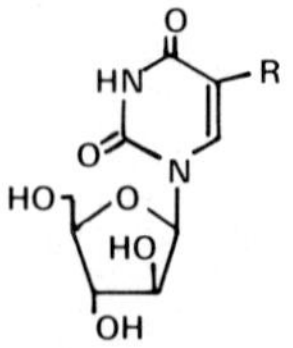

Spongouridine   R = H
Spongothymidine   R = CH₃

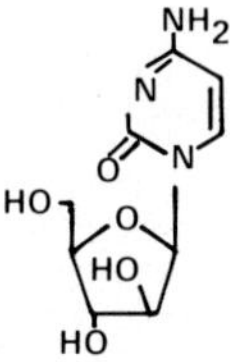

Cytarabin (Cytosar®) 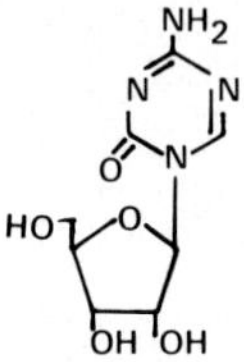   5−Azacytidine

Fig. 8

Nitrogen Mustards

X-CH₂CH₂—N—CH₂CH₂-X
                |
                R

R	X	Name
CH₃	Cl	Mechlorethamine (Mustargen®)
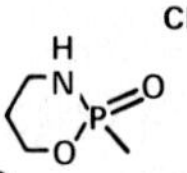 (phosphoramide ring)	Cl	Cyclophosphamide (Cytoxan®)
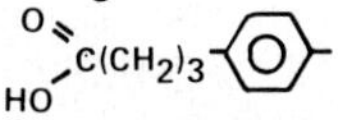 HOOC(CH₂)₃—C₆H₄—	Cl	Chlorambucil (Leukeran®)
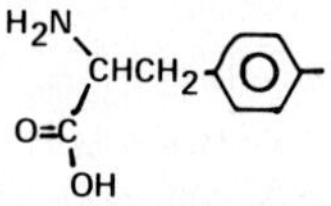 H₂N–CH(COOH)–CH₂—C₆H₄—	Cl	Melphalan (Alkeran®)

Fig. 9

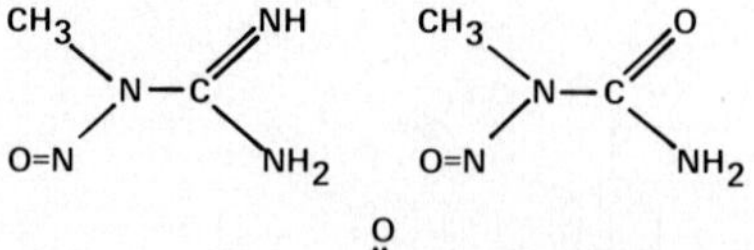

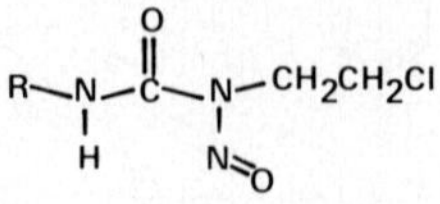

R—N(H)—C(=O)—N(CH₂CH₂Cl)(N=O)

R = CH₂CH₂Cl   Carmustine (BiCNU®)   BCNU

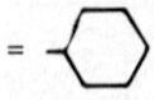

= —cyclohexyl   Lomustine (CeeNU®)   CCNU

= —cyclohexyl—CH₃   Semustine (Me-CCNU)

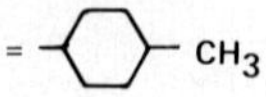

Fig. 10

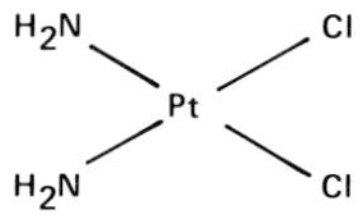

Cisplatin (Platinol®)

Fig. 11

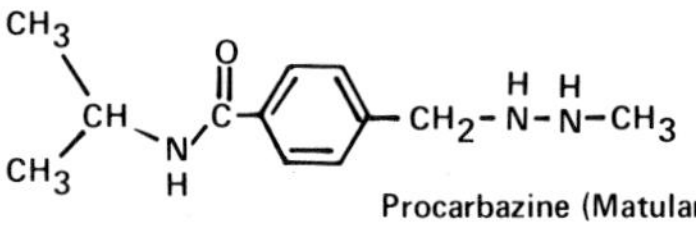

Procarbazine (Matulane®)

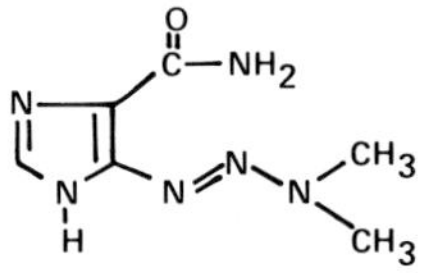

Dacarbazine (DTIC-Dome®)

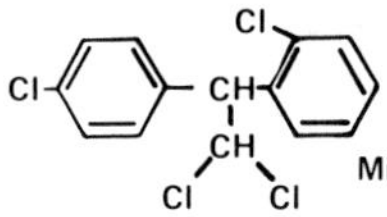

Mitotane (Lysodren®)

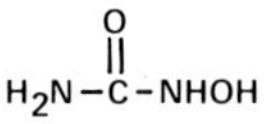

Hydroxyurea (Hydrea®)

Fig. 12

IV. EXPLOITATION OF NEW LEADS

Once a new lead has been discovered, there are a number of strategies which may be used to exploit it. In every case the goal is to produce a drug having greater activity or less toxicity. In some cases the reduction of a limiting toxicity, such as myelosuppression or cardiotoxicity, may be the goal, e.g., an adriamycin analogue which lacks the dose-limiting leukopenia or course-limiting cardiac toxicity of adriamycin would undoubtedly find a place in current chemotherapy.

The strategies for new lead exploitation from the chemist's point of view can be divided into several areas.

A. Directed Screening

The discovery of the antitumor agent adriamycin has led to extensive screening of organisms which produce anthracyclines. From such programs have emerged the antitumor agents aclacinomycin A (Fig. 13) (Oki, 1977) and carminomycin

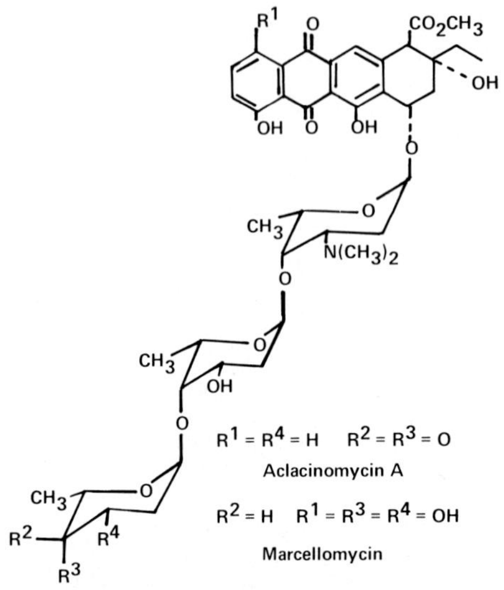

Fig. 13

$R^1 = R^4 = H$ $R^2 = R^3 = O$

Aclacinomycin A

$R^2 = H$ $R^1 = R^3 = R^4 = OH$

Marcellomycin

(Fig. 1) which are currently in clinical trials as well as a host of other analogs, including marcellomycin (Fig. 13) (Nettleton *et al.*, 1977) which is being considered for clinical trial based on its reduced leukopenia relative to the other anthracyclines. The anthracycline antitumor agents, aclacinomycin A and marcellomycin, are of special interest due to their unique mode of action—RNA synthesis inhibition (Crooke *et al.*, 1978).

The low yield of maytansine (Fig. 7) from plant sources resulted in its retarded development and stimulated a search for a microbial source. Recently, the group at Takeda (Higashide *et al.*, 1977) discovered a fermentation source for maytanacine, a compound closely related to maytansine. With supplies of maytansine available for semisynthetic work, a proper structure–activity relationship study can be carried out.

The search for new or improved sources for known antibiotics, or for new members of an interesting class of antitumor agents, is a cooperative one involving the chemist and microbiologist. The chemist supplies analytical support as well as extraction and isolation of the new agents. When a fermentation produces a complex mixture of antibiotics, the use of specific chemical assays is important.

B. Semisynthesis

There is no reason to believe that nature produces the optimal antitumor agent. New compounds which are first isolated from natural sources may often be improved upon by semisynthetic modifications. The history of β-lactam antibiotics is a good case in point. In this case, derivatives with several hundredfold improvements in activity or vast differences in spectrum were prepared semisynthetically. Historically, this appraoch to antitumor agents has not taken place, primarily due to the fact that a vacuum existed in this therapeutic area and initial leads were rushed rapidly into clinical development. The reasons were also economic due to the relatively low volume of sales to be expected for any one agent. Manufacturers felt that extensive chemical research was not economically justified in the market which existed only 10 years ago. Today the situation is changing due to the fact that there are a number of agents on the market, sales volumes have increased, and Federal Drug Administration regulations which require that a new agent not only be shown efficacious but also be better than any agent on the market before approval will be given. Today there is little excuse for marketing new antitumor agents prior to optimization of their activity–toxicity patterns.

Semisynthetic modification of lead compounds has been used to produce compounds with reduced toxicity. A good example is the podophyllotoxins. While one of the naturally occurring members of this group, α-peltatin, was given a clinical trial; no clear-cut clinical efficacy was noted (Greenspan et al., 1954). Semisynthetic modification of podophyllotoxin by the chemists at Sandoz (Keller-Juslen et al., 1971) resulted in VP-16 (etoposide) and VM-26 (teniposide) (Fig. 6) which possessed sufficiently favorable toxicity–activity ratios to warrant clinical trials.

Another example is the compound chlorozotocin (Fig. 14). The discovery of streptozotocin (Fig. 14) in fermentation broths (Herr et al., 1967) coupled with the knowledge that β-chloroethyl nitrosoureas possess superior activity led to the synthesis of chlorozotocin (Johnson et al., 1975).

The use in therapy of various hormones, both synthetic and natural, has led to attempts to improve their activity by hybridizing them with alkylating agents. This has resulted in the synthesis of prednimustine (Konyves et al., 1974) and Estracyt (Fig. 15) (Konyves and Liljekvist, 1976), which are being used in the treatment of prostatic cancer. In these cases it was hoped that the hormone carrier

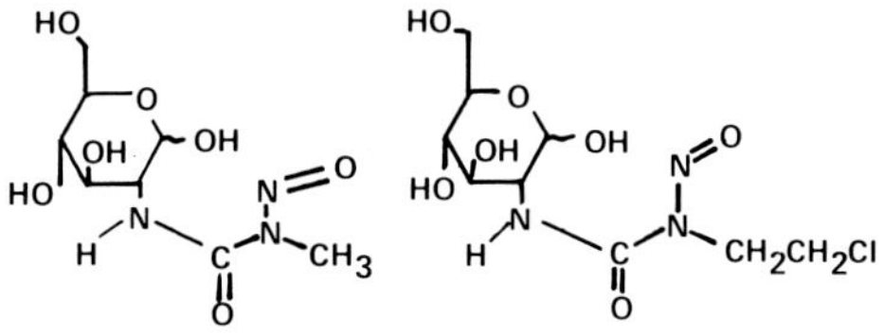

Streptozotocin (Zanosar®)   Chlorozotocin

Fig. 14

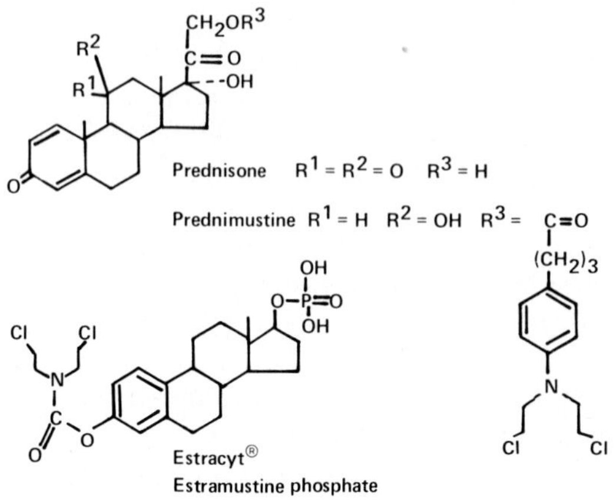

Prednisone $R^1 = R^2 = O$ $R^3 = H$

Prednimustine $R^1 = H$ $R^2 = OH$ $R^3 =$

Estracyt®
Estramustine phosphate

Fig. 15

would deliver the alkylating agent to the active site where it would be activated by hydrolysis.

At times, biosynthetic transformation of a lead structure may permit access to compounds which would be impractical to synthesize. A good example of such an approach is bleomycin in which precursor feeding experiments have resulted in the preparation of hundreds of variants, based on bleomycinic acid (Fig. 2), differing in the terminal amine (Umezawa, 1976). Similarly, the use of precursor feeding experiments has resulted in production of a number of variants of actinomycin D (Fig. 16) (Schmidt-Kastner, 1956b; Yajima *et al.*, 1972; Kusnetson *et al.*, 1974).

Recently, Claridge and Schmitz (1978) have used biotransformation to prepare a number of derivatives of anguidine (Fig. 17) one of which, 15-acetoxy-

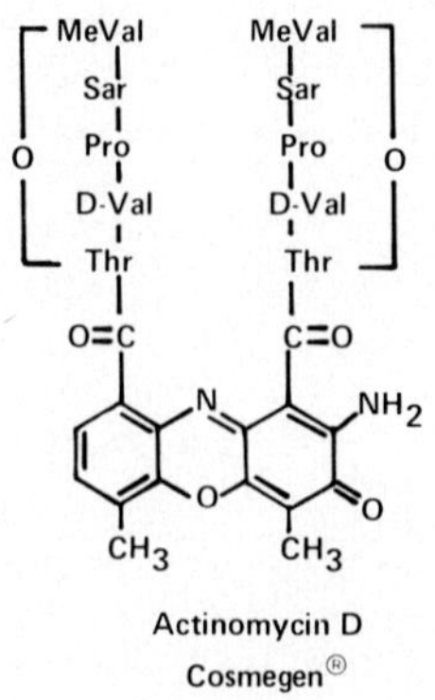

Actinomycin D
Cosmegen®

Fig. 16

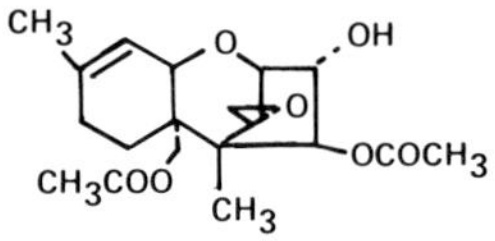

Anguidine

Fig. 17

scirpen-3α,4β-diol, was more potent and more active than anguidine itself (Claridge *et al.*, 1978). The uses of biotransformation are discussed at length in Chapter 16, this volume, by Claridge.

C. Total Synthesis

As we learn more about the structure activity relationships in a new chemotype, new synthetic targets not readily accessible via semisynthetic modification of the lead may be suggested. In some cases, an antitumor agent originally isolated from a natural source may be too scarce from that source to permit commercial exploitation and may have to be synthesized. A good case in point is the glutamine antagonist AT-125 (Fig. 18), the production of which by fermentation has proved so erratic as to make total synthesis an attractive alternate (Kelly *et al.*, 1978).

One area which has been extensively studied is the nitrogen mustards. While the toxic effects of the nitrogen mustards (Fig. 15) (especially the myelosuppression) had been known from World War I (Krumbhaar and Krumbhaar, 1919), their use as possible anticancer agents was not explored until the early 1940s (Gilman *et al.*, 1946; Goodman *et al.*, 1946; Jacobson *et al.*, 1946; Karnofsky *et al.*, 1947; Rhoads, 1947). From this early work, a family of antitumor agents, the synthesis of which was inspired by the nitrogen mustards, has come into therapeutic use.

The rationale for the synthesis of cyclophosphamide (Fig. 9) is interesting, since it is illustrative of the types of data employed by the medical chemist in analogue studies. It was hoped since the active bischloroethylamino portion had to be released via cleavage of the phosphorous–nitrogen bond, that greater selec-

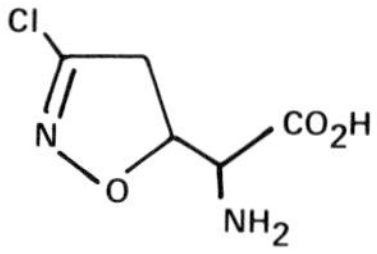

AT-125

Fig. 18

tivity for neoplastic tissue would result, given the high phosphatase and phosphamidase activity of such tissue (Calabresi and Parks, 1970). In addition to those compounds shown in Fig. 9, a large number of other nitrogen mustards has also been synthesized.

The mechanism of action of the nitrogen mustards is generally thought to be alkylation of various biomolecules (proteins and nucleic acids), primarily DNA (Brookes and Lawley, 1961; Lawley and Brookes, 1965; Wheeler and Alexander, 1965). Such linking may occur either intra- or intermolecularly (Fig. 9).

In addition to the bischloroethylamine type of cross-linking agents, a number of analogues having aziridines have been prepared, such as thiotepa and triethylene melamine (Fig. 19). These compounds are capable of forming the highly reactive ethyleneimonium ion *in vivo*.

The concept of preparing compounds capable of cross-linking with biomolecules has been extended to a number of derivatives which do not contain a central nitrogen atom such as Dibromodulcitol (DBD) and Dianhydrogalactitol (DAG) (Eckhardt *et al.*, 1963; Sellei *et al.*, 1969, Institoris *et al.*, 1967a, b), and busulfan (Galton, 1953) (Fig. 20).

One class of alkylating agents which has received a good deal of study is the nitrosoureas. The initial lead was 1-methyl-3-nitro-1-nitrosoguanidine which was discovered to have antitumor activity in a random screening program (Schepartz, 1976). An early analogue *N*-methylnitrosourea exhibited even better activity and led to the synthesis of a number of newer analogues having the *N*-nitroso-2-chloroethylamino function (Johnston *et al.*, 1963; Montgomery, 1976). From these studies a number of nitrosoureas BCNU, CCNU, and methyl-CCNU were chosen for further clinical development (Fig. 10).

The common feature of the biological alkylating agents which exhibit high antitumor activity would appear to be their ability to cross-link various biological macromolecules both inter- and intramolecularly. A number of other antitumor drugs have been suggested to work by such a mechanism as well, including, *cis*-platinum (Roberts and Pascoe, 1972; Rosenberg, 1971; Roberts, 1974; Thompson and Mansy, 1972) (Fig. 11). The exciting antitumor activity of *cis*-platinum has led to the synthesis of large numbers of analogues in which both the amine and chloro ligands have been modified. A number of these analogues are under active clinical investigation.

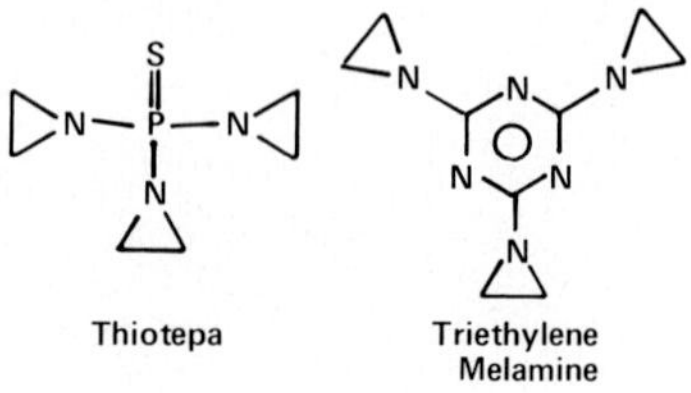

Thiotepa   Triethylene
                        Melamine

Fig. 19

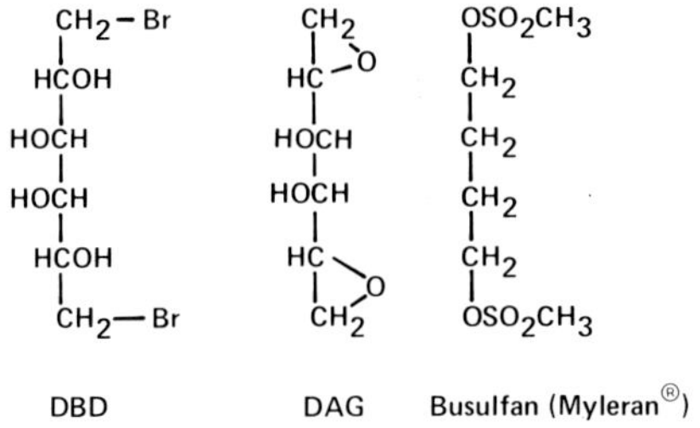

$$
\begin{array}{ccc}
\text{CH}_2-\text{Br} & \text{CH}_2 & \text{OSO}_2\text{CH}_3 \\
| & |\,\,^\diagdown\text{O} & | \\
\text{HCOH} & \text{HC} & \text{CH}_2 \\
| & | & | \\
\text{HOCH} & \text{HOCH} & \text{CH}_2 \\
| & | & | \\
\text{HOCH} & \text{HOCH} & \text{CH}_2 \\
| & | & | \\
\text{HCOH} & \text{HC} & \text{CH}_2 \\
| & |\,\,^\diagdown\text{O} & | \\
\text{CH}_2-\text{Br} & \text{CH}_2 & \text{OSO}_2\text{CH}_3
\end{array}
$$

DBD   DAG   Busulfan (Myleran®)

Fig. 20

In addition to those leads which have been discovered via a screening approach, a number of antitumor agents have been synthesized based on information of cell metabolism. With the discovery of the mechanism of action of the sulfa drugs as folic acid antagonists, the concept of using antimetabolites came into its own.

A consideration of the cases of cytosine arabinoside (ARA-C) and 5-azacytidine (Fig. 8) would be illustrative of the principles involved. If one examines the structure of cytosine riboside it is evident that the molecule may be considered as consisting of two halves; a pyrimidine and a pentofuranoside. Modification of the sugar by inversion of the 2'-hydroxyl function gave ARA-C (Walwick *et al.*, 1959) which was shown to possess antitumor activity (Evans *et al.*, 1961). Up to that time the only pyrimidine arabinosides which had been found in nature were spongouridine and spongothymidine (Bergman and Feeney, 1950; Bergman and Burke, 1955) (Fig. 8). 5-Azacytidine was originally synthesized by Piskala and Sorm (1964) and later isolated from the fermentation broths of *Streptovericillium ladakanus* by Hanka and Evans (1966) and Bergy and Herr (1966). Both ARA-C and 5-azacytidine function as antimetabolites of cytidine.

A number of analogues of pyrimidine or purine bases have been synthesized which rely on their conversion in the cell to the nucleoside for their action. Several of these have found use in chemotherapy, such as thiaguanine, 6-mercaptopurine, and 5-fluorouracil (5-FU). The 5-FU prodrug ftorafur acts as a depot form of 5-FU and is slowly hydrolyzed *in vivo* to 5-FU (Fig. 21).

There has been a prolonged interest in antimetabolites of folic acid (Fig. 22) in chemotherapy. While a large number of analogues have been synthesized, the drug currently receiving the most use is methotrexate which competitively inhibits dihydrofolate reductase (Bertino, 1963; Werkhesier, 1963). While methotrexate closely resembles the parent, Baker's antifol is an analogue with considerable structural changes (Baker, 1971). While Baker's antifol is also a competitive inhibitor or dihydrofolate reductase, there appears to be a difference in transport.

The observations that a number of antitumor drugs, e.g., adriamycin (Fig. 1) (Zunino *et al.*, 1972) and actinomycin D (Fig. 16) (Reich and Goldberg, 1964)

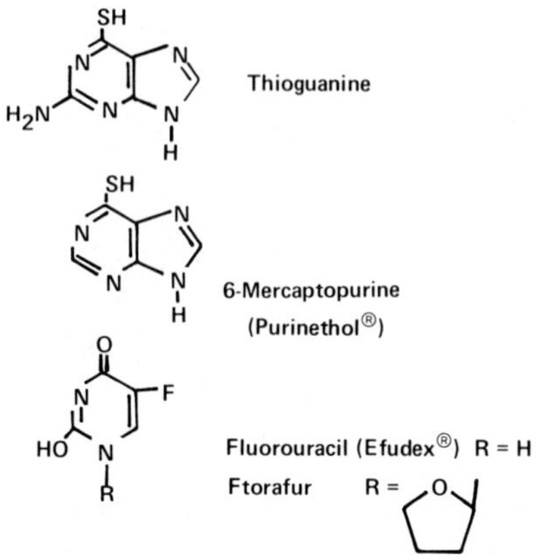

Thioguanine

6-Mercaptopurine
(Purinethol®)

Fluorouracil (Efudex®) R = H

Ftorafur   R =

Fig. 21

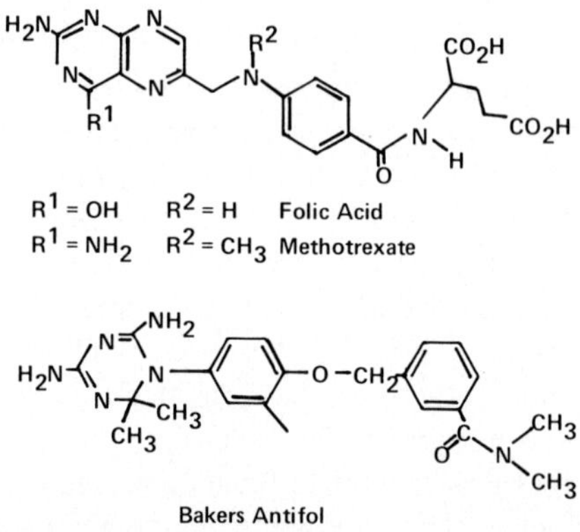

R^1 = OH   R^2 = H   Folic Acid
R^1 = NH$_2$ R^2 = CH$_3$ Methotrexate

Bakers Antifol

Fig. 22

are capable of intercalation with double-stranded DNA molecules has attracted much attention in recent years and has served as a basis for the synthesis of a number of compounds capable of intercalating with DNA in the hope that these would possess antitumor activity as well. Two of the more promising candidates which have arisen from this work are the aminoalkyl anthraquinone derivatives (Fig. 23) which show good activity against several experimental tumors (Zee-Cheng and Cheng, 1978) and the 4'(9-acridinylamino) methane sulfonanilides (AMSA) (Fig. 24) derivatives which have been synthesized by Cain and co-workers (Denny and Cain, 1978; Denny et al., 1977, 1978).

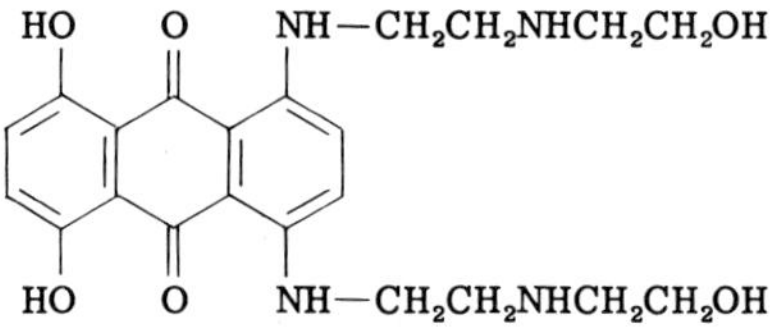

1,4-Dihydroxy-5,8-bis[2-(hydroxy-
ethyl)aminoethyl]amino-9,10-
anthracenedione (DHAQ)

Fig. 23

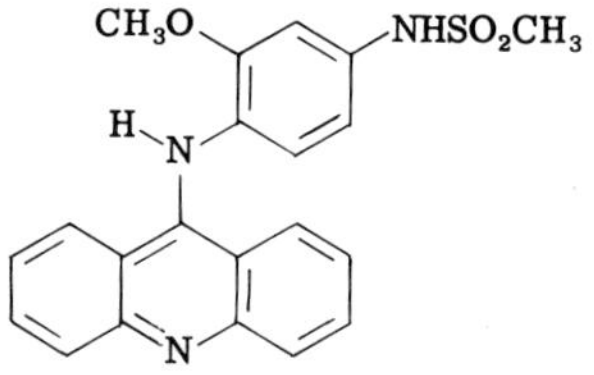

N-[4-(9-acridinylamino)-2-
methoxyphenyl]methane-
sulfonamide (m-AMSA)

Fig. 24

V. DISCUSSION

In this chapter, I have tried to outline some of the sources of new drug leads and the role of chemistry in their development as drugs. With the remarkable progress which has been made in cancer chemotherapy in the past decade, it is reasonable to assume that the type of research described will increase, especially in the areas of new lead optimization by semisynthesis and in rationally designed totally synthetic analogues.

REFERENCES

Arcamone, F., Franceschi, G., and Orezzi, P. (1968). *Tetrahedron Lett.*, pp. 3349-3356.
Arcamone, F., Cassinelli, G., Fantini, G., Grein, A., Orezzi, P., Pol, C., and Spalla, C. (1969). *Biotechnol. Bioeng.* **11**, 1101-1110.
Baker, B. R. (1971). *Ann. N.Y. Acad. Sci.* **186**, 214-226.
Bergman, W., and Burke, D. C. (1955). *J. Org. Chem.* **20**, 1501-1507.
Bergman, W., and Feeney, R. J. (1950). *J. Am. Chem. Soc.* **72**, 2809.
Bergy, M. E., and Herr, R. R. (1966). *Antimicrob. Agents Chemother.* pp. 625-630.
Bertino, J. (1963). *Cancer Med.* **23**, 1286.

Brazhnikova, M. G., Zbarsky, V. B., Ponomarkeno, V. I., and Potapova, N. P. (1974). *J. Antibiot.* **27**, 254–259.

Brookes, P., and Lawley, P. D. (1961). *Biochem. J.* **80**, 496–503.

Calabresi, P., and Parks, R. E. (1970). *In* "The Pharmacologic Basis of Therapeutics" (L. S. Goodman and A. Gilman, eds.), 4th ed., pp. 1344–1394. Macmillan, New York.

Claridge, C. A., and Schmitz, H. (1978). *Appl. Environ. Microbiol.* **36**, 63–67.

Claridge, C. A., Bradner, W. T., and Schmitz, H. (1978). *J. Antibiot.* **31**, 485–486.

Crooke, S. T., Duvernay, V. H., Galvan, L., and Prestayko, A. W. (1978). *Mol. Pharmacol.* **14**, 290–298.

Denny, W. A., and Cain, B. F. (1978). *J. Med. Chem.* **21**, 430–437.

Denny, W. A., Atwell, G. J., and Cain, B. F. (1977). *J. Med. Chem.* **10**, 1242–1246.

Denny, W. A., Atwell, G. J., and Cain, B. F. (1978). *J. Med. Chem.* **21**, 5–10.

Eckardt, S., Sellei, C., Horvath, I. P., and Institoris, L. (1963). *Cancer Chemother. Rep.* **33**, 57–61.

Evans, J. S., Musser, E. A., Mengel, G. D., Forsblad, K. R., and Hunder, J. H. (1961). *Proc. Soc. Exp. Biol. Med.* **106**, 350–353.

Galton, D. A. G. (1953). *Lancet* **1**, 208–213.

Gilman, A., Goodman, L., Lindskog, G. E., and Dougherty, S. (1946). *Science* **103**, 409–415.

Goodman, L., Wintrobe, M. M., Dameshek, W., Goodman, M. J., Gilman, A., and McLennan, M. T. (1946). *J. Am. Med. Assoc.* **132**, 126–132.

Greenspan, E., Colsky, J., Schoenbach, B., and Shear, M. (1954). *J. Natl. Cancer. Inst.* **14**, 1257–1276.

Hanka, L. J., and Evans, J. S. (1966). *Antibicrob. Agents Chemother.* pp. 619–624.

Hata, T., Sano, Y., Sugawara, R., Matsume, A., Kanamori, K., Shima, T., and Hoshi, T. (1956). *J. Antibiot. Ser. A* **9**, 141–146.

Herr, R. R., Jahnke, J. K., and Argoudelis, A. D. (1967). *J. Am. Chem. Soc.* **89**, 4808–4809.

Higashide, E., Asai, M., Ootsu, K., Tanida, S., Kozai, Y., Hasegawa, T., Kishi, T., Sugino, Y., and Yoneda, M. (1977). *Nature (London)* **270**, 721–722.

Institoris, L., Horvath, I. P., Pethes, G., and Eckhardt, S. (1967a). *Cancer Chemother. Rep.* **51**, 261–270.

Institoris, L., Horvath, I. P., and Csanyi, E. (1967b). *Arzeim. Forsch.* **17**, 145–149.

Jacobson, L. O., Spurr, C. L., Barron, E. S., Smith, T., Lushbaugh, C., and Dick, G. F. (1946). *J. Am. Med. Assoc.* **132**, 263–271.

Johnson, I. S., Wright, H. F., Svoboda, G. H., and Vlantis, J. (1960). *Cancer Res.* **20**, 1016–1022.

Johnston, T. P., McCaleb, G. S., and Montgomery, J. A. (1963). *J. Med. Chem.* **6**, 669–681.

Johnston, T. P., McCaleb, G. S., and Montgomery, J. A. (1975). *J. Med. Chem.* **18**, 104–106.

Karnofsky, D. A., Craver, L. F., Rhoads, C. P., and Abels, J. C. (1947). *In* "Approaches to Tumor Chemotherapy" pp. 319–347. Am. Assoc. Adv. Sci., Washington, D.C.

Keller-Juslen, C., Kuhn, M., von Wartburg, A., and Stahelin, A. (1971). *J. Med. Chem.* **14**, 936–940.

Kelly, R. C., Schletter, I., Stein, S. T., and Wierenga, W. (1978). *176th Meet., Am. Chem. Soc.* Abstract 092 Orgn.

Konishi, M., Saito, K., Numata, K., Tsuno, T., Asama, K., Tsukiura, H., Naito, T., and Kawaguchi, H. (1977). *J. Antibiot.* **30**, 789–805.

Konyves, I., and Lilijekvist, J. (1976). *In* "Biological Character of Human Tumors" (W. Davis and C. Maltoni, eds.), p. 98. Am. Elsevier, New York.

Konyves, I., Fex, H., and Hogberg, B. (1974). *Prog. Chemother., Proc. Int. Congr. Chemother. 8th, 1973*. Vol. III, pp. 791–795.

Krumbhaar, E. B., and Krumbhaar, H. D. (1919). *J. Med. Res.* **40**, 497–508.

Kupchan, S. M., Komoda, Y., Thomas, G. J., and Hintz, H. P. J. (1972a). *J. Chem. Soc., Chem. Commun.* p. 1065.

Kupchan, S. M., Komoda, Y., Court, W. A., Thomas, G. J., Smith, R. M., Karim, A., Gilmore, C. J., Haltiwanger, R. C., and Bryan, R. F. (1972b). *J. Am. Chem. Soc.* **94**, 1354–1356.

Kupchan, S. M., Komoda, Y., Branfman, A. R., Dailey, R. G., Jr., and Zimmerly, V. A. (1974). *J. Am. Chem. Soc.* **96**, 3706–3708.

Kupchan, S. M., Branfman, A. R., Sneden, A. T., Verma, A. K., Dailey, R. G., Jr., Komoda, Y., and Nagao, Y. (1975). *J. Am. Chem. Soc.* **97**, 5294–5295.

Kupchan, S. M., Komoda, Y., Branfman, A. R., Sneden, A. T., Court, W. A., Thomas, G. J.,Hintz, H. P. J., Smith, R. M., Karim, A., Howie, G. A., Verma, A. K., Nagao, Y., Dailey, R. G., Jr., Zimmerly, V. A., and Sumner, W. C., Jr. (1977). *J. Org. Chem.* **42**, 2349–2357.

Kusnetson, V. S., Orlova, T. I., and Silaev, A. B. (1974). *Antibiotiki (Moscow)* **19**, 295–298.

Lawley, P. D., and Brookes, P. (1965). *Nature (London)* **206**, 480–483.

Montgomery, J. A. (1976). *Cancer Treat. Rep.* **60**, 651–664.

Nettleton, D. E., Jr., Bradner, W. T., Bush, J. A., Coon, A. B., Moseley, J. E., Myllymaki, R. W., O'Herron, F. A., Schreiber, R. H., and Vulcano, A. L. (1977). *J. Antibiot.* **30**, 525–529.

Nobel, R. L., Beer, C. T., and Cutts, J. H. (1958). *Ann. N.Y. Acad. Sci.* **76**, 882–894.

Oki, T. (1977). *J. Antibiot.* **30**, S-70.

Piskala, A., and Sorm, F. (1964). *Collect. Czech. Chem. Commun.* **29**, 2060–2076.

Reich, E., and Goldberg, I. H. (1964). *Prog. Nucleic Acids Res.* **3**, 183–234.

Rhoads, C. P. (1947). *Trans. Assoc. Am. Physicians* **60**, 110–117.

Roberts, J. J. (1974). *In* "Platinum Coordination Complexes in Cancer Chemotherapy" (T. A. Connors and J. J. Roberts, eds.), p. 79. Springer-Verlag, Berlin and New York.

Robert, J. J., Pascoe, J. M. (1972). *In* "Advances in Antimicrobial and Antineoplastic Chemotherapy," Vol. II, p. 249. University Park Press, Baltimore.

Rosenberg, B. (1971). *Platinum Met. Rev.* **15**, No. 2.

Schepartz, S. A. (1976). *Cancer Treat. Rep.* **60**, 647–650.

Schmidt-Kastner, G. (1956). *Abh. Med.-Chem. Forschungsst. Farbenfabr Bayer A. G.* **5**, 463.

Sellei, C., Eckhardt, S., Horvath, I. P., Kralovánszky, J., and Institoris L. (1969). *Cancer Chemother. Rep.* **53**, 377–384.

Takita, T., Muraoka, Y., Nakatani, T., Fujii, A., Umezawa, Y., Nagawana, H., and Umezawa, H. (1978). *J. Antibiot.* **31**, 801–804.

Thompson, A. J., and Mansy, S. (1972). *Adv. Antimicrob. Antineoplast. Chemother., Proc. Int. Congr. Chemother., 7th, 1971* Vol. II, pp. 199–202.

Umezawa, H. (1976). *GANN Monogr. Cancer Res.* **19**, 3–36.

Walwick, E. R., Dekker, C. A., and Roberts, W. K. (1959). *Proc. Chem. Soc., London* p. 84.

Werkheiser, W. (1963). *Cancer Res.* **23**, 1277–1285.

Wheeler, G., and Alexander, J. A. (1965). *Cancer Res.* **29**, 98–109.

Yajima, T., Grigg, M. A., and Katz, E. (1972). *Arch. Biochem. Biophys.* **151**, 565–575.

Zee-Cheng, R. K.-Y., and Cheng, C. C. (1978). *J. Med. Chem.* **21**, 291–294.

Zunino, F., Gambetta, R., DiMarco, A., and Zacchara, A. (1972). *Biochim. Biophys. Acta* **277**, 489–498.

15

APPROACHES TO NEW DRUGS: FERMENTATION APPROACHES TO NEW DRUG DEVELOPMENT
William T. Bradner

I. INTRODUCTION

Among the cancer chemotherapeutic drugs marketed in the United States, antitumor antibiotics make a major contribution. A large majority of human tumors respond, in some degree, to treatment with some antitumor antibiotic used alone or in combination. There has been continuing long-term support for fermentation programs, in attempts to discover new chemotypes or superior analogues of existing antibiotics, even though such programs are costly and development times very long. This chapter presents a brief summary of our experiences with a fermentation program emphasizing some of the choices that

CANCER AND CHEMOTHERAPY, VOL. I

must be made at various stages, the decisions we made in past years at these points, and the results in terms of the products discovered.

II. CULTURE ISOLATION AND FERMENTATION

All of the topics listed in Table I are common to both antimicrobial and antitumor antibiotics. Information can be found in many textbooks and monographs on soil sources, collection methods, and procedures for isolation of organisms from soil and will thus not be reviewed here. Organism selection and primary fermentation will be discussed because of some of the choices that must be made in operating an antitumor antibiotic screening program.

Table II in condensed form shows the principal groups of soil microorganisms and the major classes of clinically used antibiotics (see Conover, 1971, for detailed history). It is immediately apparent that the actinomycetes are the most prolific. They are also the most thoroughly studied and thus yield duplicates of known materials at the alarming rate of above 95% of all actives in primary screening. Thus we are faced with our first major decision point in operating a

TABLE I

Culture Isolation and Fermentation

1. Soil source—collection
2. Isolation of organisms
3. Culture identification—organisms selected for fermentation
4. Primary fermentation—replication of conditions

TABLE II

Types of Microorganisms and Antibiotics

Microorganisms	Antibiotics used clinically	
	Antimicrobial	Antitumor
Actinomycetes	Aminoglycosides	Anthracyclines
	Macrolides	Bleomycins
	Polyenes	Mitomycins
		Actinomycins
		Aureolic acids
Fungi	Beta Lactams	Tricothenes
Bacteria	Polypeptides	Enzymes

primary screen. Do we choose abundance and have to sort out the knowns? Do we screen those organisms which may produce more novel materials, but where overall yield is low? Or do we screen them all?

If we choose to screen within a single class of organisms (Table III), there are advantages and disadvantages. Among the advantages are, first, that common fermentation conditions can be used which makes the operation more efficient. Second, there is a higher opportunity for discovery because of the concentration of effort. Finally, dereplication is less of a problem because the discovery of known agents will tend to be confined and techniques for avoiding them can be developed. Two disadvantages of the single class screen are (1) the narrow discovery scope and (2) the fact that the class discovery rate is fixed. This would be particularly bad if the rate was low.

The multiclass screen, which covers essentially everything which can be isolated from the soil, has the attributes shown in Table IV. In its favor are a broad discovery scope and the fact that the discovery rate is not fixed to any one group of organisms. Some drawbacks are that multiple fermentation conditions are required making the mounting of primary fermentation less efficient, the de-

TABLE III

Single Class Screen

Pro	Con
1. Common fermentation conditions 2. Higher opportunity for discovery within class (and for significance of discovery) 3. Ease of dereplication	1. Narrower discovery scope 2. Class discovery rate is fixed (may be low)

TABLE IV

Multiclass Screen

Pro	Con
1. Broad discovery scope 2. Rate not fixed	1. Requires multiple fermentation conditions (less efficient) 2. Development of procedures may be prolonged 3. Overall discovery rate may be diluted

velopment of procedures may be prolonged because of the variety required, and the overall discovery rate may be diluted. Nevertheless, we consider that the broad discovery scope is a much more compelling reason than any of the drawbacks and are now applying the multiclass screening to that portion of our program devoted to random selection of new soil isolates.

Assuming the choice of microorganisms to be screened has been made, the next decision is fermentation conditions to be used. It is obvious that several chemical and physical conditions must be defined, a few of which are shown in Table V. In fact, the permutations become very numerous when consideration is given to the many variations for each of the parameters listed.

Table VI shows the outcome of scheduling strategy for primary fermentations. In the case of antitumor antibiotics, limitations are imposed because of quantities of broth fermented and the limited capacity of the tumor test system to handle large numbers. If we assume in a modest primary screening program that 30 different fermentations could be prepared and tested per week, we must choose

TABLE V

Primary Fermentation—
Parameters to Be Considered

1. Medium
        Carbohydrate
        Nitrogen source
        Growth factors
        Salts
2. Physical conditions
        Temperature
        Aeration
        Fermentation time

TABLE VI

Primary Fermentation—Scheduling Strategy: Multiconditions versus Multicultures

Multiconditions	Multicultures
5 Media	1 Media
×	×
2 Temperature	1 Temperature
×	×
3 Days of harvest	1 Day of harvest
30 Conditions	1 Condition
1 Culture	30 Cultures cycling

between multi- (fermentation) conditions and multicultures. An extreme example of multiconditions would be to use five fermentation media, two incubation temperatures, and three different harvest days. This results in 30 conditions and thus only one culture could be studied each week. The rationale for using multiconditions is that at least one combination might promote production of a new antibiotic to an extent sufficient for detection by the primary screen, thereby reducing the number of actives missed because of low concentration.

The alternative approach is to select a single medium, temperature, and harvest time (in essence one condition) which permits fermenting and screening 30 new cultures per week. There are two reasons this is the more favorable method. First, it is possible to change conditions every few months (known as cycling) and thus enhance the chance of matching a new culture with an optimum fermentation design. There is an old principle in antibiotic screening that all leads "come around again" and that if they are not detected the first time, they will be eventually. Second, and perhaps more important, is the fact that multiconditions put heavy effort into attempts to improve the fermentation of organisms which do not produce compounds with activity.

III. PRIMARY SCREENING AND PRESCREENING

A primary screen may be defined as a biological test system which gives the first suggestion of clinical potential. It must be in animals, and it must be relevant to the disease to be treated in humans. Although antimicrobial antibiotics are accurately characterized because they are tested against their authentic targets, antitumor agents have no such equivalents. Even the animal tumor systems used at present do not have exact human counterparts. Nevertheless, activity in such systems is a requirement for a chemotherapeutic drug to be accepted for clinical trial by government agencies.

Some other characteristics of in vivo screening systems must be considered (Table VII). These systems have the advantage of differentiating toxicity to the host and the tumor, and can detect agents operating through host-mediated mechanism. Some unfavorable characteristics are (1) they are slow and inefficient, (2) each tumor type may be limited in its scope of response, and (3) quantitative sensitivity may be insufficient for detection of activity in crude fermentation broths. It is for these reasons that *in vitro* prescreens have been studied so extensively and are being increasingly employed (Bradner, 1978a).

Table VIII briefly outlines some of the prescreens which have been used in most laboratories. We have employed tissue cultures, antimicrobial effects and induction of lysogenic bacteria (ILB) most extensively. The ILB system has been particularly useful because of its high sensitivity—in some cases below 0.01 μg/ml. Sensitivity is the single most important attribute of a fermentation pre-

TABLE VII

Primary Screen Detection System (Antitumor Antibiotics)

Definition: A biological test system which gives the first suggestion of clinical potential.

1. Must be in animals
2. Must be relevant to disease in humans

Experimental animal tumors

Advantage	Disadvantage
1. Differentiates toxicity to host and tumor	1. Slow and inefficient
	2. Limited scope of response
2. Detects agents operating through host-mediated mechanisms	3. Sensitivity may be too low for screening fermentation broths

TABLE VIII

***In Vitro* Prescreens**

1. Tissue culture—cytotoxicity, cell cycle
2. Microorganisms—antimicrobial, antiphage, lysogenic induction, deficient or permeable mutants
3. Enzymatic—DNA, RNA, protein synthesis

Priority: (1) sensitivity, (2) specificity

screen. Specificity is of secondary importance since it would be moot if nothing were detected.

IV. YIELDS OF ANTITUMOR ANTIBIOTICS

As an example of a program which has employed several approaches for a number of years, our program will be discussed. During the first 9 years, 17 purified antibiotics were submitted to the National Cancer Institute (NCI) arising from our efforts with actinomycetes (Table IX). The rate for detection of confirmed actives in primary screening was approximately 2%. Following this in agreement with the NCI, we switched to screening fungi exclusively which sharply reduced our yield. The primary screen gave only 0.5% active broths. The final 2 years were devoted to a study of bacteria. No new materials were submitted to the NCI from this source and the primary screening rate was 0.3% for P-388 leukemia and 0.08% for L-1210. Since that time, we have operated a broad screen which is unrestricted regarding types of microorganisms.

TABLE IX

Yield of Antitumor Antibiotics

Microorganism	Purified antibiotics/years (rate)	
Actinomycetes	17/9	(2%)
Fungi	4/5	(0.5%)
Bacteria	0/2	4/1290 PS (0.3%)[a]
		1/1269 LE (0.08%)[a]

[a] PS, P-388 leukemia; LE, L-1210 leukemia.

Table X lists the antibiotics discovered in actinomycete fermentations. The asterisk indicates novelty. Phleomycin is listed in both columns since Dr. Umezawa (Maeda *et al.*, 1956) discovered it first, but we later independently isolated it in our own primary fermentation program. However, it was in our laboratory that the first observation of antitumor activity was made (Bradner and Pindell, 1962). Peliomycin (Price *et al.*, 1964), ossamycin (Schmitz *et al.*, 1965), and demetric acid (DeVault *et al.*, 1966), were all isolated on the basis of tissue culture activity alone. They are all highly insoluble and have little or no *in*

TABLE X

Antibiotics Discovered in Actinomycte Fermentation[a]

Isolated by Bristol[a]	Isolated in Japan
A649 (Olivomycin)	Mitomycin
Actinogan*	(Dr. Hata)
Peptinogan*	Phleomycin
Hedamycin*	(Dr. Umezawa)
Phleomycin*	Bleomycin
Peliomycin*	(Dr. Umezawa)
Ossamycin*	Macromomycin
Demetric Acid*	(Dr. Umezawa)
Mycorhodin*	Neocarzinostatin
Kundrymycin*	(Dr. Ishida)
Orpheomycin (chromomycin A$_2$)	
Borrelidin	
Valinomycin	
Figaroic acid	
Carminomycin	
Bohemic acid	
Musettamycin*, marcellomycin*	
Sibiromycin	
Tallysomycin (BBRI)*	

[a] Asterisk indicates novelty.

TABLE XI

Antibiotics Isolated from Fungal Fermentation

1. Muconomycin A
2. Anguidine
3. 5-Methoxysterigmatocystin
4. Sterigmatocystin

vivo tumor inhibitory effects. Hence, they were never considered worthy of clinical candidacy.

Fungal products are shown in Table XI. Though all were known chemicals, anguidine was not available in the United States, and the sterigmatocystins were not previously known to be strong inhibitors of tumor growth. Anguidine has completed Phase I clinical trial under NCI sponsorship and is now entering Phase II trials.

V. STRUCTURES

A few structures have been selected which will be representative of the diversity of products obtained using these fermentation approaches.

A. Hedamycin

This is a highly potent ILB active agent which is moderately inhibitory to P-388 (Bradner *et al.*, 1967) (Fig. 1). It has two amino sugars as well as the unusual feature of two ethylene oxides (Sequin *et al.*, 1975). It has been found to bind to DNA and inhibit strand separation (White and White, 1969).

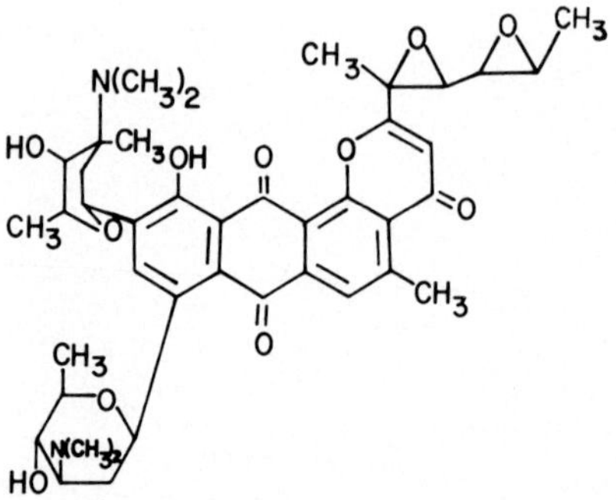

Fig. 1. Structure of hedamycin.

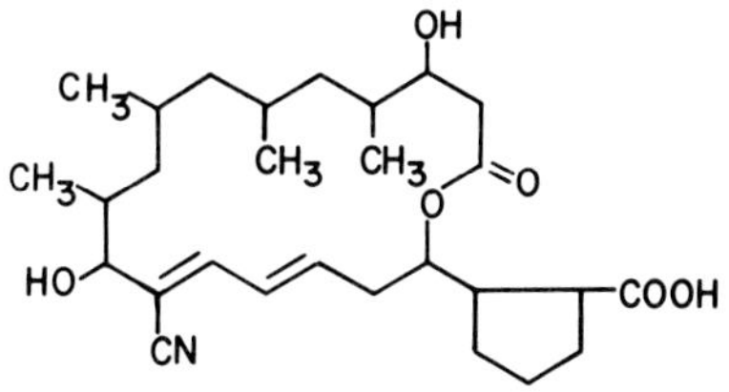

Fig. 2.   Structure of borrelidin.

B. Borrelidin

This macrolide was first discovered to protect mice against *Borrelia* infection (Berger *et al.*, 1949) (Fig. 2). Later it was rediscovered as having antitumor activity (Sugiura and Sugiura, 1958).

C. Valinomycin

This is a depsipeptide ionophore which chelates alkali metals and increases membrane transport (Poole and Butler, 1970) (Fig. 3). It is moderately effective against P-388 leukemia and has good activity against B16 melanoma. It is being studied presently by the NCI.

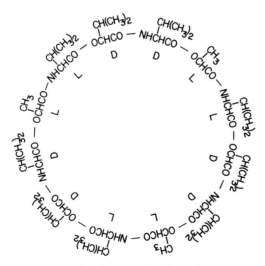

Fig. 3.   Structure of valinomycin.

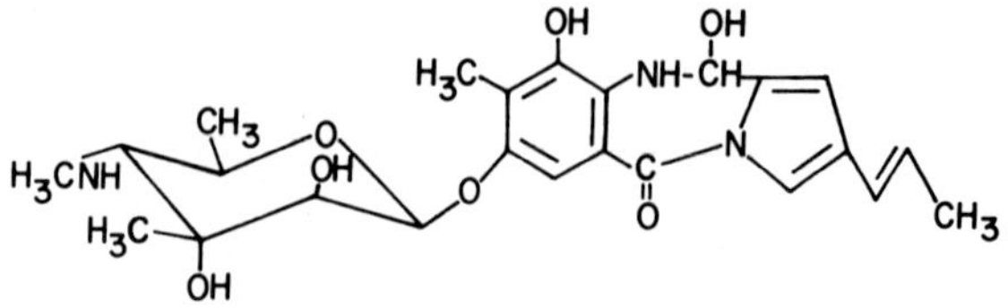

Fig. 4. Structure of sibiromycin.

D. Sibiromycin

This anthramycin class antibiotic was first isolated in the Soviet Union (Gause *et al.*, 1969) (Fig. 4). It differs from anthramycin by having a sugar attached. It is extremely toxic and has shown activity on P-388 and B16. It is a DNA inhibitor and binds to DNA with a high G-C content (Gause and Dudnik, 1972).

E. Sterigmatocystin

5-Methoxysterigmatocystin (5-MS) and sterigmatocystin have long been known as carcinogenic mycotoxins; however, we discovered that they are potent tumor inhibitors (Bradner *et al.*, 1975) (Fig. 5). One study suggests that sterigmatocystin interferes with nucleic acid metabolism by inhibiting uridine and thymidine transport. Although sterigmatocystin is 1/250 as carcinogenic as the related aflatoxin B_1, it is probably too hazardous to consider for clinical trial. Nevertheless, analogue work which might breed out this property is of interest because of the excellent antitumor activity.

F. Anguidine

This tricothene fungal toxin inhibits protein synthesis (Fig. 6). It is one of a large group of tricothecane mycotoxins, many of which have antineoplastic effects (Doyle and Bradner, 1979).

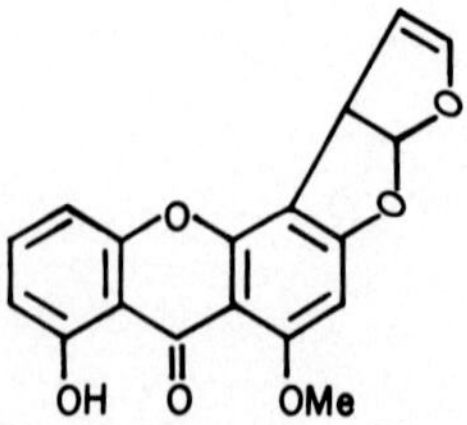

Fig. 5. Structure of sterigmatocystin.

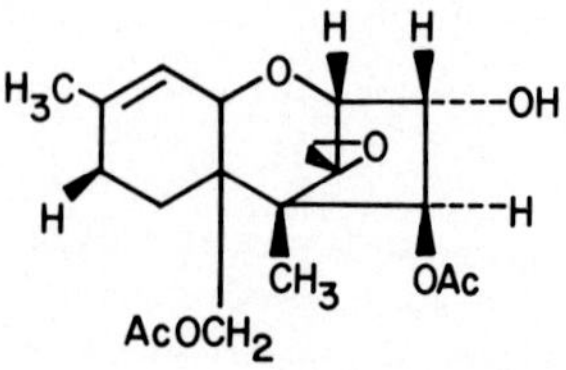

Fig. 6. Structure of anguidine.

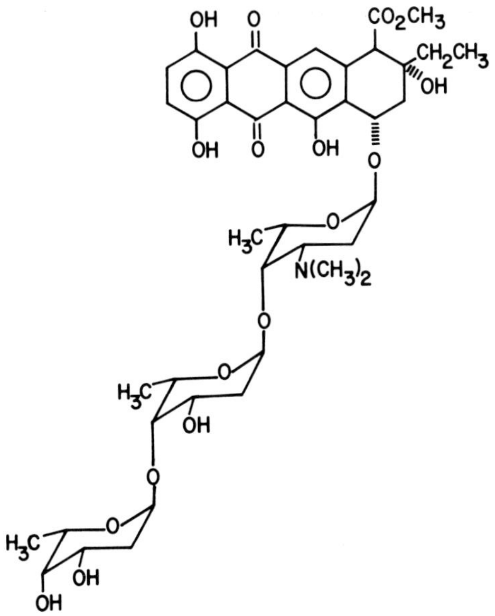

Fig. 7. Structure of marcellomycin.

G. Marcellomycin

This is a pyrromycinone trisaccharide from an anthracycline complex called bohemic acid (Fig. 7) (Nettleton *et al.*, 1977). It is effective against L-1210 leukemia (Bradner and Misiek, 1977) and is a potent RNA inhibitor particularly of peribosomal RNA synthesis (Crooke *et al.*, 1978).

H. Tallysomycin

This is the new bleomycin analogue isolated in the Bristol-Banyu Research Institute (Kawaguchi *et al.*, 1977) (Fig. 8). It differs from bleomycin chemically by some alterations in the nuclear amino acids, an added talose sugar, and the insertion of β-lysine in the side chain amine (Konishi *et al.*, 1977). The structure shown has been drawn on the basis of the recently revised structure of bleomycin lacking the β-lactam. Direct proof of this configuration of tallysomycin products is currently under investigation. Tallysomycin A has at least four times the potency of bleomycin complex in terms of both toxicity and antitumor effects *in vivo*. It also appears to cause a lower incidence of lung fibrosis than bleomycin in chronically treated mice (Bradner, 1978b). For these reasons, tallysomycin is undergoing large animal preclinical toxicology at Bristol Laboratories with plans for Phase I clinical trials if warranted by the completed toxicological profile. Hopefully, tallysomycin will represent the next generation of bleomycins.

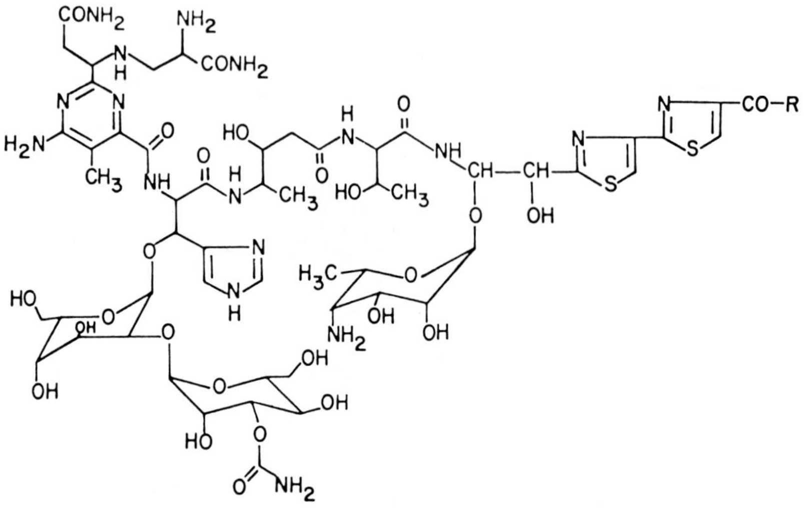

$$R = NHCH_2CH_2CH_2CHCH_2CONH(CH_2)_3NH(CH_2)_4NH_2$$
$$\qquad\qquad\qquad\quad |$$
$$\qquad\qquad\qquad NH_2$$

Fig. 8.   Structure of tallysomycin A.

VI. DISCUSSION

In this chapter, some of the strategies involved in the operation of a fermentation program for the discovery of new antitumor antibiotics have been discussed. Both scientific and logistic decisions are required in balancing the numbers and types of organisms selected, the prescreens applied, primary fermentation conditions, and *in vivo* tumor screens used as the first indicator of antitumor activity. This is only the first stage of the discovery process since chemical fractionation, purification, structural identification, and scaled-up production are following activities in antibiotic development which can span several years to complete. Thus, fermentation approaches to new antitumor drugs may seem inefficient compared to synthetic approaches. The availability of five marketed antitumor antibiotics in the United States offering a broad spectrum of effects on human neoplasms and operating through a variety of mechanisms suggest that the endeavor is worth continuing.

REFERENCES

Berger, J., Jampolsky, L. M., and Goldberg, M. W. (1949). *Arch. Biochem.* **22**, 476–478.
Bradner, W. T. (1978a). *Antibiot. Chemother. (Basel)* **23**, 4–11.

Bradner, W. T. (1978b). *In* Bleomycin: Current Status and New Developments (S. K. Carter, S. T. Crooke, and H. Umezawa, eds.), pp. 333-342. Academic Press, New York.

Bradner, W. T., and Misiek, M. (1977). *J. Antibiot.* **30,** 519-522.

Bradner, W. T., and Pindell, M. H. (1962). *Nature (London)* **196,** 682.

Bradner, W. T., Heinemann, B., and Gourevitch, A. (1967). *Antimicrob. Agents Chemother.* pp. 613-618.

Bradner, W. T., Bush, J. A., Myllymaki, R. W., Nettleton, D. E., Jr., and O'Herron, F. A. (1975). *Antimicrob. Agents & Chemother.* **8,** 159-163.

Conover, L. H. (1971). *Adv. Chem. Ser.* **108,** 33-80.

Crooke, S. T., Duvernay, V. H., Galvan, L., and Prestayko, A. W. (1978). *Mol. Pharmacol.* **14,** 290-298.

DeVault, R. L., Schmitz, H., and Hooper, I. R. (1966). *Antimicrob. Agents Chemother.* pp. 796-800.

Doyle, T. W., and Bradner, W. T. (1979). *In* "Anticancer Agents Based on Natural Product Models" (J. M. Cassady and J. D. Douros, eds.). Academic Press, New York (in press).

Gause, G. F., and Dudnik, Y. V. (1972). *Adv. Antimicrob. Antineoplast. Chemother., Proc. Int. Congr. Chemother., 7th, 1971* Vol. I, pp. 87-88.

Gause, G. F., Preobrazhenskaya, T. P., Ivanitskaya, L. P., and Soeshnikova, M. A. (1969). *Antibiotiki* **14,** 963-969.

Kawaguchi, H., Tsukima, H., Tomita, K., Konishi, M., Saito, K., Kobaru, S., Numata, K., Fujisawa, K., Miyaki, T., Hatori, M., and Koshiyama, H. (1977). *J. Antibiot.* **30,** 779-788.

Konishi, M., Saito, K., Numata, K., Tsuno, T., Asama, K., Tsukiura, H., Naito, T., and Kawaguchi, H. (1977). *J. Antibiot.* **30,** 789-805.

Maeda, K., Kosaka, H., Yagishita, K., and Umezawa, H. (1956). *J. Antibiot., Ser. A* **9,** 82-85.

Nettleton, D. E., Jr., Bradner, W. T., Bush, J. A., Coon, A. B., Moseley, J. E., Myllymaki, R. W., O'Herron, F. A., Schreiber, R. H., and Vulcano, A. (1977). *J. Antibiot.* **30,** 525-529.

Poole, D. T., and Butler, T. C. (1970). *Fed. Proc., Fed. Am. Soc. Exp. Biol.* **29,** 807.

Price, K. E., Schlein, A., Bradner, W. T., and Lein, J. (1964). *Antimicrob. Agents Chemother.* pp. 95-99.

Schmitz, H., Jibrinski, D., Hooper, I. R., Crook, K. E., Jr., Price, K. E., and Lein, J. (1965). *J. Antibiot.* **18,** 82-88.

Sequin, U., Bedford, C. T., Chung, S. K., and Scott, A. I. (1975). *Chimia* **29,** 527-528.

Sugiura, K., and Sugiura, M. M. (1958). *Cancer Res.* **18,** Part 2, 246-318.

White, H. L., and White, J. R. (1969). *Biochemistry* **8,** 1030-1042.

16

BIOTRANSFORMATION
Charles A. Claridge

I. INTRODUCTION

Microorganisms, through their highly selective complement of metabolic enzymes, are capable of performing many oxidative or reductive reactions upon selective substrates. These enzymes thus can be exploited to produce highly specific chemical transformations on complex molecules under extremely mild reaction conditions. In many instances, the microbial method of transformation can be shown to be superior to chemical modification, particularly with complex substrates, such as some of the naturally occurring antitumor agents. In the field of antitumor biology the use of this technique to modify existing antitumor agents is a relatively new development.

The beginning of microbial transformation on an industrial scale was detailed in the work of Peterson and Murray (1952), who showed that cells of the fungus *Rhizopus nigricans* would oxygenate progesterone at the 11-position to form 11α-hydroxyprogesterone in high yield (Fig. 1). The significance of this development lay in the discovery that corticosteroids were useful drugs and that their preparation by routine chemical procedures was difficult. This initial report was soon followed by the findings that many other organisms would also perform various transformations on steroids, including oxygenations at other positions on the steroid nucleus, dehydrogenations, and side chain cleavage (Iizuka and Naito, 1967; Wallen *et al.*, 1959; Charney and Herzog, 1967). Microbial transformations have been performed with other classes of compounds, including alkaloids (Iizuka and Naito, 1967; Kieslich, 1976), antibiotics (Sebek, 1974, 1975), other natural products (Kieslich, 1976; Fonken and Johnson, 1972), and antitumor agents (Rosazza, 1978). This last group of agents has only recently come under closer scrutiny as a class of substrates for microbial transformation through the interest of the National Cancer Institute in the United States.

Thus, the importance of microbial transformation in the development of new antitumor drugs should not be overlooked. During the past two decades, many new structural classes of antitumor compounds have been discovered from higher plants and microorganisms, including new kinds of alkaloids, steroids, terpenes, enzymes, and antibiotics. However, because many of these compounds are also toxic, their therapeutic value is restricted. In addition, many of these agents have relatively complex chemical structures and thus resist simple modification by standard chemical procedures. Thus, by analogy to the success in the steroid field, the idea was conceived that successful transformations of antitumor compounds could occur.

Rosazza (1978) has stated that the two major goals sought in the study of microbial transformation with antitumor compounds are the production of potentially useful metabolites possessing less toxicity than the parent compound and

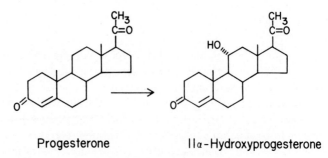

Progesterone   11α-Hydroxyprogesterone

Fig. 1.   Transformation of progesterone by *Rhizopus nigricans*.

the determination of their metabolic fate. The production of new potentially active metabolites follows the steroid transformation rationale of high selectivity and mild reaction conditions. New metabolites may be obtained in sufficient quantity for complete structure determination and testing for biological activity. Because microorganisms mimic many metabolic reactions which occur in mammalian systems, valuable information may be obtained about metabolic pathways which provide insights into mechanisms of toxicity not easily obtained with animals (Smith and Rosazza, 1975).

II. SELECTION OF ORGANISMS

Organisms to be used in a study of the biotransformation of antitumor compounds, or of any complex organic compound, can be selected in a variety of ways. In addition, once the organism has been selected, the reaction can be conducted by a number of different methods which must be examined for each substrate since these fermentations are still carried out in a highly empirical fashion. Numerous probing experiments have to be done before the most satisfactory procedures is finally found (Fonken and Johnson, 1972).

If one knows the structure of the compound under investigation, one can speculate what reactions may occur, then select organisms already reported to perform these reactions (Iizuka and Naito, 1967; Kieslich, 1976). Substrate specificity, however, will generally limit the success of this approach.

Another method of organism selection is by an enrichment procedure whereby the compound to be transformed is supplied to a source of mixed organisms (such as found in soil) as the sole source of carbon and/or nitrogen (Veldkamp, 1970; Longden and Claridge, 1976). Organisms metabolizing the added agent will multiply and can be selected out of the mixture. On occasion, organisms that will completely degrade a compound that is to be transformed can be treated with a mutagenic agent to produce a blocked mutant that will accumulate an intermediate having desirable properties (Abbott and Gledhill, 1971).

The most general method, however, of seeking organisms capable of transformation is by a random selection from among pure cultures obtained either from established culture collections or by isolation from suitable sources such as soil. By the use of pure cultures, one is always able to return to a constant source when repetitive experiments become necessary. Because of the extreme specificity of the microorganism (enzyme)–substrate reaction, organisms previously demonstrated to carry out reactions with one class of compound will not necessarily perform the same reaction with another substrate, so that this method of random screening for organism selection becomes a necessary part of biotransformation studies.

III. MICROBIAL TRANSFORMATION REACTIONS

A number of methods have been detailed for the study of microbial bio-transformations (Perlman, 1976). The most commonly used procedure is to add the antitumor agent directly to the growing culture being studied. Following a suitable incubation period, the broth is examined for the presence of a bio-transformation product, perhaps by thin-layer or high performance liquid chromatography. The appropriate assay method must be developed for each compound being studied.

A second method, which allows an investigator to maintain more control over the reaction is to add the substrate to already pregrown and washed cells suspended in a buffer medium of known pH. These "resting" cells are actively metabolizing, but not growing. The reaction can be controlled by variations in the constitution and pH of the buffer and also by the addition of various co-metabolites which may enhance the transformation (Claridge and Schmitz, 1978). A variation of this procedure in which fungal spores are used as the source of enzymes for transformation has been studied extensively by Vezina and colleagues (Vezina and Singh, 1975). Several advantages result from the use of these preparations, among which are the stability of the spores and the possibility of continued reuse, the ability to store the spores until needed, and the fact that aseptic conditions are not needed to run the reactions.

Another procedure, which has usefulness when large-scale transformations are desired, is through the isolation and purification of the appropriate enzyme, followed by immobilization on some inert support for placement in a column for continuous operation. Some enzymes prepared this way have demonstrated half-lives of several months (Bernath *et al.,* 1977). A variation of this procedure eliminates the need for isolated enzyme systems, and whole microbial cells can be immobilized for continuous and repeated use. Half-lives have been reported to be up to 600 days (Abbott, 1978).

A relatively new procedure employs solvent mixtures immiscible with water, wherein the cells remain in the aqueous phase and the substrate in the solvent phase, the reaction taking place at the interface (Buckland *et al.,* 1975). This technique has only been demonstrated in a few specialized cases, and for the most part microbial transformations are studied by the use of the first two mentioned procedures.

IV. ANTITUMOR COMPOUNDS

The remainder of this review will focus on a few examples of the transformations employing antitumor compounds as substrates. Although Kieslich (1976) has compiled a large number of microbial transformations of nonsteroid cyclic compounds, very few reports have appeared on the use of antitumor compounds as substrates for these reactions. Many new alkaloids, steroids, terpenes, antibiotics, and enzymes, all possessing antitumor activity, have been discovered in recent years. Because most of these have relatively complex chemical structures, they lend themselves as suitable substrates for transformation studies. However, inadequate supplies of many of these agents has prevented their use. Nevertheless, there are reports on the biotransformations of such diverse antitumor compounds as acronycine (Betts *et al.*, 1974; Brannon *et al.*, 1974); actinomycin (Perlman *et al.*, 1966); anguidine (Claridge and Schmitz, 1978, 1979); mycophenolic acid (Jones *et al.*, 1970); lapachol (Otten and Rosazza, 1978); papaverine (Rosazza *et al.*, 1977); rifamycin B (Lancini *et al.*, 1967); showdomycin (Ozaki *et al.*, 1972); D-tetrandrine (Davis and Rosazza, 1976); thalicarpine (Nabih *et al.*, 1977); vinblastine (Neuss *et al.*, 1974a); vindoline (Nabih *et al.*, 1978; Neuss *et al.*, 1973, 1974b); withaferin A (Rosazza *et al.*, 1978); daunomycin, *N*-acetyldaunomycin, and steffimycin (Marshall *et al.*, 1976a, b; Aszalos *et al.*, 1977); the bleomycins (Umezawa *et al.*, 1973); and olivomycins (Schmitz and Claridge, 1977). This review will outline transformations that have been studied with some of these compounds.

A. Bleomycins

The bleomycins are a group of structurally related antitumor antibiotics discovered by Umezawa *et al.* (1966). Produced by strains of *Streptomyces verticillus,* the bleomycins differ from one another in the nature of the terminal amine. The addition of a diamine or triamine to a fermentation medium causes the production of a bleomycin containing the amine added and suppresses the production of other bleomycins (Umezawa, 1976). The main structural component common to all bleomycins, bleomycinic acid, can be prepared from bleomycin B_2 (Fig. 2) with resting cells or cell-free preparations of *Fusarium anguoides* (Umezawa *et al.*, 1973). These cells will react only with bleomycin B_2, suggesting that the enzyme is specific for the agmatine and not the bleomycinic acid portion of the molecule. This new enzyme, which has been called acylagmatine amido-hydrolase, hydrolyzes not only bleomycin B_2 but also acetyl-, propionyl-, and benzoylagmatine (Takahashi *et al.*, 1975).

B. Acronycine

Acronycine is an antitumor alkaloid isolated from the bark of *Acronychia baueri,* a shrub found in Australia. Betts *et al.* (1974) have found that cells of the fungus *Cunninghamella echinulata* will hydroxylate acronycine in the 9-position in an overall 30% yield to form 9-hydroxyacronycine (Fig. 3). Brannon *et al.* (1974) also reported the formation of this analogue by cells of *Aspergillus*

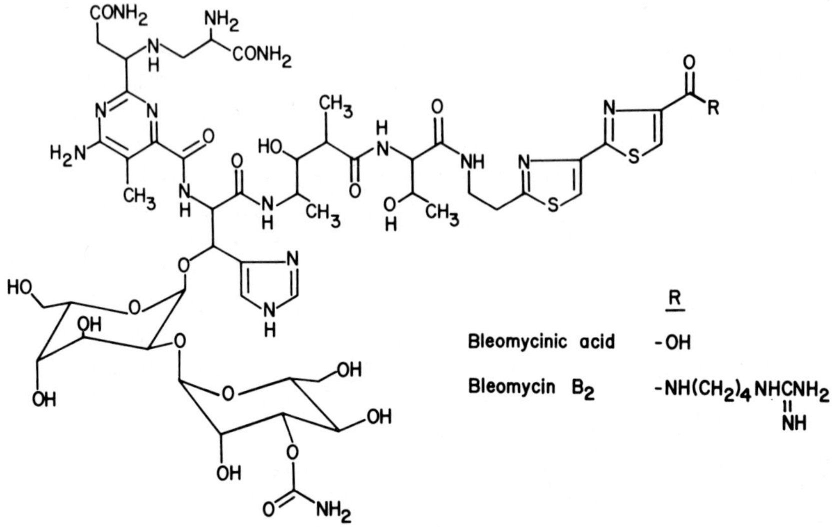

Fig. 2.   Structures of bleomycinic acid and bleomycin B$_2$.

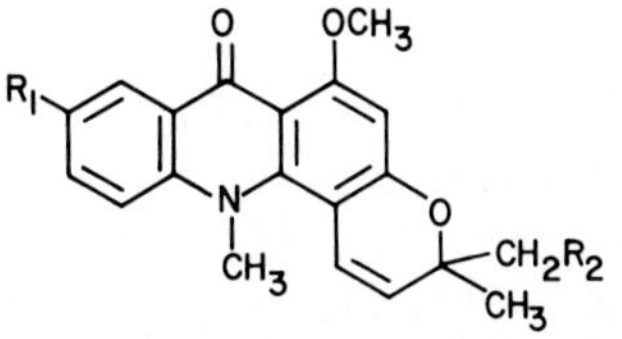

	R
Bleomycinic acid	-OH
Bleomycin B$_2$	-NH(CH$_2$)$_4$NHCNH$_2$ ‖ NH

	R$_1$	R$_2$
Acronycine	H	H
9-Hydroxyacronycine	OH	H
3-Hydroxymethylacronycine	H	OH

Fig. 3.   Structures of acronycine and analogues.

alleaceus and also of the 3-hydroxymethylacronycine (Fig. 3) by growing cells of *Streptomyces spectabilis*. Neither of these two derivatives has been reported to have activity against X5563 plasma cell myeloma or C-1498 myelogenous leukemia at levels which gave a positive response with acronycine.

C. Anthracyclines

The anthracyclines are a large family of closely related antitumor antibiotics including the clinically useful daunomycin and adriamycin (Fig. 4). Adriamycin

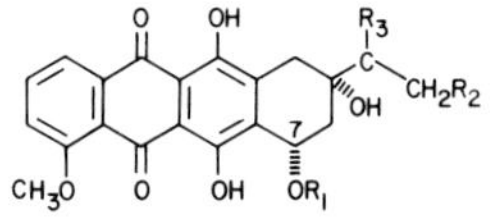

	R_1	R_2	R_3
Daunomycin	Daunosamine	H	=O
Adriamycin	Daunosamine	OH	=O
Daunomycinol	Daunosamine	H	H,OH
13 – Dihydrodaunomycin	Daunosamine	H	H,H

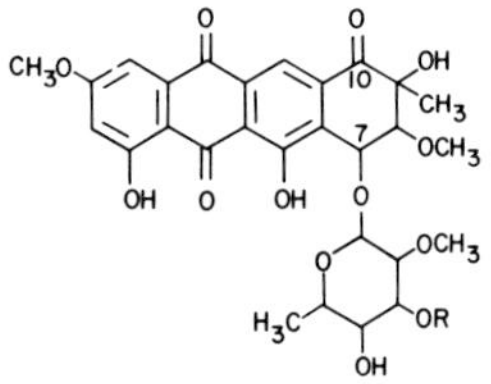

	R
Steffimycin	H
Steffimycin B	CH_3

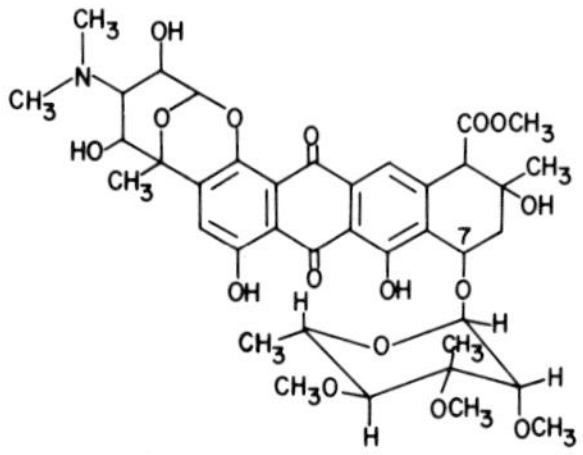

Nogalamycin

Fig. 4. Structures of some anthracycline antitumor agents.

was first discovered as the product of the fermentation of a mutant of the daunomycin-producing organism, *Streptomyces peucetius*. The mutant was able to reduce the C-14 of daunomycin to form the new compound adriamycin (Arcamone *et al.*, 1969). Because of the cumulative cardiac toxicity that apparently is manifest through clinical use of these compounds, a very large number of analogues have been synthesized, both chemically and biologically, seeking one devoid of this property.

The conversion of daunomycin to daunomycinol (Fig. 4) by *Streptomyces* and other bacterial species was first described by Florent and Lunel (1975). Daunomycinol has been reported as a mammalian metabolite of daunomycin (Aszalos *et al.*, 1977; Bachur *et al.*, 1976). Wiley and Marshall (1975) have shown transformation of several anthracyclines by anaerobically grown cultures of *Aeromonas hydrophila, Escherichia coli,* and *Citrobacter freundii*. The reductive reactions on substrates steffimycin, steffimycin B, nogalamycin, and daunomycin (Fig. 4) did not occur if the organisms were incubated in an adequate supply of oxygen. The products obtained were isolated and identified as 7-deoxysteffimycinone from the first two substrates, 7-dexoynogalarol from nogalamycin, and 7-deoxydaunomycinone from daunomycin.

Further work from the same laboratory (Wiley *et al.*, 1977) revealed that cells of *Streptomyces nogalater* (produces nogalamycin) and *Streptomyces peucetius* var. *caesius* (produces adriamycin) would catalyze the reduction of the C-10 carbonyl of steffimycinone to steffimycinol. Steffimycinol was further reduced by *Aeromonas hydrophila* to the 7-deoxy analogue. The production of 13-dihydrodaunomycin (Fig. 4) from daunomycin has also been shown to be efficiently carried out by aerobically grown cells of *Bacillus cyclooxydans* and *Cornyebacterium simplex* (Ninet *et al.*, 1976), and also by many unidentified soil microorganisms (Aszalos *et al.*, 1977).

D. Olivomycins

Schmitz and Claridge (1977) have shown that antibiotics of the olivomycin and chromomycin class were transformed when incubated with cells of *Whetzelinia sclerotiorum*. The metabolites could be isolated by methylene chloride extraction of the filtered broth followed by countercurrent distribution and column chromatography. The major products were the desisobutyryl derivatives (Fig. 5), with lesser amounts of the products having lost both the isobutyryl and acetyl groups. The deisobutyrylolivomycin A has considerable less antibacterial activity than its parent, whereas the two chromomycin pairs have similar antibacterial activity.

E. Lapachol

Lapachol, a naturally occurring naphthaquinone derivative found in the heartwood of several plants and from the roots of the Indian plant *Stereospermum suaveolens,* has activity against Walker 256 carcinosarcoma in rats, but is inactive against carcinoma 755, leukemia L-1210, and sarcoma 180. Recently Otten and Rosazza (1978) have shown that a number of fungi will form an acidic

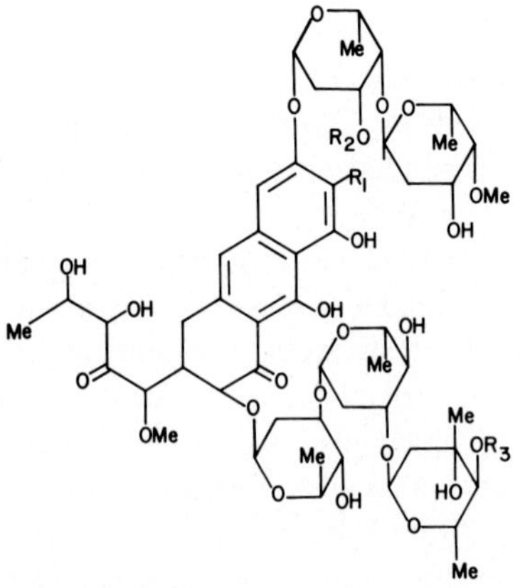

	R_1	R_2	R_3
Olivomycin	-H	-COCH$_3$	-COCH(CH$_3$)$_2$
Chromomycin	-CH$_3$	-COCH$_3$	-COCH(CH$_3$)$_2$
Desisobutyryl olivomycin	-H	-COCH$_3$	-H
Desisobutyryl chromomycin	-CH$_3$	-COCH$_3$	-H

Fig. 5. Structures of olivomycin and chromomycin and their desisobutyryl derivatives.

Lapachol Lapachol metabolite

Fig. 6. Structures of lapachol and transformed metabolite.

metabolite from lapachol (Fig. 6). A strain of *Penicillium notatum* was selected to produce sufficient transformed product so that its structure could be determined. The metabolite was identified as an intermediate formed in the Hooker oxidation of lapachol.

F. Tetrandrine

D-Tetrandrine is a plant alkaloid first isolated from *Stephania tetrandra,* a plant found in southern Europe, India, and Asia. Rosazza and his colleagues (Davis and Rosazza, 1976; Davis *et al.*, 1977) have found two major metabolites formed by cells of *Streptomyces griseus* and *Cunninghamella blakesleeana. Streptomyces griseus* selectively *N*-demethylates *d*-tetrandrine to form in 50% yield *N*-(2′)-nor-*d*-tetrandrine, whereas *C. blakesleeana* forms *N*-(2)-nor-*d*-tetrandrine in 20% yield (Fig. 7). These reactions demonstrate the extreme specificity of microbial biotransformation reactions.

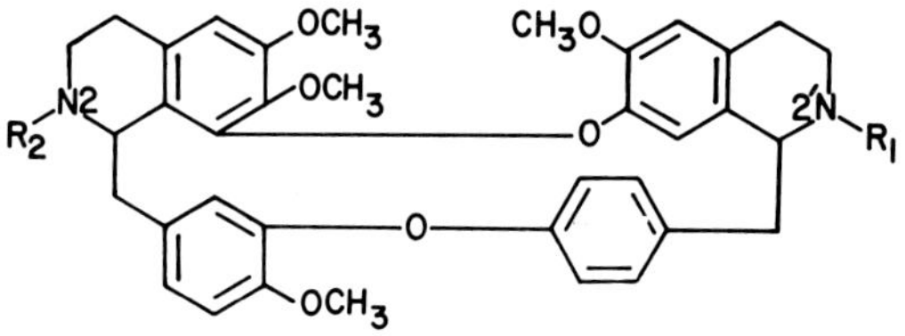

	R_1	R_2
d-Tetrandrine	CH_3	CH_3
N(2′)-nor-*d*-Tetrandrine	H	CH_3
N(2)-nor-*d*-Tetrandrine	CH_3	H

Fig. 7. Structures of tetrandrine and metabolites.

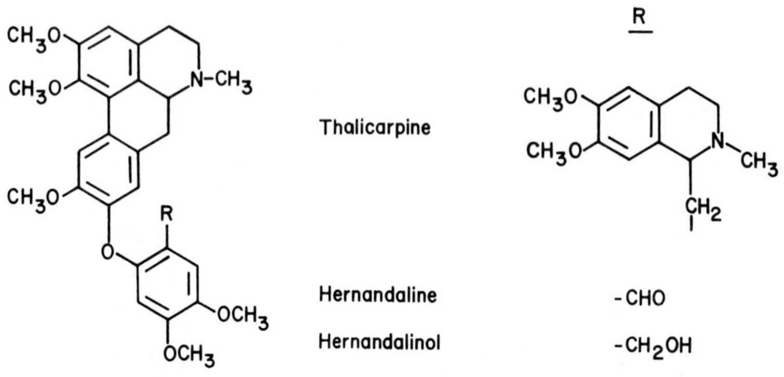

Fig. 8. Structures of thalicarpine, hernandaline, and hernandalinol.

G. Thalicarpine

Thalicarpine, another plant alkaloid which has demonstratable antitumor activity, both *in vitro* and *in vivo*, is at present undergoing clinical trials in humans. However, its use may be severely limited because of its toxicity. Rosazza and his co-workers (Nabih *et al.*, 1977) have shown that cells of *Streptomyces punipalus* will transform thalicarpine in 10% yield to a metabolite identified as hernandalinol. This latter compound can be obtained chemically by the reduction of the alkaloid hernandaline (Fig. 8). *Streptomyces punipalus* cells will also reduce hernandaline to hernandalinol, thus it is likely that hernandaline is an intermediate in this transformation of thalicarpine.

H. Withaferin A

Withaferin A is a member of a group of steroid lactones known as the withanolides isolated from *Withania somnifera* and *Acnistus arborescens*. Antitumor activity of this compound has been demonstrated against sarcoma-180 in mice.

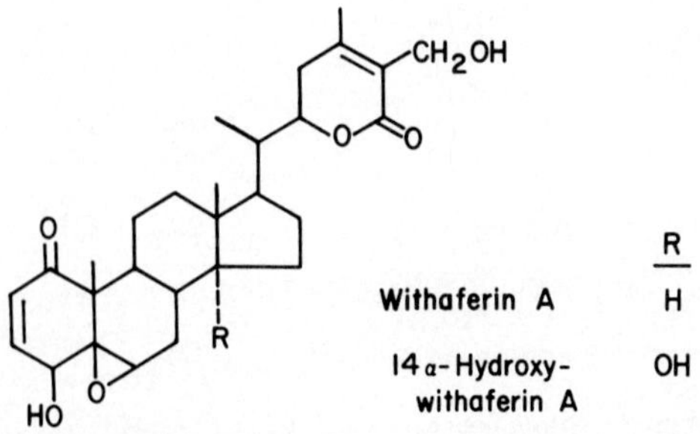

Fig. 9. Structures of withaferin A and a 14α-hydroxy analogue.

Rosazza *et al.* (1978) have shown that a number of fungi will transform withaferin A; a strain of *Cunninghamella elegans* being the best of those tested. This organism produced a metabolite identified as 14α-hydroxywithaferin A (Fig. 9). This analogue has similar activity to withaferin A when tested in the sarcoma-180 system. However, an as yet unidentified metabolite has greater activity in this same antitumor system.

I. Vinblastine and Vindoline

The two clinically important antitumor alkaloids vinblastine and vindoline (Fig. 10) are obtained from the white periwinkle, *Vinca rosea.* They are used in the treatment of Hodgkin's disease and monocytic leukemia, frequently in combination with other antitumor agents. Neuss *et al.* (1974a) showed that several species of *Streptomyces* would convert vinblastine into an aromatic ring hydroxylated product and an ether derivative. No biological activity of these metabolites was reported. This same group of workers also reported on the microbial transformation of the monomeric *Vinca* alkaloid vindoline by cells of *Streptomyces albogriseolus* and *Streptomyces cinnamonensis* to yield *N*-demethyl, deacetyl, and ether derivatives (Fig. 10) (Neuss *et al.*, 1973, 1974b; Mallett *et al.*, 1964).

Rosazza and co-workers (Nabih *et al.*, 1978) have recently reported the production of a new metabolite in 30% yield from vindoline by cells of *Streptomyces*

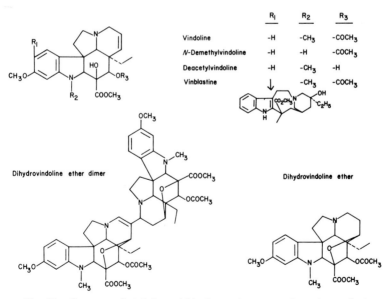

Fig. 10. Structures of vindoline, vinblastine, and some transformation products.

griseus. Isolation and characterization showed the new product to be a dimer of dihydrovindoline ether (Fig. 10).

J. Anguidine

Anguidine, a representative of a class of compounds called mycotoxins, is produced by a number of species of fungi. Many of these mycotoxins have antifungal and antitumor properties (Bamburg and Strong, 1971). Claridge and Schmitz (1978, 1979) have shown that a number of microorganisms will transform anguidine into a series of mono-, di-, and triacetoxy derivatives (Fig. 11). The cells employed were selected strains of *Acinetobacter calcoaceticus, Streptomyces griseus, Mucor mucedo* and *Fusarium oxysporum* f. sp. *vasinfectum*. The *in vivo* activity against P-388 and L-1210 leukemia in mice was determined and revealed that the 15-acetoxy analogue was much more active than the starting anguidine (Claridge *et al.*, 1979). This observation lead the way to the development of a larger series of chemically produced anguidine derivatives, many of which have even greater *in vivo* activity (T. Doyle, unpublished results).

Although this review has covered reports on direct microbial transformations of antitumor agents to form new analogues, two methods for the indirect biological formation of new derivatives should be mentioned. These techniques are referred to a mutational biosynthesis (Shier *et al.*, 1969) and directed biosynthesis (Sebek, 1974: Shibata and Uyeda, 1978). Very few reports have appeared relating these procedures to the formation of new antitumor agents, but the potential for the development of new compounds by these methods is probably greater than the field of direct biotransformation itself.

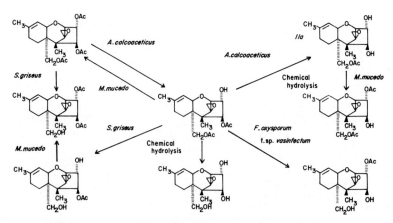

Fig. 11.   Microbial and chemical transformations of anguidine.

V. MUTATIONAL BIOSYNTHESIS

A novel method for preparing semisynthetic aminoglycoside antibiotics was developed in 1969 by Shier *et al.* by using mutants of *Streptomyces fradiae* incapable of producing the 2-deoxystreptamine portion of neomycin. When 2-deoxystreptamine was added to the medium, the antibiotic was formed. Mutants of this type have been called idiotrophic mutants (Nagaoka and Demain, 1975). Addition of 2-deoxystreptamine analogues to a fermentation of the idiotrophic mutants of a number of aminoglycoside antibiotic-producing organisms has lead to the formation of a wide variety of modified aminoglycoside antibiotics (Claridge, 1979; Nara, 1977; Shibata and Uyeda, 1978). The possibility exists for the application of this technique to a number of antitumor antibiotics produced by microorganisms. Fleck has recently reported on an idiotrophic mutant of *Streptomyces violaceus* which will not produce the anthracycline antibiotic violamycin unless the aglycone is added exogenously (Fleck, 1979). When modified aglycones were fed, new anthracyclines were formed. C. A. Claridge (unpublished results) has also developed idiotrophic mutants of two anthracycline-producing cultures: an *Actinosporangium* sp. which forms the bohemic acid complex, and a *Streptosporangium* sp. which produces the figaroic acid complex. Exogenously added aglycones restore the production of antibiotic activity.

VI. DIRECTED BIOSYNTHESIS

The addition of precursors to antibiotic fermentations leading to the formation of active antibiotic analogues has been known for a long time. New penicillins (Demain, 1966), echinomycins (Dhar *et al.*, 1971; Yoshida *et al.*, 1968), pyrrolnitrins (Hamill *et al.*, 1970), novobiocins (Walton *et al.*, 1962), polyoxins (Isono *et al.*, 1973) phleomycins (Umezawa, 1973), bleomycins (Fujii *et al.*, 1974), and actinomycins (Katz *et al.*, 1977) have been produced this way. Here also, the closer examination of more antitumor antibiotic fermentations by this method may possibly lead to the formation biosynthetically of analogues of the parent antitumor antibiotic having greater activity or less toxicity.

A combination of these two methods or the examination of mutants of antitumor antibiotic-producing organisms may lead to new products. Already cited was the work of Arcamone *et al.* (1969) on the formation of adriamycin by a mutant of *Streptomyces peucetius*. Recently, Blumauerova reported that mutants of *Streptomyces galilaeus* would produce new anthracyclines different from the normal aklavinone type (Blumauerova *et al.*, 1979). These new anthracyclines have yet to be isolated and identified and, more importantly, compared to the parent anthracycline for activity and toxicity.

VII. DISCUSSION

The development of new antitumor compounds through the use of microorganisms, either as sources of biochemical reagents or as fermentation agents, employing mutant cultures or modified growth conditions is a relatively new field that has yet to be explored to its full potential. Hopefully, new useful drugs will emerge from these programs.

ACKNOWLEDGMENT

This work was supported in part under United States Public Health Service Contract NO 1-CM-77138 from the National Cancer Institute.

REFERENCES

Abbott, B. J. (1978). *Annu. Rep. Ferment. Processes* **2**, 91–123.

Abbott, B. J., and Gledhill, W. E. (1971). *Adv. Appl. Microbiol.* **14**, 249.

Arcamone, F., Cassinelli, G., Fantini, G., Grein, A., Orezzi, P., Pol, C., and Spalla, C. (1969). *Biotechnol. Bioeng.* **11**, 1101–1110.

Aszalos, A., Bachar, N. R., Hamilton, B. K., Langlykke, A. F., Roller, P. P., Sheikh, M. Y., Sutphin, M. S., Thomas, M. C., Wareheim, D. A., and Wright, L. H. (1977). *J. Antibiot.* **30**, 50–58.

Bachur, N. R., Steele, M., Meriweather, W. D., and Hildebrand, R. (1976). *J. Antibiot.* **29**, 1199–1202.

Bamburg, J. R., and Strong, F. M. (1971). *In* "Microbial Toxins" (S. Kadis, A. Ciegler, and S. Ajl, eds.), Vol. 7, pp. 207–292. Academic Press, New York.

Bernath, F. R., Venkatasubramanian, K., and Vieth, W. R. (1977). *Annu. Rep. Ferment. Processes* **1**, 235–266.

Betts, R. E., Walters, D. E., and Rosazza, J. P. (1974). *J. Med. Chem.* **17**, 599–609.

Blumauerová, M., Královcová, E., Matějů, J., Hoštálek, Z., and Vaněk, Z. (1979). *In* "Genetics of Industrial Microorganisms" (O. K. Sebek and A. I. Laskin, eds.), p. 90. Am. Soc. Microbiol., Washington, D.C.

Brannon, D. R., Horton, H. R., and Svoboda, G. H. (1974). *J. Med. Chem.* **17**, 653–654.

Buckland, B. C., Dunhill, P., and Lilly, M. D. (1975). *Biotechnol. Bioeng.* **17**, 815–826.

Charney, W., and Herzog, H. L. (1967). "Microbial Transformations of Steroids." Academic Press, New York.

Claridge, C. A. (1979). *Econ. Microbiol.* **3**, 151.

Claridge, C. A., and Schmitz, H. (1978). *Appl. Environ. Microbiol.* **36**, 63–67.

Claridge, C. A., and Schmitz, H. (1979). *Appl. Environ. Microbiol.* **37**, 693–696.

Claridge, C. A., Schmitz, H., and Bradner, W. T. (1979). *Cancer Chemother. Pharmacol.* **2**, 181–182.

Davis, P. J., and Rosazza, J. P. (1976). *J. Org. Chem.* **41**, 2548–2551.

Davis, P. J., Wiese, D., and Rosazza, J. P. (1977). *Lloydia* **40**, 239–246.

Demain, A. L. (1966). *In* "Biosynthesis of Antibiotics" (J. F. Snell, ed.), pp. 29–94. Academic Press, New York.

Dhar, M. M., Singh, C., Khan, A. W., Arif, A. J., Gupta, C. M., and Bhaduri, A. P. (1971). *Pure Appl. Chem.* **28,** 469–473.

Fleck, W. F. (1979). *In* "Genetics of Industrial Microorganisms" (O. K. Sebek and A. I. Laskin, eds.), p. 117. Am. Soc. Microbiol., Washington, D.C.

Florent, J., and Lunel, J. (1975). German Patent 2,456,139.

Fonken, G. S., and Johnson, R. A. (1972). "Chemical Oxidations with Microorganisms." Dekker, New York.

Fujii, A., Takita, T., Shimada, N., and Umezawa, H. (1974). *J. Antibiot.* **27,** 73–77.

Hamill, R. L., Elander, R. P., Mabe, J. A., and Gorman, M. (1970). *Appl. Microbiol.* **19,** 721–725.

Iizuka, H., and Naito, A. (1967). "Microbial Transformation of Steroids and Alkaloids." Univ. Park Press, State College, Pennsylvania.

Isono, K., Crain, P. F., Odiorne, T. J., McCloskey, J. A., and Suhadolnik, R. J. (1973). *J. Am. Chem. Soc.* **95,** 5788–5789.

Jones, D. E., Moore, R. H., and Crowley, G. C. (1970). *J. Chem. Soc. C* p. 1725.

Katz, E., Williams, W. K., Mason, K. T., and Mauger, A. B. (1977). *Antimicrob. Agents & Chemother.* **11,** 1056–1063.

Kieslich, K. (1976). "Microbial Transformation of Non-Steroid Cyclic Compounds." Wiley, New York.

Lancini, G. C., Thiemann, J. E., Sartori, G., and Sensi, P. (1967). *Experientia* **23,** 899–900.

Longden, A. R., and Claridge, C. A. (1976). *Appl. Environ. Microbiol.* **32,** 188–189.

Mallett, G. E., Fukuda, D. A., and Gorman, M. (1964). *Lloydia* **27,** 334–339.

Marshall, V. P., Reisender, E. A., Reineke, L. M., Johnson, J. H., and Wiley, P. F. (1976a). *Biochemistry* **15,** 4139–4145.

Marshall, V. P., Reisender, E. A., and Wiley, P. F. (1976b). *J. Antibiot.* **29,** 966–968.

Nabih, T., Davis, P. J., Caputo, J. P., and Rosazza, J. P. (1977). *J. Med. Chem.* **20,** 914–917.

Nabih, T., Youel, L., and Rosazza, J. P. (1978). *J. Chem. Soc., Perkin Trans. 1,* p. 757.

Nagaoka, K., and Demain, A. L. (1975). *J. Antibiot.* **28,** 627–635.

Nara, T. (1977). *Annu. Rep. Ferment. Processes* **1,** 299–326.

Neuss, N., Fukuda, D. S., Mallett, G. E., Brannon, D. R., and Huckstep, L. L. (1973). *Helv. Chim. Acta* **56,** 2418–2426.

Neuss, N., Mallett, G. E., Brannon, D. R., Mabe, J. A., Horton, H. R., and Huckstep, L. L. (1974a). *Helv. Chim. Acta* **57,** 1886–1890.

Neuss, N., Fukuda, D. S., Brannon, D. R., and Huckstep, L. L. (1974b). *Helv. Chim. Acta* **57,** 1891–1893.

Ninet, L., Florent, J., Lunel, J., Abraham, A., Lombardi, B., and Tissler, R. (1976). *Abstr. Int. Ferment. Symp., 5th, 1976* (Abstract No. 17.06).

Otten, S., and Rosazza, J. P. (1978). *Appl. Environ. Microbiol.* **35,** 554–557.

Ozaki, M., Kariya, T., Kato, H., and Kimura, T. (1972). *Agric. Biol. Chem.* **36,** 451–456.

Perlman, D. (1976). *Tech. Chem. (N.Y.)* **10,** Part 1, 47–68.

Perlman, D., Mauger, A. B., and Weissbach, H. W. (1966). *Biochem. Biophys. Res. Commun.* **24,** 513–518.

Peterson, D. H., and Murray, H. C. (1952). *J. Am. Chem. Soc.* **74,** 1871–1874.

Rosazza, J. P. (1978). *Lloydia* **41,** 297–311.

Rosazza, J. P., Kammer, M., Youel, L., Smith, R. V., Erhardt, P. W., Troung, D. H., and Leslie, S. W. (1977). *Xenobiotica* **7,** 133–143.

Rosazza, J. P., Nicholas, A. W., and Gustafson, M. E. (1978). *Steroids* **31,** 671–679.

Schmitz, H., and Claridge, C. A. (1977). *J. Antibiot.* **30,** 635–638.

Sebek, O. K. (1974). *Lloydia* **37,** 381–388.

Sebek, O. K. (1975). *Acta Microbiol.* **22,** 381–388.

Shibata, M., and Uyeda, M. (1978). *Annu. Rep. Ferment. Processes* **2,** 267–297.

Shier, W. T., Rinehart, K. L., Jr., and Gottlieb, D. (1969). *Proc. Nat. Acad. Sc. U.S.A.* **63**, 198–204.

Smith, R. V., and Rosazza, J. P. (1975). *J. Pharm. Sci.* **64**, 1737–1759.

Takahashi, Y., Shirai, T., and Ishii, S. (1975). *J. Biochem. (Tokyo)* **77**, 823–830.

Umezawa, H. (1973). *Biomedicine* **18**, 459–475.

Umezawa, H. (1976). *In* "Fundamental and Clinical Studies of Bleomycin" (S. K. Carter, T. Ichikawa, G. Mathé, and H. Umezawa, eds.), pp. 3–36. Univ. of Tokyo Press, Tokyo.

Umezawa, H., Maeda, K., Takeuchi, T., and Okami, Y. (1966). *J. Antibiot., Ser. A* **19**, 200–209.

Umezawa, H., Takahashi, Y., Fujii, A., Saino, T., Shirai, T., and Takita, T. (1973). *J. Antibiot.* **26**, 117–119.

Veldkamp, H. (1970). In "Methods in Microbiology" (J. R. Norris and D. W. Ribbons, eds.), Vol. 3A, pp. 305–361. Academic Press, New York.

Vezina, C., and Singh, K. (1975). *In* "The Filamentous Fungi" (J. E. Smith and D. R. Berry, eds.), Vol. 1, pp. 158–192. Wiley, New York.

Wallen, L. L., Stodola, F. H., and Jackson, R. W. (1959). "Type Reactions in Fermentation Chemistry," ARS Bull. ARS-71-13. Agric. Res. Serv., Peoria Illinois.

Walton, R. B., McDaniel, L. E., and Woodruff, H. B. (1962). *Dev. Ind. Microbiol.* **3**, 370–375.

Wiley, P. F., and Marshall, V. P. (1975). *J. Antibiot.* **28**, 838–840.

Wiley, P. F., Koert, J. M., Elrod, D. W., Reisender, E. A., and Marshall, V. P. (1977). *J. Antibiot.* **30**, 649–654.

Yoshida, T., Kimura, Y., and Katagiri, K. (1968). *J. Antibiot.* **21**, 465–467.

17
DESIGN AND EVALUATION OF CLINICAL TRIALS OF ANTICANCER DRUGS

Stephen K. Carter

I. INTRODUCTION

Cancer chemotherapy is still a relatively new discipline. With the discovery of nitrogen mustard followed by the discovery of the antifolates and actinomycin D, the modern era of utilizing drugs to treat cancer came soon after World War II. There developed a veritable explosion of drugs available with which to treat patients with cancer, and over the years it has been shown that chemotherapy, either by itself or in combination with radiation therapy or surgery, can now be curative in at least eight or nine different malignant diseases in a certain percentage of the time (Carter *et al.*, 1977). It is the hope of the future that, by utilizing chemotherapy in a wide range of combined approaches with surgery and radiation therapy, an even greater impact against some of the major cancer killers can be made. With this brief background, the purpose of this chapter is to describe the types of clinical studies of some of the problems encountered in the development of new cancer chemotherapeutic agents.

CANCER AND CHEMOTHERAPY, VOL. I

II. BASIC CONCEPTS

All new cancer drugs go through three phases of clinical trial (Carter, 1977). The definitions of these three phases are modifications of the outline of these trials developed by the United States Food and Drug Administration (FDA). For new drugs in general, these phases are valuable from a conceptual point of view, as they focus attention on the strategies for these clinical trials. It should be recognized that there is easy movement between these phases and that there is overlap to some degree.

Table I shows the definitions of the three clinical trials, adding a fourth phase which is increasing in importance in the United States. Phase one is designed as clinical pharmacology, phase two as an efficacy screen, phase three as role delineation, and phase four as the application in medical practice. Phase four involves taking the findings which have been shown to be positive in a research setting, and demonstrating that they will be effective in the day-to-day practice of medicine.

Figure 1 introduces the concept that cancer is not one disease, but at least a hundred different diseases; cancer of the breast is very different from cancer of the lung, which is very different from the cancer of the colon. Each kind of disease that we call cancer has a different therapeutic strategy, different diagnostic patterns, different relapse patterns, and different sensitivities to various kinds of chemotherapeutic agents. Therefore, each disease, which we call cancer, has its own therapeutic strategy. The phase I trial is a modality oriented study, but by the time phase II is reached, there has to be the integration of a disease oriented strategy. Therefore, a phase II study is described as being designed for a given type of cancer and the disease strategy may modulate where this new drug evaluation may be performed.

When any drug is tested, a very complex process within the framework of the disease oriented strategy against cancer is initiated. As soon as activity is observed for a new drug in phase II studies, there is no longer an automatic move to phase III and to phase IV in the classic drug development mode. One may immediately, with an active drug, begin to study that drug in combination with other active drugs against that tumor type. The combination which is derived is

TABLE I

Clinical Trials

Phase I	Clinical pharmacology
Phase II	Efficacy screen
Phase III	Role delineation
Phase IV	Application in medical practice

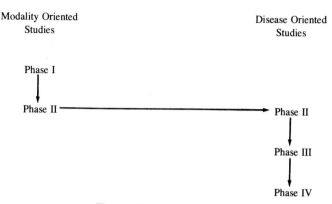

Fig. 1.   Therapeutic strategy.

new and can be viewed as a new drug. It is then placed in a pilot study composed of a combination of phase I and phase II evaluations. This particular combination may move to phase III and phase IV studies. As soon as a drug is shown to be active, it may be studied in combination with radiation therapy, immunotherapy, or surgery, and again, this starts with a pilot approach before moving into phase III and phase IV studies (Fig. 2).

The combination regimen, if active, can be put in a combined modality pilot study proceeding through the various phases. It is seen that a drug placed into clinical trial and which exhibits a level of activity becomes integrated into the great complexity of the treatment strategy for the various forms of cancer.

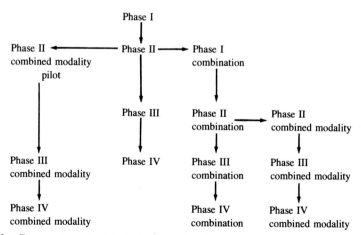

Fig. 2.   Fourteen possible clinical trials involving single agent with one combination and one combined modality approach.

III. PHASE I CLINICAL TRIALS

The ultimate goals of a phase I study for a cancer drug are the following: to determine the maximally tolerated dose, to elucidate the parameters of the toxicity, to establish whether biologic activity exists for the particular compound, and to elucidate potential therapeutic activity.

As opposed to other drugs investigated by the pharmaceutical industry, there are two obvious aspects which make cancer drugs unique. They are the concepts of the maximally tolerated dose and the normality of toxicity. Cancer chemotherapy functions to kill cancer cells in a selective fashion; ideally, a drug should kill every single cancer cell, thereby effecting a cure. It is postulated that drugs kill cancer cells by first-order kinetics. This means that a given dose of an antineoplastic drug will kill a fixed percentage of cancer cells, regardless of the number of cancer cells that a patient may harbor. That is, a given dose will kill 99.9% of a thousand cells, a million cells or a billion cells. Implicit in this is the concept that the higher the dose given, the greater the percentage of cells killed and more rapidly could total cell eradication be achieved before resistance occurs. Therefore, cancer drugs are given at the highest dose possible, with the limitation being the toxicity to the patient.

Since there has never been discovered a cancer drug which is absolutely selective for cancer cells and not normal tissue, some level of toxicity with cancer drugs is inevitable. While in other areas of drug development any level of toxicity can be cause for concern, toxicity is an essential element of current cancer chemotherapy. The critical question for any cancer drug is: What is the therapeutic index? Can meaningful therapeutic benefit be obtained from that drug at a reasonable cost in toxicity? As a result, the strategy of phase I is to establish how high a dose of the drug can be administered, so that in phase II, there is the best chance to kill a large number of cancer cells and observe drug activity. Dosed at the maximum tolerated dose (MTD), it is imperative to establish what the toxicity of the drug is and if it is predictable, reversible, and treatable.

It needs to be emphasized that a phase I trial is a therapeutic trial in a patient with cancer and that the hope and the idea of that study is to give some therapeutic benefit to that particular patient. While it is common to emphasize the clinical pharmacology aspects of the phase I study, it is in truth a trial with therapeutic intent, and many times therapeutic benefit and therapeutic response are seen in the phase I trial. On the other hand, it should not be forgotten that phase I trials are performed with advanced cancer patients who have had a great deal of extensive prior therapy. That therapeutic activity is not observed in phase I studies should not be a cause for feeling that the drug is a failure and that development should be discontinued.

Phase I studies are limited to clinical pharmacology in patients with tumors resistant to all currently available therapy. These patients should have relatively "normal" organ function and should not have received such extensive prior therapy that evaluation is difficult. The estimated survival of patients should be at least 2 months to allow complete evaluation of toxicity. Measurable disease or illness that can be evaluated is not required and a favorable clinical response, although gratifying and significant when it occurs, is not essential at this stage in terms of decision making for phase II.

As in any clinical study, the design of a phase I trial must encompass a number of critical variables, such as (1) initial dose, (2) dose schedules, (3) dose escalation procedure, (4) number of patients treated on any dose schedule, (5) data collection, (6) pharmacology, and (7) criteria for proceeding to phase II studies.

The initial dose for phase I studies may be chosen on the basis of rodent or large animal data or clinical data obtained with an analogue or from foreign clinical trials. Freireich *et al.* (1966) reviewed a large volume of experimental data and showed that there is close relationship between the LD_{10} (lethal dose for 10% of the treated animals) in rodents and the maximum tolerated dose (MTD) in man when the values are given on a milligrams per square meter basis. However, their conclusions strongly emphasize the dangers of attempting direct extrapolation of animal toxicity data to MTD in man. They did not suggest that it would be wise to convert mouse or rat LD_{10} to milligrams per square meter and start clinical trials in man at one-third this level. However, calculation of the MTD in these terms has been recommended and is used in Europe (Kenis, 1969).

The large animal dose levels that might be selected in the initial phase I dose are (1) highest nontoxic dose (HNTD), (2) toxic dose low (TDL), (3) toxic dose high (TDH), and (4) lethal dose (LD). Although one-third of the TDL in the most sensitive species, expressed in milligrams per square meter of body surface area, has been the approach for years, the critical questions remain: Is this really the best starting level? Is it safe enough? Can it be improved? Goldsmith *et al.* (1975) have done a large-scale retrospective analysis on many drugs in which this procedure was used, and it was found to be in almost all cases a safe approach, the emphasis being to achieve an initial dose which is nontoxic. From the point of view of the FDA and the current climate in our society, it would be very detrimental for the future of a drug, or a drug development program for that matter, if the first dose taken with a new drug were severely toxic. Therefore, the aim is to initiate phase I studies with a first dose that is nontoxic and then to escalate into the level of toxicity.

Commonly used schedules for cancer drugs include single dose, daily times five or ten, twice weekly, or continuous infusion. In the United States today cancer drugs are being utilized almost exclusively on intermittent schedules. The original utilization of the chronic daily schedule with cancer drugs, which was popular 20 years ago, has certainly decreased. If one goes to Japan, the Soviet

Union, or many other areas of the world, where active drug development is on-going in cancer chemotherapy, chronic daily schedules for 30 days or longer are still common.

Since the pharmacokinetics of most of the drugs are not known prior to the clinical study, most of the time the schedule chosen is based on what could be called clinical rational empericism with a very large dose of clinical convenience included. There is very little logic at this moment in time as to how the initial schedules for new cancer drugs in the United States are chosen. The daily times five schedule is now the most common and popular schedule for almost all cancer drugs. Toxicity should always be related to a given dose level on a given dose schedule for a given duration of time. Some definitions of toxic doses are in Table II.

How is dose escalation approached? A few years ago, at the National Cancer Institute, there was a great emphasis put on the modified Fibonacci search scheme approach to escalating doses (Table III). In this approach the first escalation is 100%. The second 75%, the third 50%, the fourth 33%, and so on; the concept of this modified Fibonocci search scheme approach being the use of large dose escalations initially and then progressively smaller dose increments as the toxic range comes closer. There is no longer a rigid adherence to this scheme. It is now understood that clinical intuition and knowledge of the individual parameters of clinical drug evaluation are more critical than any rigid formulation. It is interesting that in the retrospective analysis of Goldsmith et al. (1975) the number of steps to go from one-third to TDL in animals as the initial dose level in man to the MTD in man, using the Fibonocci approach were in most cases not excessive. It was found that, with only three exceptions, all the drugs analyzed required eight dose steps or less. This indicates that the Fibonocci

TABLE II

Toxicity Definitions in Phase I Study

Term	Definition
Subtoxic dose	A dose that causes *consistent* changes of hematologic or biochemical parameters and might thus herald toxicity at the next higher dose level or with prolonged drug administration (example, consistent drug-related decrease of thrombocytes without dropping below an arbitrarily defined "toxic" level of $100,000/mm^3$)
Minimal toxic dose	The smallest dose at which one or more of three patients show consistent, readily reversible drug toxicity
Recommended dose for therapeutic trial	The dose that causes moderate, reversible toxicity in most patients
Maximum tolerated dose	The highest safely tolerable dosage

TABLE III

Idealized Modified Fibonacci Search Scheme Approach to Dose Escalation in Phase I Study

Drug dose[a] (n)[a]	Percentage increase above preceding dose level
2.0n	100
3.3n	67
5.0n	50
7.0n	40
9.0n	30–35
12.0n	30–35
16.0n	35–35

[a] Starting dose = n (milligrams/square meter).

scheme is reasonable. However, there are exceptions where rigid adherence could lead to a large number of steps being needed.

IV. PHASE II CLINICAL TRIALS

Phase II studies are designed to determine whether a new drug exhibits antitumor activity worthy of further clinical evaluation. The phase II trial, which is not planned to give definitive answers on the ultimate value or role of a given drug (the purpose of the larger phase three studies), is a screen for antitumor activity and contains the imperfections of any screening system.

The efficacy of a compound must be examined in as many aspects as possible; it is not just a question of whether a drug is effective, but to what degree it is effective and how it compares with other drugs used to treat a given tumor. In the initial phase II trial, the estimated maximum tolerated dose derived in phase I studies is usually chosen to test the efficacy of the drug. In most cases, trials are conducted with only one dose and one schedule. Unfortunately, it is not possible to be certain that this dose schedule approaches the optimum with regard to therapeutic effect. Animal studies demonstrate clearly that therapeutic effect of many active agents is highly dependent on the dose schedule, and so, ideally, without comparative pharmacology for animals and man, different schedules and doses ought to be used in phase II trials. However, this is rarely feasible.

On completion of phase II clinical studies, it should be possible to make a reasonable judgment regarding the degree of efficacy and the nature of adverse effects at a particular dose schedule. Whether or not further large-scale studies should be performed rests on consideration of those factors, which can be summed up by the concept of the risk-to-benefit ratio. When efficacy is considered the critical point, as Gehan and Schneiderman (1973) have pointed out, the decision to be reached is whether the agent could be or is unlikely to be effective in $x\%$ of patients or more. An answer can usually be obtained after studying a relatively small number of patients.

The end points of the phase II study include the level of antitumor activity expressed as a numerator over a denominator or percent response. The numerator is dependent on the response criteria chosen, and the denominator is equally important in defining the results that will be reported.

Another end point is the toxicity at the active dose level, so that a therapeutic index can be determined. Phase II is a screen, and at the end of the phase II study there is the decision about whether the drug has enough activity, in a given kind of cancer, to justify larger scale trials. This is a go or no go decision, and it is perhaps the most critical juncture in the clinical flow for any anticancer drug. After many years and many dollars have been spent, the critical decision will be made, many times on 20 or 30 patients, as to whether the drug should then go on for further study in a given tumor type.

Phase II trials with drugs, for any disease site, have a wide range of possibilities above and beyond the classic drug development mode. In addition to phase II studies of new drugs, there are combinations, an established drug untested in that disease, a new schedule, or combined drug with any one of a variety of other modalities (Table IV). The modulating factor for phase II studies is the strategy for that given disease, and therefore in a drug development program careful consideration must be given to resources needed for the drugs in clinical trials. If too many drugs are enrolled in clinical trials, there can be an overload of the system with resultant inadequate trials.

Ideally, a phase II study with a new drug should be performed in every kind of cancer for which the drug could be applicable. This might entail up to forty phase II studies for a given drug and, obviously, this is not possible. What evolved at the National Cancer Institute (NCI) was the concept of signal tumors, which were

TABLE IV

Possible Phase II Drug Trials for Any Disease Site

I. New investigational agent
II. New combination regimen
III. Established active drug or regimen on new schedule
IV. Combined drug with
   a. Immunotherapy
   b. Hormonal therapy
   c. Radiotherapy
   d. Toxicity blocking agent
   e. Reductive surgery
   f. Any combination of a–e

TABLE V

Signal Tumors of the Division of Cancer Treatment Chemotherapy Program[a]

Adenocarcinoma of the breast
Adenocarcinoma of the colon
Bronchogenic carcinoma
Adenocarcinoma of the pancreas
Ovarian cancer
Malignant melanoma
Acute myelocytic leukemia
Acute lymphocytic leukemia
Lymphomatous disease
Malignant gliomas

[a] Currently in transition.

ten tumors which would be representative of the major solid tumors and hematologic malignancies mixing potentially responsive and potentially unresponsive tumors (Table V). If an adequate phase II trial was done in all ten of these signal tumors, there would be a reasonable expectation, if all were negative, that this would not be a valuable drug. It was recognized that this could still miss a drug that would be specific for functioning islet cell tumors of the pancreas, or testicular cancer which would not be included in the routine. It is a danger, but there is always that kind of danger in every screen. What the specific signal tumors should be are in evolution at NCI at this point in time. The signal tumor concept never functioned ideally, because the clinical reality is that if a new drug fails in two or three phase II studies, clinical interest is lost rapidly. It is very hard to then push clinicians to continue to do phase II studies in tumors to fill in, if you will, the boxes in a signal tumors list. It is incumbent on any drug development program to think about a reasonable list of tumors in which phase II studies are to be performed.

V. PHASE III CLINICAL TRIALS

Classically, a phase III trial for a new drug is a study in which the drug is given to large numbers of patients to determine: (1) Will the efficacy seen in phase II be confirmed? (2) Will unexpected events, such as new types of efficacy or adverse effects not previously detected occur? (3) What is the value of the drug in relation to other potential therapies for the tumor?

Phase III is a rather large challenge. It is much more than an attempt to confirm the findings of phases I and II. It is an attempt at total identification of the drug. What is not always appreciated or realized in phase III studies is the amount of effort necessary to generate and retrieve essential information. In most cases phase III trials are controlled clinical trials.

The sine qua non of a controlled study is the comparability of patient groups assigned to each treatment so that the only reasonable explanation of an observed difference is directly attributable to the treatment program. This end requires comparability of patients as they are entered into the study, as they are managed on study, and as their data are analyzed after the study is completed.

Simple randomization does not guarantee a balance of all important prognostic variables among treatments, although the larger the study the more likely there will be a balanced, random distribution of factors. If there are minor variations between the patient populations on different regimes, adjustments often can be made in the statistical analysis. Prerandomization stratification as used in phase III studies is aimed at achieving prospectively overall balance and also attempts to equally distribute the treatment programs within each stratum. The efficiency of stratification in balancing the prognostic factors is related to the number of strata and the number of patients in the study. With an excessive number of stratifications, there is a great likelihood of obtaining an unbalanced sample, and its value compared with simple randomization is diminished.

The vast majority of current phase III studies randomly allocate patients to treatment programs. The prime purpose of randomization is to eliminate conscious or unconscious investigator bias in assigning treatments. There are two basic types of control groups: patients treated concurrently, and those selected from past records and termed ''historical controls.'' Most phase III cancer trials now employ randomized concurrent control groups, and patients are prospectively and randomly assigned to a treatment program. The patient selection factors, therapy, supportive care, follow-up, and definitions of response remain essentially constant throughout the trial.

Again, this approach is not accepted by all investigators. It has been suggested that careful selection of controls from the literature, matched controls from a particular group or institution, or controls from sequential studies may provide an adequate group for comparison with a new therapy.

The final purpose in evaluating the effects of a new therapy is to demonstrate its absolute and relative efficacy and safety. Clinical trials are biological experiments carried out in heterogenous material capable of considerable variation. Because of this the measurements of effect must be analyzed statistically. The clinician, when reading reports of clinical trials, is faced with the difficulty of distinguishing results which are of clinical importance or significance from those that are not.

In the clinical context, the word ''significant'' implies that what is observed is notable, or important, or worthy of consideration in the statistical sense. It implies that the mean results in comparing two or more groups differ from each other by more than twice the standard error. It is known that such a difference could occur by chance relatively rarely (normally 5 times in 100 tests) and, therefore, the difference in results is said to be significant. Statistical significance gives a measure of probability of the observed difference being real, rather than occurring by chance. It implies also that when random samples are taken from one of the groups under study, there will not be a significant difference between them. It should not be forgotten that when there is "no significant difference" between two groups it means only that the difference is not proven rather than that there is a proven lack of difference.

Many trials are "uncontrolled" and the results are compared to some past experience or to a historical control. Often with historical controls the traditional statistical significance tests are applied. In most cases, this is done despite the fact that the comparability of the two groups compared has not been adequately demonstrated. In this case a "statistical difference" between two groups may not reflect a meaningful biological difference due to therapy, but a meaningful biological difference due to different populations being evaluated.

In the utilization of historical controls the question can always be asked: Is the improvement observed with a new therapy due to the fact that (1) patients are coming in for diagnosis and treatment earlier in their disease when treatment is likely to be more successful, (2) ancillary care has improved and therefore a better response rate is now possible, or (3) the physicians involved are better trained in the disease under study and more enthusiastic about their current study?

The use of historical controls almost assumes that you know all you will ever need to know about what comprises a response in patients. This is hardly ever true as new prognostic variables are almost constantly being uncovered or redis-covered. Historical controls may not provide comparable data for testing and evaluation. Research on immunological and biological markers may uncover new prognostic categories that are not available in the retrospective control. Using concurrent control groups, similar parameters may be followed in all patients, then all treatment groups can be equally evaluated as new characteristics appear.

What is even more disturbing is how common it is in historically controlled studies to see minimal or no matching of the known prognostic variables between the study group and the "control." In the absence of a great deal of prior work on patient characteristics—carefully assembled and treated with a high order of statistical sophistication—the clinician might be wise to continue to rely on the randomized controlled clinical trial before recommending significant changes in medical practice. This is not to deny that when the "magic bullet" comes we will not need a control to find it or that significant advances have been made with uncontrolled series. Many advances have been made, however, with less dramatic results. Looking only for the dramatic effect could be a wasteful approach which misses many opportunities for advancement.

VI. COMPARABILITY FACTORS IN CLINICAL TRIALS

The comparability factors which exist in clinical trials are very extensive and are outlined in Table VI. They begin with the patient selection factors, followed by the pretherapeutic work that is done for the patient and the staging definition. After staging there is the treatment prescription for the patient, and the delivery of therapy with the variety of factors that go into it (such as dose level, schedule, duration, titration to toxicity) which is an essential element in the equation. Then there are criteria of response, adequacy of follow-up, and data reporting techniques, including defining the numerator and the denominator. The performance status is one of the most important patient selection variables which affect prognosis and response for cancer chemotherapy studies in advanced diseases. The performance status is an evaluation of how well a given patient can function in a normal life situation. Is the patient able to do all normal activities? Is the patient hampered to some degree in doing normal activities? Can the patient perhaps do no normal activities with some degree of help? Is the patient ambulatory or nonambulatory? A variety of scales have been developed to try to quantify what is in essence a subjective determination, the performance status of the patient. The most commonly utilized one is one that was developed by Dr. David Karnofsky at Memorial Hospital, New York City. It is called the Karnofsky scale,

TABLE VI

Comparability Factors in Clinical Trials

I.	Patient selection factors
II.	Pretherapeutic work-up
III.	Staging definition
IV.	Delivery of therapy
	a. Dose level
	b. Schedule
	c. Duration
	d. Titration to toxicity
V.	Criteria of response
	a. Objective regression
	b. Survival
VI.	Adequacy of follow-up
VII.	Data reporting techniques
	a. Defining numerator
	b. Defining denominator

and it starts from 10, which is the best performance status, fully functional, and goes down to 1 in which the patient is nearly moribund and clearly nonambulatory.

In every advanced solid tumor situation in which it has been evaluated, the performance status is an important prognostic indicator of survival length and response to active drug treatment. In bronchogenic carcinoma, it may be the most potent variable of all and should be a stratification variable in every comparative clinical trial in advanced disease patients.

In an idealized trial, if drug A gives a median survival of 20 weeks, and drug B gives a median survival of 4 weeks, the impression could be that drug A is clearly superior to drug B, as it gives five times the survival. If the data show, however, that all patients treated with drug A had a performance scale of 8 to 10, and all the patients treated with drug B had a performance scale of 1 to 4, then what is being seen are not differences in drug effect, but differences due to imbalances of a patient selection factor in the trial. It is absolutely essential, before we analyze the clinical trial data from any study and make decisions based on it, that we have an awareness of what the important prognostic variables for response are for the disease treated.

The potential heterogeneity in selection factors that patients with given kinds of cancer bring to a clinical trial is one of the major reasons for the utilization of randomization techniques to attempt to assure comparability. Besides randomization, some clinicians and statisticians employ stratification before randomization, so that one separates out subsets of patients that have particular prognostic groupings and then randomizes inside those groups.

Table VII details data summarized from M. D. Anderson Hospital on chemotherapy of ovarian cancer with established active drugs in patients who have had prior therapy. As can be seen, there is almost no response for the best drugs, when prior drug treatment has been given. Therefore, in ovarian cancer

TABLE VII

Response to Second Trial Chemotherapy in Ovarian Cancer[a]

Drug	No. Rx	No. response	Percent response
1. Melphalan	71	8	11.3
2. 5-FU	46	1	2.2
3. Adriamycin	27	0	0
4. Hexamethylmelamine	12	1	8.3
5. Actinomycin D + 5-fluorouracil + cyclophosphamide	145	9	6.2

[a] Data of Stanhope et al. (1977).

TABLE XIII

Responses That Are Less Than "Partial"

1. Improvement
2. Stable disease
3. Minor response
4. Mixed response
5. Poor partial response
6. Partial failure

there is a problem in therapeutic strategy because if phase II study is restricted to patients who have been treated with melphalan, adriamycin, or hexamethylmelamine, then the new drug will have to be an extremely active drug if any activity is going to be seen. From these data it is clearly that a drug as active as adriamycin would be missed in ovarian cancer if it were tested only in patients who had prior treatment with alkylating agents.

A critical variable in data analysis is the definition of tumor response. In advanced disease, criteria of response are not uniform and a wide variety of definitions exist. In Table VIII are shown some "response" terms used that are less than a 50% shrinkage, which most investigators define as the minimal shrinkage for partial response. Most investigators measure a lesion in two perpendicular diameters and take the product of these two measurements. A few investigators take the sum. If the latter is used, a 50% decrease is a much more demanding criteria than if products are used (Table IX). Partial regression is the

TABLE IX

Difference between Product and Sum of Perpendicular Diameters of a Tumor Lesion

First measurement
   10 by 10
      Product = 100
      Sum   = 20

Second measurement
   7 by 7
      Product = 49 = partial response
      Sum   = 14 = "improvement"

Third measurement
   5 by 5
      Product = 25 = PR
      Sum   = 10 = PR

most critical variable for chemotherapy of advanced disease at this point in time. Unfortunately for many of the major kinds of cancer partial regressions are all that are observed in most circumstances. Other variables inside the 50% shrinkage requirement are the minimal duration that should be observed for shrinkage, and whether if four lesions are measured is the shrinkage of one or all four needed for response to be called. Unfortunately the measuring of lumps and bumps and the measuring of X-ray shadows with calipers and rulers is not as precise a science as might be thought. This difficulty is illuminated by a study reported by Moertel and Hanley (1976). An experiment was performed with balls of varying sizes placed under foam rubber. The balls were placed under the foam rubber and investigators of the Eastern Cooperative Study Group came in with their calipers and were asked to measure the size of the "lesion." Their measurements were put on a flow sheet exactly as if they were doing a clinical study. Without telling sixty-four of these investigators, they were asked to come back a second time to measure the same lesion they had measured earlier. What they found when they had the same investigator measure the same lesion two sequential times was that 19% of the time the difference was greater than a 25% shrinkage, and that in about 8% of the time it was greater than a 50% shrinkage, which is the classic definition of objective response (Table X). This indicates that there exists a background level of investigator variability and that utilization of less stringent criteria, that is only 25% shrinkage, should be avoided because with 25% shrinkage definition the background level of investigator variability in measurement begins to approach 20%, which is considered meaningfully active for some diseases. In the same series when two separate investigators made the same measurements, the variability was 25% for a 25% shrinkage, and 31% for a 25% growth (Table XI).

Survival is another end point used in drug studies. From a clinical point of view there are a variety of ways of looking at survival (Table XII). The percent surviving in a fixed period of time, perhaps 5 years or 1 year, median survival,

TABLE X

Measuring Error in Objective Response Determination[a]

No. of repeat same investigator evaluations	No. of investigators who reported objective response	
	≥25% shrinkage	≥50% shrinkage
64	12 (18.8%)	5 (7.8%)

[a] From Moertel and Hanley (1976).

TABLE XI

Erroneously Declared Objective Responses When Two Different Investigators Measure Tumor Which Has Remained the Same Size[a]

No. of different investigator pairings	No. of pairings who report objective responses	
	≥25% shrinkage	≥50% shrinkage
1920	497 (24.9%)	130 (6.8%)
	Progression	
	≥25%	≥50%
	growth 604 (31.5%)	*growth* 342 (17.8%)

[a] Data from Moertel and Hanley (1976).

TABLE XII

Survival Calculations

1. Percent surviving at a fixed period
2. Median
3. Mean
4. Survival curve

mean survival, or the survival curve can all be used. Each of these has weaknesses and strengths, and ideally one would like to have all of these kinds to make a full evaluation of survival. What is the zero point for determining survival? (Table XIII) The end point of survival is fixed, as it is easily established when a patient dies. When does the calculation start? It can be when symptoms

TABLE XIII

Zero Points for Survival Determination

1. Date of first symptions
2. Date of diagnosis
3. Date of initiation of primary treatment
4. Date of completion of treatment
5. Date of recurrence of disease
6. Date of initiation of secondary treatment
7. Date of completion of secondary treatment
8. Date of secondary treatment failure

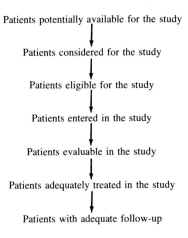

Patients potentially available for the study

↓

Patients considered for the study

↓

Patients eligible for the study

↓

Patients entered in the study

↓

Patients evaluable in the study

↓

Patients adequately treated in the study

↓

Patients with adequate follow-up

Fig. 3. Patient flow in clinical trials.

begin, or at the date of diagnosis, the date when primary treatment was started, etc. Obviously there are all ranges of zero point, and if there is not comparability of zero points, there is difficulty in analyzing various studies.

A critical aspect in the evaluation of trials concerns defining the denominator. All patients that enter a clinical trial are part of a flow (Fig. 3). Within the flow are a variety of possible choices for the denominator in a response rate calculation.

TABLE XIV

Cytosine Arabinoside in the Treatment of Acute Myeloblastic Leukemia[a]

Number of cases entered	44
Number of cases evaluable	36
Number of cases with adequate trials	24
Number of complete responders (CR)	9
Number of partial responders (PR)	4
Number of hematologic improvement (HI)	1

Response rate

$$\frac{\text{No. of CR}}{\text{No. of entered}} = \frac{9}{44} = 20\%$$

or

$$\frac{\text{No. of CR} + \text{PR} + \text{HI}}{\text{No. of adequate trials}} = \frac{14}{24} = 60\%$$

[a] Modified from Bodey et al. (1969).

An example of the problem of defining the denominator is shown in a study of Bodey *et al.* (1969) on cytosine arabinoside treatment for acute myeloblastic leukemia (Table XIV). Forty-four cases were entered. There were 36 evaluable cases and 24 adequate trials (defined as being able to receive two complete courses of the treatment). There were nine complete responders, four partial responders, one hematologic improvement and ten failures. What is the response rate? Table XIV shows that by stringing out the three potential denominators vertically and the three potential numerators horizontally, there are nine possible response rates that can be delineated from the data and they range from 20% to 60%. Of course what this cries out for is a certain degree of standardization for any trial of how we define evaluable patients versus those entered, how we adequately define treated patients, what criteria of responses we use, and which of these response criteria we will utilize for our numerator.

VII. CONCLUSIONS

There is a competitive bottleneck in clinical trials (Fig. 4). All the modalities have new developments that require clinical trial resources. The potential interactions between all of these new developments are staggering in number. Therefore, the number of patients in a clinical research should be maximized. These patients constitute a precious resource, and they should be placed only into trials properly designed to answer the questions posed. The questions need to be developed within a multidisciplinary framework. The medical oncologist, surgical oncologist, radiation oncologist, pathologist, immunologist, and statistician all have to work together as a team.

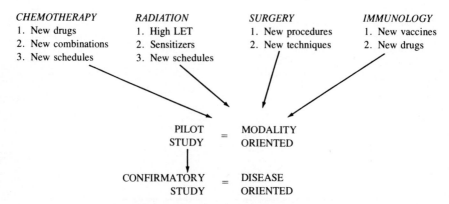

Fig. 4.   The competitive bottleneck in clinical trials.

REFERENCES

Bodey, G. P., Freireich, E. J., Monto, R. W., and Hewlett, J. S. (1969). *Cancer Chemother Rep., Part I* **53**, 59–66.

Carter, S. K. (1977). *Cancer* **40**, 544–557.

Carter, S. K., Bakowski, M., and Hellman, K. (1977). "Chemotherapy in Cancer." Wiley, New York.

Freireich, E. J., Gehan, E. A., and Rall, D. P. (1966). *Cancer Chemother. Rep.* **50**, 219–244.

Gehan, E. A., and Schneiderman, M. A. (1973). *In* "Cancer Medicine" (J. F. Holland, E. Frei, eds.), pp. 499–519. Lea & Febiger, Philadelphia, Pennsylvania.

Goldsmith, M. A., Slavik, M., and Carter, S. K. (1975). *Cancer Res.* **35**, 1354–1364.

Kenis, Y. (1969). *Recent Results Cancer Res.* **21**, 54–61.

Moertel, C. G., and Hanley, J. A. (1976). *Cancer* **38**, 388–394.

Stanhope, C. R., Smith, J. P., and Rutledge, F. (1977). *Gynecol. Oncol.* **5**, 52–58.

INDEX